# Handbook of
# Bone Marrow Transplantation

# Handbook of
# Bone Marrow Transplantation

*Edited by*

**Jacob M Rowe** MD
Professor and Director
Department of Hematology & BMT
Rambam Medical Center and Technion
Haifa, Israel

*and* Adjunct Professor of Medicine
University of Rochester
Rochester, NY, USA

**Hillard M Lazarus** MD
Professor of Medicine
Ireland Cancer Center
Case Western Reserve University
Cleveland, Ohio, USA

**Angelo M Carella** MD
Professor and Coordinator
MOA Hematology and Autologous BMT
Azienda Ospedale San Martino
Genoa, Italy

MARTIN DUNITZ

© Martin Dunitz Ltd 2000

First published in the United Kingdom in 2000 by

Martin Dunitz Ltd
The Livery House
7–9 Pratt Street
London NW1 0AE

Tel:        +44-(0)20-7482-2202
Fax:        +44-(0)20-7267-0159
E-mail:     info@mdunitz.globalnet.co.uk
Website:    http://www.dunitz.co.uk

A CIP catalogue record for this book is available from the British Library

ISBN 1-85317-889-6

Distributed in the United States by:
Blackwell Science Inc.
Commerce Place, 350 Main Street
Malden, MA 02148, USA
Tel: 1-800-215-1000

Distributed in Canada by:
Login Brothers Book Company
324 Salteaux Cresent
Winnipeg, Manitoba R3J 3T2
Canada
Tel: 1-204-224-4068

Distributed in Brazil by:
Ernesto Reichmann Distribuidora de Livros, Ltda
Rua Coronel Marques 335, Tatuape 03440-000
Sao Paulo,
Brazil

Composition by Wearset, Boldon, Tyne and Wear.
Printed and bound in Great Britain by Biddles Ltd. Guildford and King's Lynn.

# Contents

# Preface

Over the past three decades, bone marrow transplantation has been established as a curative form of therapy for various acquired hematological malignancies and congenital immune deficiencies, as well as inborn errors of metabolism.

The early success of allogeneic transplantation followed over two decades of classic and painstaking studies in animals that established the feasibility and durability of engraftment across histocompatibility barriers. Although autologous marrow grafts were used as early as the 1950s, it is only in the past two decades that they have been established for the therapy of both hematologic malignancies and solid tumors.

Extraordinary scientific developments over the past decade, based on genetic marking, adoptive immunotherapy, and further developments in the establishment of tolerance, have enabled more transplants to be performed in more diseases and with far greater success. The importance of improvements in supportive care cannot be over-emphasized.

The new millennium brings with it a new era of advances in stem cell selection devices, newer methodologies for more efficient mobilization of stem cells, allogeneic transplants from alternative donors, and novel preparative regimens.

A greater understanding of the biology of tolerance in engraftment has also permitted transplantation in older adults using less toxic pretransplant regimens, and gene transfer lies at the center of potential future developments in such transplantation. Many of these advances are thoroughly reviewed in this manual. Progress has been so rapid that many publications are almost out of date by the time they are published. An attempt has been made in this text to bring the latest information to readers in as rapid a time as is possible, with the hope that these and other new developments will further enhance our understanding of the biology and feasibility of basic and clinical transplantation, and ultimately lead to a greater percentage of patients that are cured. The courage and faith of these patients has sustained all those involved in bone marrow transplantation, and it is to these extraordinary individuals that this volume is dedicated.

*Jacob M Rowe*
*Hillard M Lazarus*
*Angelo M Carella*

# Contributors

**Claudio Anasetti MD**
Division of Clinical Research
Fred Hutchinson Cancer Research
Center
1100 Fairview Avenue North
Seattle, WA 98109–1024
USA

**Andrea Bacigalupo MD**
Department of Hematology
Azienda Ospedale San Martino
Viale Benedetto XV 6
16132 Genoa
Italy

**Andrea Banfi MD**
Centro di Biotecnologie Avanzate
Istituto Nazionale per la Ricerca sul
Cancro
Largo Rosanna Benzi 10
16132 Genoa
Italy

**William Bensinger MD**
Division of Clinical Research
Fred Hutchinson Cancer Research
Center
1100 Fairview Avenue North
Seattle, WA 98109–1024
USA

**Giovanni Berisso MD**
Department of Hematology
Ospedale San Martino
Viale Benedetto XV 6
16132 Genoa
Italy

**James E Butrynski MD**
Division of Clinical Research
Department of Medicine
University of Washington
Fred Hutchinson Cancer Research
Center
1100 Fairview Avenue North
Seattle, WA 98109–1024
USA

**Ranieri Cancedda MD**
Centro di Biotecnologie Avanzate
Istituto Nazionale per la Ricerca sul
Cancro
Largo Rosanna Benzi 10
16132 Genoa
Italy

**Angelo M Carella MD**
MOA Hematology & Autologous BMT
Azienda Ospedale San Martino
Largo Rosanna Benzi 10
16132 Genoa
Italy

Joachim Deeg MD
Division of Clinical Research
Fred Hutchinson Cancer Research
Center
1100 Fairview Avenue North
Seattle, WA 98109–1024
USA

Peter Dreger MD
Second Department of Medicine
Christian-Albrechts Universität Kiel
D-24116 Kiel 1
Germany

Maria Galloto MD
Centro di Biotecnologie Avanzate
Istituto Nazionale per la Ricerca sul
Cancro
Largo Rosanna Benzi 10
16132 Genoa
Italy

Sergio Giralt MD
University of Texas
MD Anderson Cancer Center
1515 Holcombe Blvd, Box 065
Houston, TX 77030
USA

John A Hansen MD
Division of Clinical Research
Fred Hutchinson Cancer Research
Center
1100 Fairview Avenue North
Seattle, WA 98109–1024
USA

Christof von Kalle MD
Department I of Internal Medicine
Hematology/Oncology
Universitätsklinikum Freiburg
Hugstetterstrasse 55
D-79106 Freiburg
Germany

Hillard M Lazarus MD
Ireland Cancer Center
University Hospitals of Cleveland
Case Western Reserve University
Cleveland, OH 44106
USA

Paul J Martin MD
Division of Clinical Research
Fred Hutchinson Cancer Research
Center
1100 Fairview Avenue North
Seattle, WA 98109-1024
USA

Dana C Matthews MD
Division of Clinical Research
Pediatric Hematology/Oncology
University of Washington
Fred Hutchinson Cancer Research
Center
1100 Fairview Avenue North
Seattle, WA 98109–1024
USA

Roland Mertelsmann MD PhD
Department I of Internal Medicine
Hematology/Oncology
Universitätsklinikum Freiburg
Hugstetterstrasse 55
D-79106 Freiburg
Germany

Arthur J Molina MD
Transplantation Biology Program
Division of Clinical Research
Fred Hutchinson Cancer Research
Center
1100 Fairview Avenue North
Seattle, WA 98109-1024
USA

Andrew L Pecora MD
Hackensack University
Medical Plaza
20 Prospect Avenue, 4th Floor
Hackensack, NJ 07601
USA

Effie W Petersdorf MD
Division of Clinical Research
Fred Hutchinson Cancer Research
Center
1100 Fairview Avenue North
Seattle, WA 98109–1024
USA

Rodolfo Quarto MD
Laboratorio di Differenziamento
Cellulare
Centro di Biotecnologie Avanzate
Istituto Nazionale per la Ricerca sul
Cancro
Largo Rosanna Benzi 10
16132 Genoa
Italy

Annamaria Raiola MD
Department of Hematology
Ospedale San Martino
Viale Benedetto XV 6
16132 Genoa
Italy

Jacob M Rowe MD
Professor and Director
Department of Hematology & BMT
Ramban Medical Center and
Technion
Haifa  31096
Israel

Jean E Sanders MD
Division of Clincial Research
Fred Hutchinson Cancer Research
Center
1100 Fairview Avenue North
Seattle, WA 98109–1024
USA

Norbert Schmitz MD
Second Department of Medicine
Christian-Albrechts Universität Kiel
D-24116 Kiel 1
Germany

Patrick J Stiff MD
Hematology/Oncology
Loyola University Stritch School of
Medicine Cancer Center
2160 South First Avenue
Maywood, IL 60153
USA

Rainer F Storb MD
Transplantation Biology Program
Division of Clinical Research
Fred Hutchinson Cancer Research
Center
1100 Fairview Avenue North
Seattle, WA 98109-1024
USA

Ann E Woolfrey MD
Division of Clinical Research
Fred Hutchinson Cancer Research
Center
1100 Fairview Avenue North
Seattle, WA 98109–1024
USA

# 1

# CD34$^+$ cell selection and ex vivo expansion in autologous and allogeneic transplantation

Andrew L Pecora

## INTRODUCTION

Hematopoietic stem and progenitor cells are characterized by their cell surface expression of a variety of antigens, particularly CD34.[1,2] Hematopoietic cells expressing CD34 are readily collected from the blood following mobilization using hematopoietic growth factors with or without chemotherapy, or from bone marrow.[3,4] CD34$^+$ cells contained in harvested marrow or in blood collected using apheresis, are capable of reconstituting hematopoiesis in patients treated with myeloablative therapy.[5–7] The kinetics of hematopoietic recovery in patients treated with myeloablative therapy has been found to be largely dependent on the source and quantity of CD34$^+$ cells infused.[8–11] In fact, CD34$^+$ cells collected from the blood of patients treated with mobilization therapy and used to restore hematopoiesis in autologous and allogeneic transplant recipients have been shown to result in more rapid hematopoietic recovery, lower morbidity and lower total cost when compared with bone-marrow-derived CD34$^+$ cells.[12–14] Moreover, subsets of less-differentiated CD34$^+$ cells (i.e. CD33$^-$ and CD38$^-$ populations) contained in blood and marrow stem cell products have now been identified as the source of both early and sustained hematopoietic recovery in autologous and allogeneic transplant recipients.[11,15,16]

The clear identification that CD34$^+$ cells in blood and marrow effect engraftment has resulted in investigations to isolate and expand the number of these cells.[1] A variety of techniques are under study, some of which have been validated in clinical trials.[17–32] The goals of this effort in cell engineering are twofold. The first is to maintain or improve the hematopoietic reconstitutive capacity of a stem cell product. The second is to reduce or eliminate unwanted cells and material from the stem cell product, including the cryoprotectant, cells capable of contributing to disease relapse in autologous transplantation, and immune effectors that cause morbidity in allogeneic transplantation. These efforts can be represented in a relationship equation that has been termed the

1

'stem cell product quality equation':

$$\text{stem cell product quality} = \frac{\text{hematopoietic reconstitutive capacity}}{\text{number of unwanted cells}}$$

CD34$^+$ cell selection and ex vivo expansion offer transplant physicians new tools to reduce the morbidity associated with stem cell transplantation and potentially improve its effectiveness in disease eradication by improving the hematopoietic reconstitutive capacity and eliminating unwanted cells from stem cell products.

## CD34$^+$ CELL SELECTION METHODOLOGY

The CD34 antigen, a 115 kDa type 1 integral membrane glycoprotein, is expressed on nearly all hematopoietic cells, and has been demonstrated to be an ideal target for monoclonal antibody binding.[1,2,33,34] These observations have led to the development of devices capable of selectively collecting antibody-labeled CD34$^+$ cells and a move away from the use of non-specific isolation techniques, including centrifugation and elutriation.[35,36] Two approaches to the isolation, of CD34$^+$ cells labeled with an anti-CD34 monoclonal antibody (termed 'positive selection') have received US FDA approval for use in patients receiving bone marrow or blood stem cells.

The first was the Ceprate SC stem cell collection system (Cellpro, Bothell, WA).[37] Using an avidin–biotin immunoadsorption technique, biotinylated anti-CD34 antibody-labeled bone marrow or blood stem cells are passed through a column containing avidin-coated beads. Unbound cells are washed away, and then the bound CD34$^+$ cells are eluted using mechanical agitation (Figure 1.1). The avidin–biotin interaction utilized to bind CD34$^+$ cells has a very high dissociation constant ($K_D = 10^{-15}$). This property allows CD34$^+$ cells to be collected during a continuous flow through the column. Upon mechanical agitation, the attached cells break away from the antibody, leaving the intact antibody–avidin complex behind, fixed to the column. In fact, enzyme-linked immunosorbent assays (ELISA) have revealed less than 80 ng of antibody remaining in most selected products, explaining the absence of the development of a human anti-mouse antibody in over 300 patients analyzed to date.[38–43] The Ceprate system received FDA approval principally based on results from a trial demonstrating that infusion of CD34$^+$-selected stem cells was associated with a marked reduction in toxicity when compared with the infusion of non-selected products.[37] Selection reduces the quantity of dimethyl sulfoxide (DMSO) infused, which is known to cause nausea, vomiting, diarrhea, and at times hypotension, bronchospasm and seizure activity.[44–46]

The other approach to selection involves the use of immunomagnetic beads.[17] Here murine monoclonal antibodies directed against the class I CD34 antigen have been chosen for labeling CD34$^+$ cells because of the near absence of class I expression on leukemic cells.[47] Following a 15 minute incubation of

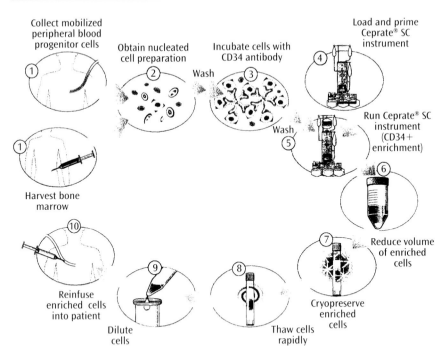

**Figure 1.1**
Avidin–biotin CD34$^+$ cell selection technique. Reproduced with permission from Marcel Dekker Inc, from Berenson RJ, Shpall EJ, Auditore-Hargreaves K et al, *Cancer Invest* 1996; **14:** 589–96.[37]

CD34$^+$ cells with a class I murine anti-CD34 antibody, immunomagnetic beads coated with antimurine immunoglobulin (IgG, usually of sheep origin) are then mixed together, in this so-called indirect method, forming rosette complexes. An alternative method, the direct method, involves mixing immunomagnetic beads with the murine anti-CD34 monoclonal antibody prior to incubation with CD34$^+$ cells. Regardless of the binding method used, the immunomagnetic bead–monoclonal antibody–CD34$^+$ cell complexes are then passed over a strong magnetic field that binds the rosette complexes. Two devices, the Isolex semi-automated device (SA) and the automated Isolex 300i (Nexell, Inc), have both been shown to provide an adequate magnetic field for this purpose (Figure 1.2).

In the presence of the magnetic field, cells not bound by the rosette complexes are removed using a wash buffer. A minimum of two washes is required to ensure that non-targeted cells that are non-specifically attached to the rosette complexes or to the magnetic chamber wall are removed from the selected product. Release of the CD34$^+$ cells from the rosette complex can then be accomplished by using an enzymatic treatment or alternatively a competitive binding approach using an oligopeptide.[48,49] The enzymatic approach

Diagram of the Isolex® 300i Magnetic

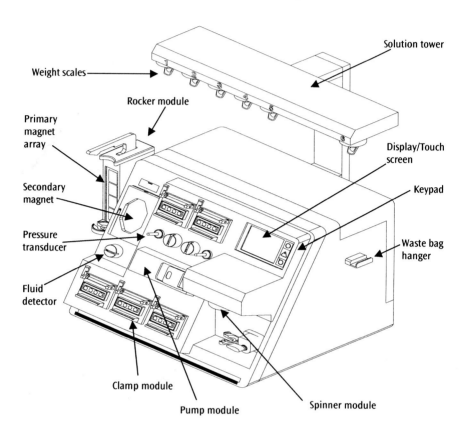

Figure 1.2
Immunomagnetic CD34⁺ cell selection technique.

utilizes the proteolytic enzyme chymopapain, which is incubated with the rosette complexes, resulting in cleavage of a portion of the CD34 antigen from its cell surface. Following reapplication of the magnetic field, the remaining immunomagnetic complexes, devoid of CD34⁺ cells, bind to the magnet. CD34⁺ cells are then readily recovered using a gentle washing technique.

   The enzymatic release approach causes damage to the CD34 antigen, limiting accurate quantification of CD34⁺ cells recovered after the selection process.[50] Therefore a more specific approach has been developed that does not alter the post-selection expression of the CD34 antigen. This method of release is based on competitive binding of an epitope-specific oligopeptide with the antigen-binding site of murine anti-CD34 antibody.[48] During a 30 minute incubation performed at ambient temperature, the oligopeptide displaces CD34$^+$ cells from the immunomagnetic bead complex without affecting expression of the CD34 antigen. Exposure of the product once more to the magnetic field results in binding of the immunomagnetic beads to the wall of the magnetic chamber. Routine collection of CD34$^+$ cells is then accomplished using a gentle wash technique. With this method, released cells retain their normal surface antigen pattern. Therefore immediate and accurate post-selection quantification is possible.

The Miltenyi selection system (CliniMax) uses a similar immunomagnetic approach; however, the magnetic particles to which CD34$^+$ cells bind are smaller than immunomagnetic beads.[51] Use of small magnetic particles has the potential advantage of obviating the need for the release step used in immunomagnetic bead systems. Further clinical trials and regulatory scrutiny are clearly needed prior to approval of the routine infusion of CD34$^+$ cells bound by these small magnetic particles.

The incremental cost associated with the use of selection has led to efforts to limit the number of selection procedures performed. One approach has been to store, overnight, an apheresis product and pool it with the subsequent day's product. A recent study has demonstrated that pooled apheresis products, once selected, maintain their hematopoietic reconstitutive capacity.[52] Specifically, the rate of myeloid and lymphoid engraftment following infusion of selected pooled products was similar when compared with infused products that were selected on the day on which they were collected. Others have explored the possibility of selecting CD34$^+$ cells from cryopreserved apheresis products (Preti RA, personal communication). In this preclinical study, 10 selections were performed using cryopreserved blood stem cells (hydroxyethyl starch and 5% DMSO) stored for more than 18 months at $-95\ °C$. These products, which were thawed at 37 °C and immediately diluted with a $Ca^{2+}/Mg^{2+}$-free solution of buffered saline containing 1.0% human serum albumin, were CD34$^+$-selected and then assessed for recovery and viability. Postselection recovery of $79.6 \pm 11.0\%$ of the CD34$^+$ cells in the starting product was observed, and a near 100% viability was demonstrated on propidium iodide exclusion. Moreover, $72.3 \pm 10.9\%$ of starting colony-forming units granulocyte–macrophage (CFU-GM) were recovered. This approach warrants testing in clinical trials, especially if further laboratory experiments find pooling of thawed cryopreserved products, aimed to limit the number of selection procedures, to be viable.

## MALIGNANT CELL PURGING USING CD34$^+$ CELL SELECTION

Controversy persists regarding the clinical relevance of autograft purging, despite reports indicating that contaminating malignant cells are clearly capable of contributing to disease relapse and numerous clinical trials demonstrating improved outcomes in autologous stem cell recipients receiving malignant-cell-free stem cell products.[53–57] The question remains, however, whether malignant cells contaminating a stem cell product solely indicate residual in vivo chemotherapy-resistant disease and thus their removal would not significantly impact on transplant treatment outcome. Nonetheless, the efficacy of CD34$^+$ cell selection for malignant cell purging of stem cell products in autologous transplant recipients has been extensively evaluated.

Immunocytochemistry has revealed that up to 48% of patients even with early stage breast cancer will have bone marrow contamination at the time of diagnosis.[58–60] Similarly, dependent on the presence of marrow contamination and the number of apheresis procedures performed, the incidence of blood stem cell product contamination approaches 50%.[61] The presence of contaminating breast cancer cells in marrow and blood prior to autologous transplant has been associated with poor outcomes.[62] Removal of these contaminating cells thus provides a strategy to test the effect on outcomes of autologous transplant treatment. It remains unknown, however, whether a threshold number of contaminating malignant cells is required to cause relapse in the autologous setting. Thus the extent to which stem cells need to be depleted of malignant cells is also unknown.

Blood-derived stem cell products usually contain a total nucleated cell number of $(1–2) \times 10^{10}$ cells. Several investigators have determined that the frequency of malignant cell contamination is usually in the range of 1–10 malignant cells per 100 000 hematopoietic cells in cases of advanced malignancy, including breast cancer.[63–66] Therefore a stem cell product, if contaminated, will contain as many as $(1–10) \times 10^5$ malignant cells. To be completely effective, it appears that purging techniques will need to remove 5 $\log_{10}$ of contaminating cells. CD34$^+$ selection results in passive malignant cell purging between 2 and 3.6 $\log_{10}$.[66,67] However, by adding a second step, termed 'negative selection', using the Isolex 300i and a panel of anti-epithelial antibodies coated with immunomagnetic beads, removal of 5 $\log_{10}$ of malignant cells has been achieved in patients with metastatic breast cancer.[68] Long-term follow-up of existing study results, as well as further phase III clinical trials, will be needed to determine the effect of 5 $\log_{10}$ purging capability in breast cancer patients.

A similar strategy has been employed in an attempt to improve the outcomes for autologous blood and marrow transplant recipients with advanced myeloma, lymphoma and chronic lymphocytic leukemia.[56,67,69] A 2–3.5 $\log_{10}$ depletion was observed in each study, with many patients having residual, albeit greatly reduced, numbers of contaminating malignant cells. To date, none of these studies have shown a direct benefit in disease-free or overall survival when patients receiving CD34$^+$-selected products are compared with patients receiving unselected products. These results indicate that CD34$^+$ selection alone will probably not significantly improve outcomes in autologous transplant recipients with advanced disease and heavily contaminated stem cell products. More rigorous purging (5 $\log_{10}$) using positive followed by negative selection techniques in advanced-disease patients or applying positive selection in early-disease patients (i.e. those with locally advanced breast cancer) may be more appropriate, but obviously needs confirmation through further clinical study. In addition, CD34$^+$ cell selection used as a component of a minimal residual disease treatment strategy, with removal of 3 log$_{10}$ or more of viable contaminating tumor cells from the stem cell product, may potentially improve the efficacy of immune-based effectors now being evaluated in the post-transplant setting.[70]

## CD34$^+$ CELL SELECTION IN ALLOGENEIC TRANSPLANTATION

Application of blood stem cell transplantation in the allogeneic setting had been somewhat delayed because of concerns regarding the potential adverse effect of cytokine mobilization on healthy donors and the risk of acute and chronic graft versus host disease (GvHD) due to a 1 log$_{10}$ greater inoculum of T cells compared to marrow recipients. Recently, mobilization of stem cells has been shown to be safe and effective.[71-73] Moreover, allogeneic blood-derived stem cell transplant recipients have improved clinical outcomes, including survival, when compared with marrow recipients.[14] In fact, several new studies indicate that allogeneic blood stem cell grafts may not cause excessive GvHD if appropriate GvHD prophylaxis is used and a threshold CD34$^+$ blood stem cell dose is not exceeded.[74-77] CD34$^+$ cell selection is a new strategy being tested to prevent GvHD.

Depletion of T cells from the donor inoculum using other methodologies has been shown to reduce the incidence and severity of GvHD, but at the expense of a higher incidence of disease relapse and, in some settings, an increase in graft failures.[78-80] Investigators have observed a 2–3 log$_{10}$ depletion of CD3$^+$ T cells following CD34$^+$ selection.[81] Typically, $(1–5) \times 10^9$ T cells are contained within a mobilized blood stem cell product. Following CD34$^+$ selection, $(1–10) \times 10^6$ T cells would be expected, providing the allogeneic recipient with enough T cells for engraftment ($>1 \times 10^6$ or $>1 \times 10^5$/kg patient body weight) but a reduced likelihood of experiencing acute GvHD. Results from ongoing clinical trials are needed to establish the merit of this approach.

## DENDRITIC CELLS GENERATED FROM CD34$^+$ STEM CELLS

Dendritic cells, the professional antigen-presenting cells of the human immune system, are under intense study to determine their role in applied immune therapies for cancer patients.[82,83] One of the several technical problems associated with the study of dendritic cells in this application is their low frequency in blood (0.1–1.0%), resulting in new strategies to isolate and expand these cells.[84] CD34$^+$ cells obtained from marrow, blood and cord blood are all capable of generating dendritic cells if cultured with appropriate cytokines and in the proper environment.[85–92] Thus, CD34$^+$ cell selection of mobilized blood using the Isolex technology has been performed in an attempt to reduce culture volumes and enhance the starting population of CD34$^+$ cells for dendritic cell expansion. In one study, this approach resulted in the expansion of functional dendritic cells even when serum free medium was used.[84] Ongoing research efforts will further elucidate the role dendritic will play in clinical therapy, however, isolation and expansion of these cells have clearly been enhanced by using CD34$^+$ cell selection.

## HEMATOPOIETIC AND IMMUNE RECONSTITUTION USING CD34$^+$-SELECTED STEM CELLS

Early clinical studies using CD34$^+$ selection involved bone marrow from autologous transplant recipients. In the first clinical trial reported, 13 patients received a minimum of $1.0 \times 10^6$ CD34$^+$-selected marrow-derived cells, and all engrafted.[93] Subsequently, a prospective phase III randomized trial involving breast cancer patients comparing routine marrow harvest versus CD34$^+$ selected marrow was performed.[94] In this trial, 94 eligible patients were randomized, and engraftment (defined by recovery of 500 neutrophils/μl by day 20) was equivalent in both groups of patients. Moreover, toxicity measured by predetermined cardiovascular endpoints was significantly reduced in patients receiving CD34$^+$-selected products – presumably a result of limiting the quantity of cryoprotectant infused along with the selected product.

In the largest prospective phase III comparative trial to date, 134 patients with multiple myeloma were randomized to receive either CD34$^+$-selected or unselected mobilized blood-derived stem cells.[67] Days to neutrophil recovery were similar in both groups, with an observed median of 12 days to achieve 500 neutrophils/μl. In addition, the median number of red blood cell transfusions was the same (4) in each group. Using intention-to-treat analysis, however, patients receiving selected products experienced a significant increase in median days to platelet engraftment (11 versus 9 days; $p = 0.003$) and platelet transfusions (3 versus 2; $p = 0.004$). Of note, multiple regression analysis performed in this study revealed that the time to platelet engraftment was significantly influenced by the number of CD34$^+$ cells per kilogram in the infused product and by the platelet count at the time of randomization. When 108 of the randomized patients, all of whom received at least $2.0 \times 10^6$ CD34$^+$ cells/kg, were compared, no difference was observed between the selected and unselected groups in median days to platelet engraftment or platelet transfusion requirements. Thus this trial demonstrates that in myeloma patients, CD34$^+$ cell selection does not adversely affect engraftment rates or transfusion requirements if an adequate dose of CD34$^+$ cells is infused.

In two Pre-ECOG studies, 101 women with metastatic breast cancer were treated with sequential high-dose chemotherapy and rescued with mobilized because malignant cells contained in the stem cell product are capable of growth, once infused.[96,97] Several investigators are now evaluating new techniques that involve the isolation of CD34$^+$ blood-derived stem cells following routine cytokine or chemotherapy and cytokine mobilization. In one study, 10 patients with advanced cancer who were eligible for high-dose chemotherapy received combination chemotherapy (ifosfamide, cisplatin and epirubicin) with granulocyte colony-stimulating factor (G-CSF) in order to mobilize peripheral blood progenitor cells.[98] Collected in a single leukapheresis, CD34$^+$ cells were then positively selected using immunoadsorption columns (Ceprate SC System). A starting inoculum of $11 \times 10^6$ CD34$^+$ cells was incubated in RPMI 1640 median (Zeromed-Biochrom, Berlin, Germany), 2% autologous plasma, recombinant human stem cell factor (SCF), recombinant human interleukin (IL)-1β, recombinant human IL-3, recombinant IL-6 and recombinant human erythropoietin. The CD34$^+$ cells were cultured in tissue flasks (175 cm$^2$; Falcon, Heidelberg, Germany) in a total volume of 100 ml per flask, and were incubated at 37 °C in a humidified atmosphere consisting of 5% carbon dioxide. Expanding cells were fed with 100 ml of fresh cytokine supporting medium on the 7th day of culture. Non-adhering cells were collected from the flask on the 12th day of culture, washed with 0.9% saline, and then resuspended in 100 ml of normal saline with 1% human albumin. Patients in this study received high-dose chemotherapy consisting of etoposide, ifosfamide and carboplatin, after which the ex vivo expanded CD34$^+$ cells were infused. There were no toxic effects observed during the infusion of these ex vivo expanded cells. Hematopoietic recovery occurred promptly, with a recovery of 500 neutrophils/µl in a median of 13 days (range 11–15 days) and a platelet count recovery of 20 000 cells/µl in a median of 12 days (range 11–15 days). The results of this study have subsequently been criticized, however, because the chemotherapy regimen used was not truly myeloablative. Nonetheless, this was the first demonstration that CD34$^+$ cells are capable of undergoing long-term culture and are safe to re-administer following aggressive chemotherapy.

Unselected peripheral blood progenitor cells are also capable of being expanded ex vivo. In a recent study involving 24 patients with breast cancer, blood-derived progenitor cells were mobilized with G-CSF with or without recombinant human SCF.[99] Unselected progenitor cells were cultured in gas-permeable bags containing 1 liter of serum free median with G-CSF, SCF and thrombopoietin along with an unidentified factor termed 'development factor'. Patients received high-dose chemotherapy consisting of cyclophosphamide, thiotepa and carboplatin. This high-dose chemotherapy regimen had previously been demonstrated to clearly be myeloablative. In addition to receiving expanded cells, cryopreserved unexpanded cells were administered to patients at a dose of $5 \times 10^6$ CD34 cells/kg. The duration of neutropenia, which ranged from two to nine days, was found to be inversely proportional to the expanded cell dose (cells/kg) administered. Strikingly, 10 patients (42%) achieved a neutrophil count above 500 cells/µl by six days post-transplant. Moreover 11 patients did not experience neutropenic fevers (46%) or require broad-spectrum antibiotics. Thus this study demonstrates that the addition of non-selected progenitor cells expanded ex vivo to unselected cryopreserved progenitor cells decreases the duration of neutropenia associated with a true myeloablative regimen and therefore, increases the hematopoietic reconstitutive capacity of a blood-derived stem cell graft.[99]

Using a different approach, other investigators have evaluated the safety and effectiveness of expanding a small volume of bone marrow ex vivo using the Aastrom Replicell system.[100,101] This system provides a perfusion–stromal-based environment where small volumes (approximately 80 ml) of marrow have been shown to be capable of undergoing extensive expansion as measured by an increase in total nucleated cell and CFU-GM content. Single-use growth chambers are perfused with media containing PIXY321 (a fusion protein of granulocyte–macrophage colony-stimulating factor and IL-3), Flt3 ligand, recombinant human erythropoietin, and a continuous gas mixture of nitrogen, oxygen and carbon dioxide. Breast cancer patients receiving myeloablative (Stamp V) chemotherapy were shown to recover 500 neutrophils/µl in a median of 18 days (range 13–22 days) and 20 000 platelets/µl in a median of 22 days (range 19–27 days), which is similar to a group that had previously undergone autologous bone marrow transplantation and that received a full bone marrow harvest. In addition to increasing the hematopoietic reconstitution of capacity of a small volume of bone marrow, ex vivo expansion in this system has been shown to reproducibly reduce the number of tumor cells contained within the starting marrow inoculum.[100]

Approximately 10–15% of patients scheduled to undergo autologous stem cell transplantation will not mobilize an adequate quantity of CD34$^+$ cells to safely proceed. Efforts aimed at acquiring an adequate CD34$^+$ cell dose from this patient population have met with limited success.[102] Recently, the addition of a small volume of bone marrow (80 ml), expanded ex vivo using the Aastrom Replicell system to a seemingly subtherapeutic dose of CD34$^+$ blood stem cells $((0.2–1.0) \times 10^6$ CD34 cells/kg), has resulted in engraftment rates of neutrophils and platelets equivalent to earlier series in which patients received a CD34$^+$ blood stem cell dose of $2.5 \times 10^6$/kg or more.[103] Thus, in addition to reducing or eliminating contaminating tumor cells from the stem cell product, application of ex vivo expansion in autologous transplantation has the potential to increase the hematopoietic reconstitutive capacity of a stem cell product, leading to the possibility of proceeding with an autologous stem cell transplant in the setting of a poor mobilizer.

Expansion of the application of allogeneic transplantation has been limited by the lack of appropriate HLA-compatible donors as well as the severity of GvHD encountered with increasing HLA disparity between donor and host. Umbilical cord blood has been shown to be capable of reconstituting hematopoietic and immune function in children and adults treated with myeloablative therapy.[104–107] Ex vivo expansion of cord blood has now been evaluated by several investigators in the hope of increasing the quantity of nucleated cells infused, which has been shown to be the best correlate to prompt and stable engraftment following an unrelated cord blood transplant.[107] A recent report describing the outcomes of two large adult patients, both of whom had high-risk chronic myelogenous leukemia (blast crisis and accelerated phase), without HLA-identical siblings or matched unrelated donors, but having available cord blood units with a seemingly subtherapeutic quantity of nucleated cells (approximately $1 \times 10^7$ total nucleated cells/kg). Using the Aastrom Replicell system, a portion of the cord blood units available for each patient was expanded ex vivo and infused along with the portion of the cord blood units not expanded. Both patients engrafted promptly and remain in long-term clinical and cytogenetic remissions (>1 year). Another approach being evaluated to expand cord blood ex vivo requires CD34+ cell selection before expansion.[108] In a trial, following CD34+ selection using either the Isolex 300i (Nexell, Inc) or the CliniMax system (Miltenyi Biotech, Inc), selected stem cells were placed in 1 liter Teflon culture bags with defined medium containing recombinant SCF, recombinant human G-CSF, and recombinant human thrombopoietin. The cultures were incubated for 10 days in 100% humidified 5% $CO_2$ at 37 °C. Expansion of CD34+ cells from both systems resulted in a 20-fold increase of CFU-GM, with a median 44-fold expansion of total nucleated cells. These data demonstrated the possibility of selecting a small fraction of frozen cord blood stem cells using clinical-scale CD34 selection devices followed by successful ex vivo expansion. Using this approach in a series including 19 patients scheduled for unrelated cord blood transplant, CD34+ cells from 40% of the thawed cord blood product were isolated using the Isolex 300i device (Nexell, Inc). The isolated CD34+ cells were then expanded as described. Following myeloablative therapy, patients received both expanded and unexpanded cord blood products infused on day 0. Engraftment of neutrophils to 500 cells/µl was observed in a median of 25 days (range 15–35 days) and of platelets to 20 000 cells/µl in a median of 58 days (range 27–91 days). While preliminary, these data suggest that ex vivo expansion of cord blood may in fact increase access of this approach to large adult patients.[109]

## SUMMARY

The ability to isolate and expand the cells capable of reconstituting hematopoiesis and immunity following myeloablative therapies holds great promise to improve the outcomes of cancer patients treated with autologous and allogeneic transplantation. Moreover, selection and expansion capabilities have the potential of being useful in treating a variety of serious medical disorders outside of the field of oncology. Abrogation of autoimmunity and induction of tolerance for solid organ transplantation are just two of the many possible applications of these techniques. Demonstration of efficiency and safety of these and other applications, however, requires the completion and maturation of ongoing clinical trials. Nonetheless, it appears that the use of unmodified, poorly defined cell populations to treat human illness is rapidly becoming a therapy of the past. Collectively these efforts will, it is hoped, lead to the application of a revised stem cell product quality equation resulting in abrogation of neutropenia, complete elimination of cells capable of causing harm, and infusion of other cells capable of eradicating minimal residual disease:

$$\text{stem cell product quality} = \frac{\text{hematopoietic reconstitutive capacity}}{\text{number of unwanted cells}} \times \frac{\text{targeted}}{\text{effectors}}$$

## REFERENCES

1. Civin CI, Strauss LC, Brovall C et al, Antigenic analysis of hematopoiesis. III Hematopoietic progenitor cell surface antigen defined by a monoclonal antibody raised against KG-1A cells. *J Immunol* 1984; **133**: 157–65.

2. Krause DS, Fackler MJ, Civin CI et al, CD34: structure, biology and clinical utility. *Blood* 1996; **87**: 1–13.

3. Sheridan WP, Begley CG, Juttner CA et al, Effect of peripheral blood progenitor cells mobilized by filgrastim (G-CSF) on platelet recovery after high-dose chemotherapy. *Lancet* 1992; **339**: 640–4.

4. Demirer T, Buckner CD, Storer B et al, Effect of different chemotherapy regimens on peripheral-blood stem-cell collections in patients with breast cancer receiving granulocyte colony-stimulating factor. *J Clin Oncol* 1997; **15**: 684–90.

5. Weaver CH, Hazelton B, Birch R et al, An analysis of engraftment kinetics as a function of the CD34 content of peripheral blood progenitor cell collections in 692 patients after the administration of myeloablative chemotherapy. *Blood* 1995; **10**: 3691–9.

6. Chao NJ, Shriber JR, Grimes K et al, Granulocyte colony-stimulating factor 'mobilized' peripheral-blood progenitor cells accelerate granulocyte and platelet recovery after high dose chemotherapy. *Blood* 1993; **81**: 2031–5.

7. Watts MJ, Sullivan AM, Jamieson E et al, Progenitor-cell mobilization after low-dose cyclophosphamide and granulocyte-stimulating factor: and an analysis of progenitor-cell quantity and quality and

factors predicting for these parameters in 101 pre-treated patients with malignant lymphoma. *J Clin Oncol* 1997; **15**: 535–46.

8. Siena S, Bregni M, Brando B et al, Flow cytometry for clinical estimation of circulated hematopoietic progenitors for autologous transplantation in cancer patients. *Blood* 1991; **77**: 400–9.

9. Hartmann O, Gaelle LE, Corroller A et al, Peripheral blood stem cell and bone marrow transplantation for solid tumors and lymphomas: haematological recovery and costs. *Ann Intern Med* 1997; **126**: 600–7.

10. Bensinger W, Appelbaum F, Rowley S et al, Factors that influence collection and engraftment of autologous peripheral-blood stem cells. *J Clin Oncol* 1995; **13**: 2547–55.

11. Pecora AL, Preti RA, Gleim GW et al, CD34+ CD33− cells influenced days to engraftment and transfusion requirements in autologous blood stem-cell recipients. *J Clin Oncol* 1998; **16**: 2093–104.

12. Smith TJ, Hillner BE, Schmitz N et al, Economic analysis of a randomized clinical trial to compare filgrastim-mobilized peripheral blood progenitor-cell transplantation and autologous bone marrow transplantation in patients with Hodgkin's and non-Hodgkin's lymphoma. *J Clin Oncol* 1997; **15**: 5–10.

13. To LB, Roberts MM, Haylock DN et al, Comparison of haematological recovery times and supportive care requirements of autologous recovery phase

peripheral blood stem cell transplants, autologous bone marrow transplants and allogeneic bone marrow transplants. *Bone Marrow Transplant* 1992; **9**: 277–84.

14. Bensinger W, Martin P, Clift R et al, A prospective, randomized trial of peripheral blood stem cells (pBSC) or marrow (BM) for patients undergoing allogeneic transplantation for hematological malignancies. *Blood* 1999; **94**(Suppl 1): 368a.

15. Copelan EA, Ceselski SK, Ezzone SA et al, Mobilization of peripheral-blood progenitor cells with high-dose etoposide and granulocyte colony-stimulating factor in patients with breast cancer, non-Hodgkin's lymphoma, and Hodgkin's disease. *J Clin Oncol* 1997; **15**: 759–65.

16. Waller EK, Lynn M, Worford L et al, The number of CD34$^+$ CD38$^-$ cells in the craft predicts the kinds of hematopoietic reconstitution following autologous or allogeneic bone marrow transplant (BMT). *Blood* 1997; **90**(Suppl): 394a.

17. Chang M, Richards G, Rembaum A, Polyacrolein microspheres: preparation and characteristics. *Methods Enzymol* 1985; **112**: 150–5.

18. Farley TJ, Ahmed A, Fitzgerald M et al, Optimization of CD34+ cell selection using immunomagnetic beads: implications for use in cryopreserved peripheral blood stem cell collections. *J Hematother* 1997; **6**: 53–60.

19. Berenson RJ, Bensinger WI, Hill RS et al, Engraftment after infusion of CD34+ marrow cells in patients with breast cancer or neuroblastoma. *Blood* 1991; **77**: 1717–22.

20. Somolo G, Sniecinski I, Odom-Maryon T et al, Effect of CD34$^+$ selection and various schedules of stem cell reinfusion and granulocyte colony stimulating factor priming on hematopoietic recovery after high-dose chemotherapy for breast cancer. *Blood* 1997; **89**: 1521–8.

21. Aversa F, Tabilio A, Terenci A et al, Successful engraftment of T-cell-depleted haploidentical (3-low side) incompatible transplants in leukemia patients by addition of recombinant human granulocyte colony-stimulating factor-mobilized peripheral blood progenitor cells to bone marrow inoculum. *Blood* 1994; **84**: 3948–55.

22. Bensinger WI, Buckner CD, Shannon-Dorcy K et al, Transplantation of allogeneic CD34+ peripheral blood stem cells in patients with advanced hematological malignancy. *Blood* 1996; **88**: 4132–8.

23. Lemoli RM, Fortuna A, Motta MR et al, Concomitant mobilization of plasma cells and hematopoietic progenitors into peripheral blood of multiple myeloma patients: positive selection and transplantation of enriched CD34+ cells to remove circulating tumor cells. *Blood* 1996; **87**: 1625–34.

24. Link J, Arseniev L, Bahre O et al, Transplantation of allogeneic CD34+ blood cells. *Blood* 1996; **87**: 4903–9.

25. Harwick AR, Law P, Kulinshi D et al, Development of a large-scale immunomagnetic separation system for harvesting CD34 cells from bone marrow. *Prog Clin Biol Res* 1992; **377**: 583–9.

26. Shpall EJ, Jones RB, Bearman SI et al, Transplantation of CD34+ enriched autologous marrow into breast cancer patients following high-dose chemotherapy: influence of CD34+ peripheral-blood progenitors and growth factors on engraftment. *J Clin Oncol* 1994; **12**: 28–36.

27. Gorin NC, Lopez M, Laprote JP et al, Preparation and successful engraftment of purified CD34+ bone marrow progenitor cells in patients with non-Hodgkin's lymphoma. *Blood* 1995; **85**: 1647–54.

28. Vogel W, Behringer D, Scheding S et al, Ex vivo expansion of CD34+ peripheral blood progenitor cells: implications for the expansion of contaminating epithelial tumor cells. *Blood* 1996; **88**: 2707–13.

29. Brugger W, Henschler R, Heimfeld S et al, Positively selected autologous blood CD34+ cells in unseparated peripheral blood progenitor cells mediate identical hematopoietic engraftment after

high-dose VP16, ifosfamide, carboplatin and epirubicin. *Blood* 1994; **84**: 1421–6.

30. Schiller G, Vescio R, Freytes C et al, Transplantation of CD34+ peripheral blood stem cells after high-dose chemotherapy for patients with advanced multiple myeloma. *Blood* 1995; **86**: 390–7.

31. Watts MJ, Sullivan AM, Jamieson E et al, Progenitor-cell mobilization after low-dose cyclophosphamide and granulocyte colony-stimulating factor: an analysis of progenitor-cell quantity and quality as factors predicting for these parameters in 101 pre-treated patients with malignancy. *J Clin Oncol* 1997; **15**: 535–46.

32. Koller MR, Palsson MA, Manchel I et al, Long-term culture-initiating cell expansion is dependent on frequent media exchange combined with stromal and other accessory cell effects. *Blood* 1995; **86**: 1784–9.

33. Tindle RW, Nichols RAB, Catovsky D et al, A novel anti-myeloid monoclonal antibody BI-3C5 recognizes early myeloid and some lymphoid precursors and sub-classifies human acute leukemias. *Hybridoma* 1984; **3**: 106.

34. Andrews RJ, Singer JW, Bernstein ID et al, Monoclonal antibody 12-8 recognizes as 115-kd molecule present on both unipotent and multipotent hematopoietic colony forming cells and their precursors. *Blood* 1986; **67**: 842–5.

35. Noga SJ, Cremo CA, Duff SC et al, Large scale separation of human bone marrow by counterflow centrifugation elutriation. *J Immunol Meth* 1986; **92**: 211–18.

36. Noga SJ, Donnenberg AD, Schwartz CL et al, Development of a simplified counterflow centrifugation elutriation procedure for depletion of lymphocytes from human bone marrow. *Transplantation* 1986; **41**: 220–29.

37. Berenson RJ, Shpall EJ, Auditore-Hargreaves K et al, Transplantation of CD34+ hematopoietic progenitor cells. *Cancer Invest* 1996; **14**: 589–96.

38. Berenson RJ, Bensinger WI, Kala-

masz D et al, Positive selection of viable cell populations using avidin–biotin immunoadsorption. *J Immunol Meth* 1986; **91**: 11–19.

39. Berenson RJ, Bensinger WI, Kalamasz D et al, Avidin–biotin immunoadsorption: a technique to purify cells and its potential application. In: *Progress in Bone Marrow Transplantation* (Gale RP, Shamplin R, eds). Alan R Liss: New York, 1987: 423–8.

40. Berenson RJ, Andrews RJ, Bensinger WI et al, Antigen CD34+ marrow cells engraft lethally irradiated baboons. *J Clin Invest* 1988; **81**: 951–5.

41. Wynter EA, Coutinho LH, Piet S et al, Comparison of purity and enrichment of CD34+ cells from bone marrow, umbilical cord and peripheral blood using fire separation systems. *Stem Cells* 1996; **13**: 524–32.

42. Berenson RJ, Bensinger WI, Kalamasz D et al, Transplantation of stem cells enriched by immunoadsorption. In: *Advances in Bone Marrow Purging and Processing* (Worthington-White DA, Gee AP, Gross S, eds). Wiley-Liss: New York, 1992: 449–59.

43. Berenson RJ, Bensinger WI, Hill R et al, Stem cell selection – clinical experience. In: *Advances in Bone Marrow Purging and Processing* (Gross S, Gee A, Worthington-White DA, eds). Wiley-Liss: New York, 1994: 403–14.

44. Hameroff SR, Otto CW, Kanel J et al, Acute cardiovascular effects of dimethylsulfoxide. *Ann NY Acad Sci* 1983: **411**: 94–9.

45. Shlafer M, Matheni JL, Karo AM et al, Cardiac chronotropic mechanism of dimethylsulfoxide: inhibition of acetylcholinesterase and antagonism of negative chronotrope biatropine. *Arch Int Pharmacodyn Ther* 1976; **221**: 21–31.

46. Samoszuk M, Reid M, Toy P et al, Intravenous dimethylsulfoxide therapy causes severe hematolysis mimiking a hemolytic transfusion reaction. *Transfusion* 1983; **23**: 405.

47. Sutherland DR, Keating A, The CD34 antigen: structure, biology, and

potential clinical applications. *J Hematother* 1992; **1**: 131–42.

48. Silvestri F, Banavali S, Savignano C et al, CD34 cell selection: focus on immunomagnetic beads and chymopapain. *Int J Artif Organs* 1993; **16**(Suppl 5): 96–101.

49. Preti RA, Nadasi S, Murawski J et al, Single step positive/negative purging for breast cancer using the Isolex 300i magnetic cell separator. *Blood* 1997; **90**(Suppl): Abst 4306.

50. Rubbi CP, Patel D, Rickwood D et al, Evidence of surface antigen detachment during incubation of cells with immunomagnetic beads. *J Immunol Meth* 1993; **166**: 223–41.

51. Brandt JE, Bartholomew AM, Fortman JD et al, Ex vivo expansion of autologous bone marrow CD34+ cells with porcine microvascular endothelial cells results in a graft capable of rescuing lethally irradiated baboons. *Blood* 1999; **94**: 106–13.

52. Lazarus H, Pecora AL, Shay T et al, CD34+ selection of hematopoietic blood cell collections and autotransplantation in lymphoma: overnight storage of cells at 4°C does not affect outcome. *Bone Marrow Transplant* 2000; **25**: 559–66.

53. Brenner MK, Rill DR, Moen RC et al, Gene-marking to trace origin of relapse after autologous bone marrow transplantation. *Lancet* 1993; **341**: 85–90.

54. Rill DR, Santata VM, Roberts WM et al, Direct demonstration that autologous bone marrow transplantation for solid tumors can return a multiplicity of tumor organic cells. *Blood* 1994; **84**: 380–3.

55. Deisseroth AB, Zu Z, Claxton D et al, genetic marking shows that Ph⁺ cells present in autologous transplants of CML contribute to relapse after ABMT in CML. *Blood* 1994; **83**: 3068–72.

56. Gribben JG, Freedman AS, Neuberg D et al, Immunologic purging of marrow assessed by PCR before autologous bone marrow transplantation for B cell lymphoma. *N Engl J Med* 1991; **325**: 1525–33.

57. Sharp JG, Kessinger A, Mann S et al, Outcome of high-dose therapy and autologous transplantation in non-Hodgkin's lymphoma based on the presence of tumor in the marrow or infused hematopoietic harvest. *J Clin Oncol* 1996; **14**(1): 214–19.

58. Kirk SJ, Cooper GG, Hoper M et al, The prognostic significance of marrow micrometastases in women with early breast cancer. *Eur J Surg Oncol* 1990; **16**: 481–5.

59. Mansi JL, Easton D, Berger U et al, Bone marrow micrometastases in primary breast cancer: prognostic significance after 6 years follow-up. *Eur J Cancer* 1991; **27**: 1552–5.

60. Diel IJ, Kaufmann M, Goerner R et al, Detection of tumor cells in bone marrow of patients with primary breast cancer: a prognostic factor for distant metastases. *J Clin Oncol* 1992; **10**: 1534–9.

61. Pecora AL, Preti RA, Lazarus HM et al, Breast cancer cell contamination of blood stem cell products in patients with metastatic breast cancer: predictors and clinical outcomes. *Blood* 1999; **94**(Suppl): 665a.

62. Schulze R, Schulze M, Wischnik A et al, Tumor cell contamination of peripheral blood stem cell transplants and bone marrow in high-risk breast cancer patients. *Bone Marrow Transplant* 1997; **19**: 1223–8.

63. Franklin WA, Shpall EJ, Archer P et al, Immunocytochemistry detection of breast cancer cells in marrow and peripheral blood of patients undergoing high-dose chemotherapy with autologous stem cell support. *Breast Cancer Res Treat* 1996; **41**: 1–7.

64. Ross AA, Cooper BW, Lazarus HM et al, Detection and viability of tumor cells and peripheral blood stem cell collections from breast cancer patients using immunocytochemical and clonogenic assay techniques. *Blood* 1993; **82**: 2605–11.

65. Moss TJ, Ross AA, The risk of tumor cell contamination and peripheral stem cell collections. *J Hematother* 1992; **1**: 225–32.

66. Pecora AL, Lazarus H, Stadtmauer E et al, Induction chemotherapy prior to sequential high dose chemotherapy compared to no induction increases the rate of complete response and duration of progression free survival in women with metastatic breast cancer. *Proc Am Soc Clin Oncol* 1999; **18**: 123a.

67. Vescio R, Schiller G, Stewart AK et al, Multicenter phase III trial to evaluate CD34+ selected vs unselected autologous peripheral blood progenitor cell transplantation in multiple myeloma. *Blood* 1999; **93**: 1–13.

68. Preti RA, Pecora AL, Jennis A et al, Blood stem cell (BSC) transplantation in metastatic breast cancer using CD34+ selection with or without negative selection for tumor cells using the Isolex 300i cell separation system. *Blood* 1998; **92**(Suppl): 492a.

69. Scime R, Indovina A, Santoro A et al, PBSC mobilization, collection and positive selection in patients with chronic lymphocytic leukemia. *Bone Marrow Transplant* 1998; **22**: 1159–65.

70. Reddish MA, McClean GD, Poppena S et al, Pre-immunotherapy serum (CA27.29 MUC-1) mucin levels and CD69+ lymphocytes correlate with the effect of serotope siayl TnKLH cancer vaccine in active specific immunotherapy. *Cancer Immunol* 1996; **42**: 303–9.

71. Pavletic S, Bishop M, Tarantolo S et al, Hematopoietic recovery after allogeneic blood stem-cell transplantation compared with bone marrow transplantation in patients with hematologic malignancies. *J Clin Oncol* 1997; **15**: 1608–16.

72. Dreger P, Haferlach T, Eckstein V et al, G-CSF-mobilized peripheral blood progenitor cells for allogeneic transplantation: safety and kinetics of mobilization, and composition of the graft. *Br J Haematol* 1994; **87**: 609–13.

73. Bensinger WI, Weaver CH, Appelbaum FR et al, Transplantation of allogeneic peripheral blood stem cells mobilized by recombinant human granulocyte colony-stimulating factor. *Blood* 1995; **85**: 1655–8.

74. Ringden O, Renberger M, Runde V et al, Peripheral blood stem cell transplantation from unrelated donors: a comparison with marrow transplantation. *Blood* 1999; **94**: 455–64.

75. Korbling M, Huh YO, Dorett A et al, Allogeneic blood stem cell transplantation: peripheralization and yield of donor-derived primitive hematopoietic progenitor cells (CD34$^+$ Thy-1$^{dim}$) and lymphoid subsets and possible predictors of engraftment in graft vs host disease. *Blood* 1995; **86**: 2842–50.

76. Schmitz N, Dreger P, Suttorp M et al, Primary transplantation of allogeneic peripheral blood progenitor cells mobilized by filgrastim (granulocyte colony-stimulating factor). *Blood* 1995; **85**: 1666–72.

77. Solano C, Martinez C, Brunet S et al, Chronic graft-vs-host disease after allogeneic peripheral blood progenitor cell or bone marrow transplantation from matched related donors. A case-controlled study. *Bone Marrow Transplant* 1998; **22**: 1129–35.

78. Ash RC, Casper JT, Chitambar CR et al, Successful allogeneic transplantation of T-cell depleted bone marrow from closely HLA-matched unrelated donors. *N Engl J Med* 1990; **322**: 45–94.

79. Ash RC, Horowitz MM, Gale RP et al, Bone marrow transplantation from related donors other than HLA-identical siblings: effects of T cell depletion. *Bone Marrow Transplant* 1991; **7**: 443–52.

80. Kernan NA, Bartsch G, Ash RC et al, Analysis of 462 unrelated marrow transplants facilitated by the National Marrow Donor Program. *N Engl J Med* 1993; **328**: 593–602.

81. Andrews RG, Bryant EM, Bartelmez SH et al, CD34+ marrow cells, the void of T and B lymphocytes, reconstitutes stable lymphopoiesis and myelopoiesis in lethally irradiated allogeneic baboons. *Blood* 1992; **80**: 1693–701.

82. Steinman RM, Dendritic cells and immuno-based therapies. *Exp Hematol* 1996; **24**: 859–64.

83. Engelman EG, Dendritic cells in the

treatment of cancer. *Biol Blood Marrow Transplant* 1996; **2**: 115–21.

84. Kowalkowski KL, Alzona MT, Aono FM et al, Ex vivo generation of dendritic cells from CD34+ cells in gas-permeable containers under serum-free conditions. *J Hematother* 1998; 7: 403–11.

85. Caux C, Saeland S, Favre C et al, Tumor necrosis factor alpha strongly potentiates interleukin-3 and granulocyte–macrophage colony-stimulating factor-induced proliferation of human CD34+ hematopoietic progenitor cells. *Blood* 1990; 75: 2292–8.

86. Caux C, Durand I, Moreau I et al, Tumor necrosis factor alpha cooperates with interleukin-3 in the recruitment of subsets of human CD34+ progenitors. *J Exp Med* 1993; 177: 1815–22.

87. Caux C, Massacrier C, DeZutter-Dambuyant C et al, Human dendritic Langerhans cells generated in vitro from CD34+ progenitors can prime naïve CD4+ T cells and process soluble antigen. *J Immunol* 1995; 155: 5427–33.

88. Caux C, Vanbervliet B, Massacrier C et al, CD34+ hematopoetic progenitors from human cord blood differentiate along two independent dendritic cell pathways in response to GM-CSF plus TNF alpha. *J Exp Med* 1996; 184: 695–9.

89. Santiago-Schwarz F, Belilos E, Diamond B et al, TNF in combination with GM-CSF enhances the differentiation of neonatal cord blood stem cells into dendritic cells and macrophages. *J Leukocyte Biol* 1992; 52: 274–83.

90. Santiago-Schwarz F, Divaris, Kay C et al, Mechanisms of tumor necrosis factor–granulocyte–macrophage colony-stimulating factor-induced dendritic cell development. *Blood* 1993; 82: 3019–23.

91. Reid CDL, Stakpoole A, Meager A et al, Interaction of tumor necrosis factor with granulocyte–macrophage colony-stimulating factor and other cytokines in the regulation of dendritic cell growth in vitro from early biotin CD34+ progenitors in human bone marrow. *J Immunol* 1992; 149: 2681–8.

92. Young JW, Szabolcs P, More MAS et al, Identification of dendritic cell colony-forming units among normal human CD34+ bone marrow progenitors that are expanded by c-kit ligand and yield pure dendritic cell colonies in the presence of granulocyte/macrophage colony-stimulating factor and tumor necrosis factor alpha. *J Exp Med* 1995; 182: 1111–17.

93. Strunk D, Rappersberger K, Egger C et al, Generation of human dendritic cells/Langerhans cells from circulating CD34+ hematopoietic progenitor cells. *Blood* 1996; 87: 1292–9.

94. Shpall EJ, Le Maistre CF, Holland K et al, A prospective randomized trial of buffy coat vs CD34-selected autologous bone marrow support in high-risk breast cancer patients receiving high-dose chemotherapy. *Blood* 1997; 90: 4313–20.

95. Stockerl-Goldstein KE, Brown JM, O'Brien RM et al, Increased transplant-related mortality following high-dose sequential chemotherapy in autologous hematopoietic stem cell transplantation (AHCT) using the Ceprate SC stem cell concentration system for multiple myeloma (MM). *Blood* 1999; 94(Suppl): 608a.

96. Brugger W, Bross KJ, Glatt M et al, Mobilization of tumor cells and hematopoietic progenitor cells into peripheral blood of patients with solid tumors. *Blood* 1994; 83: 636–40.

97. Shpall EJ, Jones RB, Release of tumor cells from bone marrow. *Blood* 1994; 83: 623–5.

98. Brugger W, Heimfeld S, Berensen RJ et al, Reconstitution of hematopoiesis after high-dose chemotherapy by autologous progenitor cells generated ex vivo. *N Engl J Med* 1995; 333: 283–7

99. Paquette RL, Dugan ST, Karpfe A et al, Ex vivo expanded unselected peripheral blood progenitor cells reduce post-transplant neutropenia in a dose-dependent manner. *Blood* 1999; 94: (Suppl 1): 556a.

100. Lundell B, Ramikumar K, Smith AK et al, Clinical scale expansion of cryopreserved cell volume whole bone marrow

aspirates produce sufficient cells for clinical use. *J Hematother* 1999; **8**: 115–27.

101. Stiff PJ, Oldenberg D, Hsi E et al, Successful hematopoietic engraftment following high-dose chemotherapy using only ex vivo expanded bone marrow grown in Aastrom (Strummel-based) bioreactors. *Proc Am Soc Clin Oncol* 1997; **16**: 88a.

102. Weaver CH, Tauer K, Zhen B et al, Second attempts at mobilization of peripheral blood stem cells in patients with initial low CD34+ cells yields. *J Hematother* 1998; **7**: 241–9.

103. Pecora AL, Preti RA, Jennis A et al, Aastrom Replicell system expanded bone marrow enhances hematopoietic recovery in patients receiving low doses of G-CSF primed blood stem cells. *Blood* 1998; **92**(Suppl): 126a.

104. Gluckman E, Broxmeyer HE, Auerbach AD et al, Hematopoietic reconstitution in a patient with Fanconi's anemia by means of umbilical-cord blood from an HLA-identical sibling. *N Engl J Med* 1989; **321**: 1174–8.

105. Kurtzberg J, Laughlin M, Graham ML et al, Placental blood as a source of hematopoietic stem cells for transplantation into unrelated recipients. *N Engl J Med* 1996; **335**: 157–66.

106. Wagner JE, Rosenthal J, Sweetman R et al, Successful transplantation of HLA-matched and HLA-mismatched umbilical cord blood from unrelated donors: analysis of engraftment and acute graft-vs-host disease. *Blood* 1996; **88**: 795–802.

107. Rubinstein P, Carrier C, Andromachi S et al, Outcomes among 562 recipients of placental-blood transplants from unrelated donors. *N Engl J Med* 1998; **339**: 1565–77.

108. McNiece I, Jones R, Bearman S et al, Rapid engraftment of neutrophils using ex vivo expanded PBPC correlates with total nucleated cells and not CD34 cells. *Blood* 1999; **94**(Suppl): 554a.

109. Shpall EJ, Quinones R, Jones R et al, Transplantation of adult and pediatric cancer patients with cord blood progenitors expanded ex vivo. *Blood* 1999; **94**(Suppl): 721a.

# 2

# Peripheral blood stem cell mobilization: Contemporary issues and early studies using Flt3 ligand

Patrick J Stiff

## BACKGROUND

Peripheral blood stem cells (PBSC) are universally accepted as the optimal stem cell source for patients undergoing autologous transplants,[1-4] and their use is increasing in the allogeneic setting as well.[5,6] While the transition from bone marrow (BM) to PBSC transplants occurred only over the past five to seven years, initial preclinical PBSC transplant studies actually began nearly 25 years ago, with the first PBSC clinical trials now nearly 20 years old. The rationale for initiating these studies in the 1970s is still valid today, with the goals being the development of a simple, less expensive alternative to marrow harvesting, the ability to infuse tumor-free grafts, and to have a transplant option for those who had received prior pelvic irradiation or had malignant cells in their iliac crest aspirates. Much has been learned in the past 20 years, as summarized in Table 2.1, and is the subject of this review. In the year 2000, with PBSC transplants firmly established as the standard of care, the goal of ongoing research is still to deliver tumor-free grafts, with current efforts exploring ex vivo purging techniques that require a larger number of stem cells than an unmanipulated graft, and strategies to increase the number of patients eligible to receive a transplant by improving stem cell mobilization in the heavily pretreated, 'hard-to-mobilize' patient population. This review will focus on current issues of stem cell mobilization and the early clinical experience with the use of a novel hematopoietic growth factor, Flt3 ligand (Flt3L), to accomplish these goals.

Pluripotent hematopoietic stem cells (HSC), capable of restoring hematopoiesis after lethal BM injury, have long been known to circulate in the blood of animals and non-human primates.[7-9] Their usual concentration in the blood, however, is approximately two logs lower than that in BM.[7] Considering the minimum numbers of colony-forming units granulocyte–macrophage (CFU-GM) per kilogram needed to reliably reconstitute patients after an autologous BM transplant ($5 \times 10^4$/kg), it was realized early that from 6 to 20

---

### Table 2.1  PBSC mobilization: current concepts

- Cytokine/chemotherapy combinations mobilize more PBSC than cytokines alone.
- Used alone, G-CSF mobilizes more PBSC than GM-CSF.
- Combined with chemotherapy PBSC yields are similar using G-CSF and GM-CSF.
- Patients who have received more than six months of alkylating agent therapy, fludarabine, or chemotherapy and radiotherapy have up to a 30% chance of not being able to proceed to transplant after standard mobilization techniques owing to inadequate stem cell dose ($<1 \times 10^6$ CD34$^+$ cells/kg).
- There is a dose–response effect for G-CSF in PBSC mobilization in both minimally treated and heavily pretreated patients.
- An early-acting cytokine (SCF or Flt3L) with a late-acting cytokine (G-CSF/GM-CSF) yields more PBSC than G-CSF alone, especially in heavily pretreated patients.

*Abbreviations:* PBSC, peripheral blood stem cell; G-CSF, granulocyte colony-stimulating factor; GM-CSF, granulocyte–macrophage CSF; SCF, stem cell factor.

---

aphereses would be required to collect enough HSC during the steady state, for a successful transplant.[7]

Studies in the late 1970s and early 1980s indicated that committed HSC, as measured by the CFU-GM and burst-forming unit erythroid (BFU-E) assays, could be mobilized into the circulation during the recovery phase after aggressive chemotherapy.[10–12] In these early studies, the magnitude of PBSC expansion after chemotherapy, as measured by the CFU-GM assay, was 20-fold. That these cells represented a cell population capable of restoring hematopoiesis after lethal BM injury was subsequently shown in several animal models. Storb et al[13] demonstrated complete hematopoietic reconstitution in lethally irradiated non-human primates who were cross-circulated with unirradiated animals. By apheresing dogs during the rebound period after chemotherapy, Abrams et al[11] showed that the 11-fold increase in CFU-GM over baseline represented a 12.5-fold increase in the ability of these cells to reconstitute lethally irradiated dogs, further documenting that pluripotent stem cells were also mobilized. In addition, in Appelbaum's studies,[1] although the BM nucleated cell dose required to restore hematopoiesis was 24 times higher for peripheral blood as compared with BM transplants, the CFU-GM dose was identical. Subsequent studies, in which committed stem cell concentrations were measured in the peripheral blood of patients after several cycles of aggressive chemotherapy for small cell lung cancer, suggested that sufficient PBSC could be collected after this form of 'mobilization' for an autologous transplant, from only two aphereses.[12]

The first reported PBSC clinical trial suggested that patients could be rescued from high-dose BCNU-based preparative regimens by stem cells collected during the rebound after chemotherapy, with a particularly rapid engraftment of neutrophils, but with some delay in platelet recovery.[14,15] The timing for these aphereses was critical, with optimal yields seen with a peripheral monocytosis of over 30% and a white blood cell count (WBC) in the range of only 1000–1500/μl. Others performed aphereses in the steady state and documented engraftment after autologous transplantation.[16,17] Research in this area slowed until the early to mid 1990s, when two discoveries were made. The first was the demonstration that recombinant hematopoietic growth factors can mobilize PBSC cells into the circulation, even without concomitant chemotherapy.[18] Secondly, the discovery of a simple, accurate marker of primitive stem cell numbers, with development of the CD34 assay,[19] insured that stem cell numbers could be accurately quantified within hours of request. By their ability to mobilize more primitive HSC than were possible to collect from a BM harvest, cytokines facilitated more rapid hematopoietic engraftment following transplants than with a BM transplant, in both the autologous and allogeneic settings.[18,20–22] Consistent, predictable engraftment has also been demonstrated as numerous clinical trials have established the 'ideal' PBSC $CD34^+$ cell dose to rapidly reconstitute hematopoiesis as $5 \times 10^6$/kg, while the minimum safe dose to proceed to transplant is $1 \times 10^6$/kg.[23–27] Most research is now directed at obtaining the ideal $CD34^+$ cell dose in all patients, in a setting where patients are infused with tumor-free grafts.

## STEM CELL MOBILIZATION USING CYTOKINES

Both granulocyte and granulocyte–macrophage colony-stimulating factors (G-CSF and GM-CSF) are approved in the USA for use in the mobilization of PBSC. Presumably by downmodulation of adhesion molecules such as very late activation antigen 4 (VLA-4),[28] cytokines 'mobilize' stem cells from the BM to the peripheral blood up to 5–60 times over steady-state levels. The amount of stem cell mobilization can vary based on the cytokine used, with G-CSF at a standard dose of 10 μg/kg/day mobilizing more $CD34^+$ cells/kg than GM-CSF at 250 mg/m²/day (approximately 5 μg/kg), the amount of prior stem cell damage as outlined below, and the dose and schedule of the cytokine. These agents work best when administered as a continuous intravenous infusion, or subcutaneously, and studies appear to indicate a dose and schedule effect for G-CSF. In general, a doubling of the dose of G-CSF leads to a near doubling of the number of CFU-GM or $CD34^+$ cells mobilized, at least in healthy individuals.[29–31] Higher doses, especially those above 20 μg/kg/day, are associated with more bone pain and/or headache, but are rarely severe enough to prevent continuation of mobilization. Preliminary data also suggest that if the subcutaneous route is selected, one-half of the dose administered every 12 hours may be superior to a single daily injection.[32] A dose–response effect of GM-CSF has not been fully explored. Apheresis usually begins on the fourth or fifth day after cytokine administration is initiated, with the number of $CD34^+$ cells collected peaking on either that or the following day. Thereafter, a fairly rapid drop in PBSC numbers ensues over the next several days, with very few collected after the first three days of apheresis. Sufficient CD34$^+$ cells can, however, usually be collected for a safe transplant, usually after two to three days of apheresis in healthy donors or minimally pretreated patients such as those typically transplanted for breast cancer. When infused after high-dose therapy, these stem cells lead to a more rapid recovery of neutrophils and platelets, and to shorter hospital stays, and are not associated with a higher rate of relapse, as compared with autologous BM transplants.[20–22] However, approximately 5% of normal donors fail to mobilize, and up to approximately 30% of certain patient groups fail to mobilize the minimum safe dose of $1 \times 10^6$ CD34$^+$ cells/kg after repeated aphereses, when standard doses of these cytokines are used for stem cell mobilization.[25,33–36]

Because in vitro studies suggested that GM-CSF increases the colony-stimulatory activity of G-CSF, it has been suggested that the combination of the two agents, especially when used sequentially, may permit the collection of a larger number of CD34$^+$ cells.[37] In one of the earliest studies of G-CSF/GM-CSF combinations, Winter et al[38] showed that, in contrast to adding GM-CSF sequentially to G-SCF, the addition of G-CSF after a six-day exposure to GM-CSF increased CFU-GM apheresis yields 80 times. There are some data indicating that the combination of G-CSF and either simultaneous or sequential use of GM-CSF leads to either higher numbers of total CD34$^+$ cells/kg collected using G-CSF alone, or higher numbers of a primitive subset of CD34$^+$ cells, namely those that are also CD38$^-$.[38–40] These data come from small series, and in many of the trials of GM-CSF plus G-CSF, cytokines are given at their full doses but have not been compared with a higher dose of G-CSF, an agent that does mobilize more PBSC at higher doses, as noted below. It appears that the primitive PBSC subpopulation may contribute greatly to early engraftment, and most studies do suggest a higher primitive PBSC cell number with G-CSF/GM-CSF combinations.[38–40] Therefore it is appropriate to investigate G-CSF and GM-CSF combinations further, and this remains an area of active investigation.

## STEM CELL MOBILIZATION USING CHEMOTHERAPY AND CYTOKINES

The initial rationale for combining chemotherapy with cytokines for stem cell mobilization is the well-described effect of PBSC mobilization by chemotherapy alone, the frequent need to cytoreduce disease pretransplant, and the beneficial effect of cytokines to reduce the complications associated with neutropenic fevers. Chemotherapy followed by either G-CSF or GM-CSF in general mobilizes more PBSC than either cytokines or chemotherapy alone, although a randomized comparison of the differing strategies has not been performed.[41–46] For example, in an early sequential comparison, Socinski et al[41] demonstrated an 18-fold increase in CFU-GM after GM-CSF alone, but, in combination with chemotherapy, a 60-fold rise was seen. Unlike mobilization from the steady state, there is no difference in the amount of PBSC mobilization obtained with chemotherapy/G-CSF combinations as compared with GM-CSF-containing combinations. The ability of PBSC collected after chemotherapy/cytokine mobilization to promote rapid hematopoietic engraftment in the transplant setting appears identical to that of cells mobilized with a cytokine alone. Unlike steady-state mobilization, there does not appear to be a dose–response effect with either cytokine when used for PBSC mobilization after chemotherapy. One-half the dose used to mobilize PBSC from the steady state (e.g. G-CSF at 5 µg/kg/day) appears optimal following chemotherapy. The higher yields make chemotherapy/cytokine combinations potentially more attractive for patients with pre-existing BM damage from prior therapy. However, there are no data to suggest that a chemotherapy/cytokine combination is superior to a cytokine alone in these heavily pretreated patients. In fact, as noted below, CD34$^+$ cell yields appear to be similar for the two methods, but more complications are reported for patients failing initial mobilization with either method who are re-mobilized with chemotherapy/cytokine combinations.[36] The requirement for patients to be in a state of remission before transplant, pre-approval from third party payors in the USA, the added costs of a longer course of cytokines, and the costs of the chemotherapy itself have led most physicians in the USA to mobilize with cytokines alone. Outside the USA, chemotherapy/cytokine combinations are routinely used, primarily because of their higher PBSC yields.

While not completely studied, the dose and specific cytotoxic agents used for mobilization appear to affect the quantity of PBSC mobilized. For single-agent cyclophosphamide, dose appears important, with 7 g/m$^2$ administered with GM-CSF leading to a near 100-fold increase in blood CFU-GM.[43] While yields increase with dose, so do the complications and costs associated with severe pancytopenia.[43,47] Most groups now use less-myelosuppressive combinations of chemotherapeutic agents, obtaining similar or higher PBSC yields than seen with high-dose cyclophosphamide. Certain combinations such as those that are paclitaxel-based appear superior to others, although this impression comes from uncontrolled retrospective analyses.[48,49]

## HARD-TO-MOBILIZE PATIENTS

Transplanting patients with optimal PBSC doses of $5 \times 10^6$ CD34$^+$ cells/kg leads to neutrophil engraftment at 8–10 days after transplant, and platelet recovery at 10–12 days. With almost any dose of CD34$^+$ cells above $1 \times 10^6$/kg, neutrophil engraftment is rapid and consistent, but there is a significant dose–response relationship between CD34$^+$ cells/kg and engraftment of platelets, with up to 30% of patients not engrafting platelets if they receive only $1 \times 10^6$ CD34$^+$ cells/kg.[25,50,51] Until CD34$^+$ cell doses reach $5 \times 10^6$/kg, from 10% to 30% of patients do not engraft platelets by day 28 post-transplant.

While most investigators agree that the optimal CD34$^+$ cell dose is $5 \times 10^6$/kg, only a fraction of any center's patients reach this target, largely because of extensive prior therapy. The risk factors associated with an inability to reach the optimal dose have been studied by various groups in univariate or multi-variate analyses,[51-56] and are outlined in Table 2.2. Overall, stem cell mobilization is inversely related to the amount of prior chemotherapy and radiotherapy a patient receives. Among the most important factors are prior radiotherapy and chemotherapy, more than 6–11 cycles, courses or months of alkylating agent therapy, the use of particular alkylating agents such as melphalan, BNCU and cisplatin, BM involvement by fibrosis or tumor, and, as stated above, the use of cytokines alone versus chemotherapy and cytokines for mobilization. In particular, patients being considered for transplants in second or third remission with a diagnosis of Hodgkin's or non-Hodgkin's lymphoma or ovarian cancer will have as much as a 30% chance of failing to mobilize a minimum safe dose of CD34$^+$ cells ($1 \times 10^6$/kg) to permit a transplant, using standard mobilization strategies.[34,35] In addition, the absolute number of CFU-GM/kg or the relative proportion of primitive subsets of CD34$^+$ cells may also be important in more accurately determining engraftment potential of borderline PBSC doses.[34,57]

Strategies for poor mobilizers have until recently focused on individual patients who mobilize poorly. These include, BM harvesting[34] or re-mobilization,[36,44,58,59] usually with higher cytokine doses, or, in the case of those who were initially mobilized with cytokines alone, the combination of chemotherapy and cytokines. BM harvesting in poor mobilizers, recently examined in two non-comparative studies,[34,35] does not appear to improve engraftment of platelets. In the study by Watts et al,[34] six out of ten patients who received

---

**Table 2.2  Factors associated with poor CD34$^+$ cell mobilization**

1. Prior radiotherapy to BM-bearing sites[35,48,52,55]
2. Prior stem cell cytotoxic therapy:[26,27,35,49,54,56,59,63,85]
   - nitrogen mustard
   - melphalan
   - BCNU
   - high-dose Ara-C
   - platinum compounds
   - fludarabine
3. Number of cycles of prior therapy (>6–11)[52,54,56,59]
4. Number of prior chemotherapy regimens (>2)[35,48,85]
5. BM involvement with tumor[48,52]
6. Specific diseases[26,35,52,54,62,63,85]
   - non-Hodgkin's lymphoma and Hodgkin's disease
   - ovarian carcinoma

autologous BM in addition to an inadequate PBSC harvest of fewer than $1 \times 10^6$ CD34$^+$ cells/kg still did not engraft platelets by day 28, as compared with five out of six transplanted with their inadequate PBSC alone. In a similar analysis performed as part of a multicenter trial, of 19 patients who mobilized fewer than $1 \times 10^6$ CD34$^+$ cells/kg, nine underwent BM harvesting. These nine who received the BM and PBSC had the same engraftment characteristics as the ten who received PBSC alone.[35] While not conclusive, these data suggest a limited role for marrow harvesting to supplement inadequate stem cell collections.

Re-mobilization is thus currently the main strategy used to increase PBSC cell doses for poor mobilizers. In general, studies have indicated that re-mobilization using the same strategy as the initial one usually yields the same PBSC dose. In a recent study by Weaver et al,[36] patients who collected fewer than $2 \times 10^6$ CD34$^+$ cells/kg were defined as poor mobilizers, and were required to undergo re-mobilization prior to transplantation. Whether or not patients were initially mobilized with chemotherapy plus cytokines or with cytokines alone, the PBSC re-mobilization yields were identical whether chemotherapy plus cytokines or cytokines alone were used. These results strongly suggest that re-mobilization with G-CSF alone is the preferred method, based on similar CD34$^+$ cell yields/kg for the two methods, and a higher risk of hospitalization for those mobilized with the cytokine/chemotherapy combinations. However, this conclusion should be interpreted with caution, since in this series, 30 out of 44 (68%) of those re-mobilized with G-CSF alone received doses of more than 10 µg/kg/day, with some receiving doses as high as 32 µg/kg/day. In a subsequent randomized trial from the same group, it was discovered that the dose of G-CSF was important for poor mobilizers, with 30 µg/kg/day being the optimal dose for this group.[49]

Our group at the Loyola University Medical Center recently analyzed data on poor mobilizers seen over a five-year period.[59] A summary of the analysis is shown in Table 2.3. Setting the minimum threshold at $2 \times 10^6$ CD34$^+$ cells/kg, 29 out of 473 (6.1%) of the autotransplants performed at this institution qualified. This represents a smaller percentage of poor mobilizers than seen at other centers, largely because clinical trials ongoing during this period explored cytokine combinations or high-dose G-CSF for the initial mobilization. Of the entire group of 29 patients, 18 had lymphoma, which represented 10% of all lymphomas treated during the five-year period (18/181). Only 3% of breast cancer and 4% of myeloma patients fit into this group, but 27% of testicular cancer patients qualified. Of the entire group of 29, 41% had received prior radiotherapy, the median number of chemotherapy cycles was 8, and 66% had received prior platinum. Re-mobilization was done using G-CSF, primarily at a total dose of 32 µg/kg/day given as 16 mg/kg twice daily. CD34$^+$ cell yields increased from a total of $0.71 \times 10^6$/kg for the entire first mobilization (median four aphereses) to $1.78 \times 10^6$/kg for the second mobilization (median three aphereses). Twenty-four patients reached the target with the second mobilization; one underwent a BM harvest, and four a third mobilization. The

**Table 2.3  Re-mobilization with dose-escalated G-CSF: the Loyola experience**

| | |
|---|---|
| Number of patients: | 29 |
| Percentage of all BMT patients: | 6.1% |
| Disease: | |
| Lymphoma: | 62% |
| Central nervous system: | 25% |
| Breast: | 14% |
| Testicular: | 10% |
| Initial mobilization (medians): | |
| Total dose: | $0.71 \times 10^6$ CD34$^+$ cells/kg |
| Number of aphereses: | 4 |
| Second mobilization (medians): | |
| Total dose: | $1.78 \times 10^6$ CD34$^+$ cells/kg |
| Number of aphereses: | 3 |
| Neutrophil engraftment: | 11 days (range 9–39 days) |
| Platelet engraftment: | 13 days (range 8–28 days) |

yield for the third mobilization was poor; with only $0.9 \times 10^6$/kg for a median of three aphereses. All 29 patients successfully underwent their transplant, with median times to neutrophil engraftment of 11 days (range 9–39 days) and to platelet engraftment of 13 days (range 8–28 days).

Taken together, these data suggest that re-mobilization using dose-escalated G-CSF may be of value; however, this needs to be evaluated prospectively. It is of note that in both studies the amount of bone pain associated with high-dose G-CSF in the poor-mobilizer group appears to be less than that of normal donors who have received high-dose G-CSF.

While re-mobilization appears to be of value for those who do not meet minimum thresholds, the costs of providing this care are significant, averaging $8000–10 000 per patient.[60] A more appropriate strategy may be to identify groups likely to be poor mobilizers and develop novel therapies to enhance PBSC mobilization for these patients. Prospective studies have, in fact, identified two strategies that may be of value: an initial mobilization using dose-escalated G-CSF,[33,61,62] and combinations of an early- and a late-acting cytokine.[33,35,63] Dose-escalated G-CSF was evaluated in a sequential analysis of patients undergoing transplants for advanced ovarian cancer at our institution.[33,61] Approximately 25% of this group failed to meet minimum CD34$^+$ cell targets using standard cytokine-only mobilization methods. The study group of 26 patients who received twice-daily G-CSF at 16 µg/kg were compared with 18 who had previously been mobilized by a single daily dose of 10 µg/kg/day. The high-dose group achieved the $2 \times 10^6$ CD34$^+$ cells/kg target

96% of the time in three aphereses, as compared with 86% in the standard-dose group. In a cost analysis that considered the costs of aphereses, transfusions, and hospital length-of-stay differences, the total costs of the two groups were identical. In addition, by achieving an optimal CD34$^+$ cell dose/kg, delayed engraftment of platelets was eliminated. This approach is being evaluated prospectively.

To decrease the proportion of poor mobilizers, the second alternative is to combine an early- and a late-acting cytokine. To date, the combination of G-CSF and stem cell factor (SCF) has been the most extensively evaluated.[33,35,63] The combination in preclinical models mobilized more PBSC than either agent alone,[64] and this was verified in an early clinical trial in patients with minimally pretreated breast cancer.[25] A subsequent phase III trial in breast cancer confirmed the benefit, with a high proportion of patients achieving the $5 \times 10^6$ CD34$^+$ cells/kg target – and doing so in fewer aphereses.[65] At the same time as the initial clinical trial in breast cancer, a similar phase I/II trial was undertaken in patients with relapsed, chemosensitive non-Hodgkin's lymphoma.[63] Taking into consideration the amount of prior therapy, there was a difference for those who had received heavy prior therapy defined as two or more cycles of procarbazine, nitrosoureas, melphalan, or nitrogen mustard, or 7 g or more of high-dose Ara-C. Those treated with 10 μg/kg/day of G-CSF mobilized only $0.28 \times 10^6$ CD34$^+$ cells/kg after three aphereses, as compared with $1.76 \times 10^6$/kg from those who received SCF at any dose (5–20 μg/kg/day) plus the same dose of G-CSF, in a retrospective analysis. As a result, platelet engraftment was significantly longer in the G-CSF group by 10 days: 23 versus 12.5 days.

A subsequent prospective, randomized trial in heavily pretreated patients with Hodgkin's disease and non-Hodgkin's lymphoma has recently been reported.[35] This trial compared G-CSF (10 μg/kg/day) with the same dose of G-CSF with 20 μg/kg/day of SCF. In contrast to the first trial, patients underwent repeated aphereses (a maximum of five) until they reached a target of $5 \times 10^6$ CD34$^+$ cells/kg. Compared with the G-CSF-alone group, those receiving the combination had a higher rate of achieving the $5 \times 10^6$ CD34$^+$ cells/kg target (44% versus 17%), a higher median CD34$^+$ cell dose (3.6 versus $2.4 \times 10^6$/kg), and a smaller percentage who did not meet the minimum safe CD34$^+$ cell dose ($1 \times 10^6$/kg) to proceed to transplant (16% versus 26%). This has represented until recently the only prospective, randomized trial data, verifying the benefits of combining an early- and a late-acting cytokine for mobilization of high-risk groups. While there are allergic-like reactions due to mast cell stimulation and degranulation, associated with SCF administration, with adequate premedications these are not life-threatening.[35,65] At this time, however, SCF is not yet available for routine clinical use in the USA.

# Flt3L AS A STEM CELL MOBILIZING AGENT

## Preclinical data

Flt3L ('fms-like tyrosine kinase 3 ligand'), a naturally occurring glycoprotein that stimulates primitive hematopoietic stem cells through the Flt3 receptor, is a member of the tyrosine kinase receptor family, which also includes the c-Kit locus, the receptor for SCF.[66–69] As such, it has similar in vitro and in vivo characteristics to SCF,[70,71] with the exception that it does not cause proliferation or stimulation of mast cells,[71,72] and it may have a greater stimulatory effect on lymphoid stem cells, in particular early B cells.[66–71] It also expands and stimulates natural killer (NK) cells and antigen-presenting cells or dendritic cells. In contrast to SCF, Flt3L has no appreciable effect on erythropoiesis or megakaryocytopoiesis when evaluated as a single agent.[71] In vitro colony assays, however, have demonstrated synergy with a variety of early- and late-acting cytokines, including thrombopoietin, interleukin (IL)-3, GM-CSF and G-CSF. Like SCF, early animal studies indicated that Flt3L mobilized PBSC,[73,74] an activity that is enhanced by the concomitant use of G-CSF or GM-CSF.[75–77] In addition, via its effect on tumor-specific immune cell enhancement, it caused significant remissions and cures in certain animal tumor systems.[78,79]

In initial murine studies, animals injected with Flt3L had increases in their WBC and spleen size.[73,74] The increase in WBC was seen in all white cell lineages: monocytes, lymphocytes and granulocytes. CFU-GM and multilineage colonies increased in the BM and blood, as did colony-forming units spleen (CFU-S). BFU-E increases were less than those seen for CFU-GM. In addition to the hematopoietic effects, Flt3L led to significant increases in CD11c$^+$ dendritic cells in the peripheral blood, spleen and lymph nodes and NK cells in the blood, BM, spleen, liver, and thymus. These cells were fully functional and were capable of priming an antigen-specific T-cell immune response in vivo. NK cells generated by Flt3L had an enhanced response to IL-2 as measured by proliferation and the development of lymphokine-activated killer activity.

When administered to non-human primates, Flt3L not only mobilized stem cells, but also expanded their numbers in the BM.[80] When administered for 14 days, the numbers of BM CD34$^+$ cells increased from 0.75% to 2.11% on day 11, while the number of blood CD34$^+$ cells increased 12–14-fold. There was a dose-dependent rise in PBSC numbers in this model, with doses of Flt3L of 400 μg/kg/day leading to sustained mobilization for at least three weeks. As seen in the murine model, there were significant increases in blood monocytes and lymphocytes (both CD20$^+$ and CD2$^+$CD56$^+$) but only a twofold increase in blood neutrophils. The only clinical side-effects were mild lymphadenopathy and splenomegaly.

Initially tested in a murine model, administration of Flt3L in combination with a committed myeloid cytokine demonstrated synergy of PBSC mobilization.[75,76] Animals receiving an Flt3L-containing combination for up to 10 days[76] had significant increases in PBSC mobilization as compared with those receiving committed cytokines alone. The greatest increase over baseline was seen in those receiving the simultaneous administration of Flt3L and G-CSF (a 200-fold increase), as compared with G-CSF alone (a 17-fold increase) or Flt3L alone (a 36-fold increase). Mobilization using the combination continued for a longer period than was seen with G-CSF alone, with the peak occurring on the final day of cytokine administration (day 10). In this model, the rise was less significant for the combination of Flt3L and GM-CSF. However, while Flt3L and G-CSF are both highly active in mice, human GM-CSF typically exhibits low activity in non-primate animals. The mobilized PBSC from Flt3L combinations were as effective in rescuing animals after lethal irradiation as those mobilized by G-CSF alone.

The combinations of Flt3L and G-CSF or GM-CSF were also evaluated in a non-human primate model.[77] As compared with Flt3L alone, which produced at the end of a 10-day course of subcutaneous administration an absolute number of $(54 \pm 17) \times 10^3$ CD34$^+$ cells/ml of blood, those treated with Flt3L and G-CSF had $(270 \pm 47) \times 10^3$ CD34$^+$ cells/ml and those with Flt3L and GM-CSF had $(384 \pm 275) \times 10^3$ CD34$^+$ cells/ml. This degree of mobilization was in the range such that a single apheresis procedure would be sufficient to perform a transplant. Increases in dendritic cells were comparable in all three groups, with increases also seen in NK cells (10.2-fold) and CD25$^+$ cells (12.5-fold). There were no adverse effects associated with the administration of the cytokines.

## Phase I human data

Initial human Flt3L trials were conducted in healthy volunteers.[81,82] The dose levels studied were 1, 5, 10, 25, 50, 75, and 100 μg/kg given subcutaneously, as a single injection, with a placebo control group. Pharmacokinetic analysis indicated a terminal half-life of 1.5–2 days in the 21 subjects (3 at each level). A slight sore throat in a single patient at the first level and an injection-site reaction after the highest dose in one subject were the only adverse effects. Daily dosing for 14 days was then studied at 10, 25, 50, 75, and 100 μg/kg/day. The only adverse reaction was local injection-site reaction, primarily erythema (with edema, induration, or pruritus in some subjects), which occurred in 11 out of 15 receiving active drug. Six subjects experienced mild (grade I) lymphadenopathy.

By the completion of the 14-day course of therapy, the total WBC increased two- to threefold, with a marked increase in monocytes (to 15-fold). A dose-dependent drop in platelets of approximately 20% was seen by the end of the 14-day course of treatment, similar to that seen in G-CSF controls. Platelet counts rebounded quickly after the drug was stopped, reaching maximal levels of approximately $3.5 \times 10^5$/μl by day 28. Dendritic cells rose to as much as 15% of mononuclear cells in the blood, reaching levels of nearly 1000/μl on day 15 of therapy. Some slight increases were seen in lactate dehydrogenase

(LDH), aspartate aminotransferase (AST), and alanine aminotransferase (ALT). No significant (grade III/IV) clinical adverse effects were seen. There was a dose-dependent rise in blood CD34$^+$ cells, starting on day 7 of administration, which continued as the drug was given for the 14-day period, and continued to rise for several days after drug discontinuation. At doses of more than 10 μg/kg/day, the CD34$^+$ cell numbers/μl approximated those levels typically seen with G-CSF alone. Unlike G-CSF, the peak was both delayed (day 18 after initiation) and more prolonged.

Flt3L was next tested in combination with G-CSF or GM-CSF in a phase I fashion, in 72 normal volunteers.[83] Endpoints were to assess the safety of the combinations, as well as the extent of PBSC mobilization. The control arm was G-CSF administered at 10 μg/kg/day, and the combinations included G-CSF at either 5 or 10 μg/kg/day or GM-CSF at 5 μg/kg/day. Flt3L doses ranged from 10 to 100 μg/kg/day. There were no grade IV adverse effects, and only one grade III clinical effect, namely abdominal pain possibly related to a study drug in a patient receiving Flt3L (10 μg/kg) and GM-CSF (5 μg/kg). Grade I/II injection site reactions were common in all groups, but most common in the Flt3L/GM-CSF group. One subject had elevated liver enzymes (grade III), felt likely to be due to study drugs (Flt3L and GM-CSF), which normalized quickly after the drug was discontinued.

CD34$^+$ cell blood concentrations for the Flt3L combinations were approximately 1.5–2.0 times greater than that seen for G-CSF alone. PBSC mobilization was more sustained, particularly for the Flt3L/GM-CSF combinations, lasting up to a week after the drugs were stopped. The GM-CSF/Flt3L CD34$^+$ cell peak occurred later than typically seen with G-CSF alone, peaking on approximately day 9 of cytokine administration. In addition, there was a dose–response effect with Flt3L, with 50 μg/kg in combination with GM-CSF (5 μg/kg being more active than 10 μg/kg of Flt3L). Dendritic cell mobilization for the combinations was more significant than that seen with Flt3L alone, with the largest increase being seen in the Flt3L/GM-CSF group, which was nearly threefold higher than with either Flt3L alone or the Flt3L/G-CSF combination.

## Phase II trial data

Two randomized phase II clinical trials evaluating the mobilization potential of Flt3L in combination with either G-CSF or GM-CSF were reported at the 1999 American Society of Hematology meeting.[84,85] Based on the normal-volunteer phase I data, the Flt3L dose chosen for these trials was 50 μg/kg/day. The study designs were identical between the two groups, with mobilization using standard doses of G-CSF (10 μg/kg/day) used as the control. The schema are shown in Figure 2.1. For the GM-CSF/Flt3L and G-CSF/Flt3L combinations, Flt3L was administered for the first three days, with the second cytokine starting on the first day and continuing through the completion of the aphereses. The two trials differed in that one (breast cancer)[84] tested the combinations in

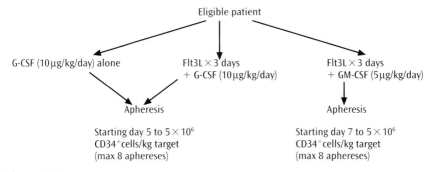

Figure 2.1

Schema of randomized trial of GM-CSF/Flt3L or G-CSF/Flt3L in heavily treated lymphoma or ovarian cancer patients or in minimally pretreated breast cancer patients.

minimally pretreated patients, while the other (lymphoma and ovarian cancer)[85] preselected patients who had been 'heavily pretreated'. To be eligible for the latter trial, patients had to have been treated with at least two prior regimens, or one fludarabine-containing regimen, to have received at least seven total cycles of chemotherapy, or to have BM involvement with tumor.

The group receiving the Flt3L/GM-CSF combination started apheresis on day 7 of cytokine administration, while the group receiving the G-CSF combination and the G-CSF control group started on day 5. Patients underwent daily 12-liter aphereses to a target CD34$^+$ cell dose of $5 \times 10^6$/kg or to a maximum of eight aphereses, unless, after five aphereses, yields were less than $0.4 \times 10^6$/kg. The primary endpoints were the number of aphereses needed to collect $5 \times 10^6$ CD34$^+$ cells/kg and the volume of blood needed to be processed for this cell dose. Secondary endpoints were the toxicities of the therapies, and the long-term survival of the patients mobilized with the Flt3L combinations.

For the breast cancer trial,[84] 27 control patients mobilized with G-CSF alone were compared with 24 receiving GM-CSF and Flt3L, and 24 receiving G-CSF and Flt3L. A total of $2 \times 10^6$ CD34$^+$ cells/kg was collected in 81% of the control group, 92% of the GM-CSF/Flt3L group, and 96% of the G-CSF/Flt3L group. Looked at differently, 67% of the control patients reached a target of $2.5 \times 10^6$ CD34$^+$ cells/kg in four or fewer aphereses, as compared with 75% of the GM-CSF/Flt3L group and 92% of the G-CSF/Flt3L group. The toxicity of the mobilization regimen was similar in the three groups, except that injection-site reactions were reported only in the two Flt3L-containing combinations. Engraftments of platelets and neutrophils, as expected, were not significantly different among the three groups. The trial design, treatment, and endpoints for the hard-to-mobilize trial were the same as for the breast cancer trial,[85] but, as expected, the CD34$^+$ cell yields were lower in these heavily pretreated patients. A total of $2 \times 10^6$ CD34$^+$ cells/kg were collected in 63% of the control group, 92% of the GM-CSF/Flt3L group, and 74% of the G-CSF/Flt3L group. The CD34$^+$ cell dose of $2.5 \times 10^6$/kg was reached in five or fewer aphereses in 46% of the control group, 79% of the GM-CSF/Flt3L group, and 48% of the G-CSF/Flt3L group. Interestingly, 25% of the G-CSF control group and 17% of the G-CSF/Flt3L group failed to meet the minimum CD34$^+$ cell dose of $1 \times 10^6$/kg, similar to the G-CSF control group, who received the same mobilizing dose of G-CSF in the G-CSF/SCF trial in heavily pretreated lymphoma patients. A comparison of the results is shown in Table 2.4. In the Flt3L study, all patients in the GM-CSF/Flt3L group, however, reached the $1 \times 10^6$ CD34$^+$ cells/kg minimum cell dose to proceed to transplant. The benefits of the combinations seemed to be related to the sustainability of mobilization, which was not seen with those mobilized with G-CSF alone. Like the breast cancer trial, engraftment rates were similar between the three groups, as was the toxicity of the study drugs. These trials suggest that there may be only a modest benefit in breast cancer patients for the Flt3L combinations as compared with G-CSF in these easier-to-mobilize patients; however, the magnitude of the benefit in the heavily pretreated patient group appears more significant.

### Table 2.4  Combinations of early- and late-acting cytokines for hard-to-mobilize patients

|  | SCF + G-CSF | Flt3l + GM-CSF |
|---|---|---|
| Patient group | Hodgkin's disease + non-Hodgkin's lymphoma | Non-Hodgkin's lymphoma + ovarian cancer |
| Phase of study | Randomized phase II | Randomized phase II |
| Total number of patients | 102 | 71 |
| Maximum number of aphereses | 5 | 8 |
| Percentage reaching $1 \times 10^6$ CD34$^+$ cells/kg | | |
|     Control group | 74% | 75% |
|     Study group | 86% | 100% |
| Percentage reaching $5 \times 10^6$ CD34$^+$ cells/kg | | |
|     Control group | 17% | – |
|     Study group | 44% | – |
| Percentage reaching $3 \times 10^6$ CD34$^+$ cells/kg | | |
|     Control group | – | 42% |
|     Study group | – | 79% |

## CONCLUSIONS

PBSC mobilization in the minimally pretreated patient is accomplished quickly with a short course of G-CSF alone, or during the rebound after chemotherapy combined with either low-dose G-CSF or GM-CSF. With more-aggressive therapy being given to patients with lymphomas, Hodgkin's disease, testicular cancer, and ovarian cancer, the percentage of those coming to transplant heavily pretreated, and thus in the poor-mobilizer group, is likely to increase. Strategies designed to increase the percentage of transplant candidates reaching not only a minimum safe PBSC dose but also equally rapid hematopoietic engraftment on the first mobilization attempt is needed. This approach is likely to be more cost-effective than re-mobilization, and less costly and morbid than the complications associated with delayed hematopoietic engraftment. The recent preliminary data utilizing GM-CSF combined with Flt3L in the heavily pretreated group appear to indicate the first combination that virtually eliminates the outlier group who fail to reach the minimum target for a safe transplant. Further studies are urgently needed in this high-risk group.

## REFERENCES

1. To LB, Haylock DN, Simmons PJ et al, The biology and clinical uses of blood stem cells. *Blood* 1997; **89**: 2253–8.

2. Shpall EJ, Cagnoni DJ, Bearman ST et al, Peripheral blood stem cells for autografting. *Annu Rev Med* 1997; **48**: 241–51.

3. Appelbaum FR, The use of bone marrow and peripheral blood stem cell transplantation in the treatment of cancer. *CA Cancer J Clin* 1996; **46**: 142–64.

4. Nemanaitis J, Cytokine-mobilized peripheral blood progenitor cells. *Semin Oncol* 1996; **23**(Suppl 4): 9–14.

5. Korbling M, Przepiorka D, Huh YO et al, Allogeneic blood stem cell transplantation for refractory leukemia and lymphoma: potential advantage of blood over bone marrow allografts. *Blood* 1995; **85**: 1659–65.

6. Russell JA, Luider J, Weaver M et al, Collection of progenitor cells for allogeneic transplantation from peripheral blood or normal donors. *Bone Marrow Transplant* 1995; **15**: 111–15.

7. Abrams RA, Deisseroth AB, Prospects for accelerating hematopoietic recovery following myelosuppressive therapy by using autologous cryopreserved hematopoietic stem cells collected solely from the peripheral blood. *Exp Hematol* 1979; 7(Suppl 5): 107.

8. Fleidner TM, Flad HD, Bruch C et al, Treatment of aplastic anemia by blood stem cell transfusion: a canine model. *Hematologicia* 1976; **61**: 141.

9. Appelbaum FR, Hematopoietic reconstitution following autologous bone marrow and peripheral blood mononuclear cell infusions. *Exp Hematol* 1979; 7(Suppl 5): 7–11.

10. Richman CM, Weiner RS, Yankee RA, Increase in circulating stem cells following chemotherapy in man. *Blood* 1976; 47: 1031–9.

11. Abrams RA, McCormack K, Bowles C, Deisseroth AB, Cyclophosphamide treatment expands the circulating hematopoietic stem cell pool in dogs. *J Clin Invest* 1989; **67**: 1392.

12. Stiff PJ, Murgo AJ, Wittes RE et al, Quantification of the peripheral blood colony forming unit-culture rise following chemotherapy: Could leukocyto-

phereses replace bone marrow for autologous transplantation? *Transfusion* 1983; 23: 500–3.

13. Storb R, Graham TC, Epstein RB et al, Demonstration of hematopoietic stem cells in the peripheral blood of baboons by cross circulation. *Blood* 1977; 50: 537–42.

14. Stiff P, Koester A, Hindman T et al, Leukapheresis of peripheral blood stem cells (PBSC) increased following chemotherapy: quantification and autologous transplantation after intensive chemotherapy. *Blood* 1983; 65(Suppl 1): 230.

15. Stiff PJ, Koester AR, Eagleton LE et al, Autologous stem cell transplantation using peripheral blood stem cells. *Transplantation* 1987; 44: 585–8.

16. Kessinger A, Armitage JP, Landmark JD, Weisenburger DD, Reconstitution of human hematopoietic function with autologous cryopreserved circulating stem cells. *Exp Hematol* 1986; 14: 192–6.

17. Kessinger A, Armitage JO, Landmark JD et al, Autologous peripheral hematopoietic stem cell transplantation restores hematopoietic function following marrow ablative therapy. *Blood* 1988; 71: 723–7.

18. Sheridan WP, Begley CG, Jutner CA et al, Effect of peripheral-blood progenitor cells mobilised by filgrastim (G-CSF) on platelet recovery after high dose chemotherapy. *Lancet* 1992; 339: 640–4.

19. Krause DS, Fackler MJ, Civin CI, Moy WS, CD34: structure, biology and clinical utility. *Blood* 1996; 87: 1–13.

20. To LB, Roberts MM, Haylock DN et al, Comparison of hematological recovery times and supportive care requirements of autologous recovery phase peripheral blood stem cell transplants, autologous bone marrow transplants and allogeneic bone marrow transplants. *Bone Marrow Transplant* 1992; 9: 277–84.

21. Ager S, Scott MA, Mahendra P et al, Peripheral blood stem cell transplantation after high dose chemotherapy in patients with malignant lymphoma: a retrospective comparison with autologous bone marrow transplantation. *Bone Marrow Transplant* 1995; 16: 79–83.

22. Schmitz N, Linch DC, Dreger P et al, Randomized trial of filgrastim-mobilized peripheral blood progenitor cell transplantation versus autologous bone marrow transplantation in lymphoma patients. *Lancet* 1996; 347: 353–7.

23. Weaver CH, Hazelton B, Birch R et al, An analysis of engraftment kinetics as a function of CD34 content of peripheral blood progenitor cell collections in 692 patients after the administration of myeloablative chemotherapy. *Blood* 1995; 86: 3961–9.

24. Sola C, Maroto P, Salazar R et al, High-dose chemotherapy (HDC) and peripheral blood stem cell (PBSC) autologous transplantation: influence of the number of infused CD34+ cells in hematopoietic recovery and support measures required. *Proc Am Soc Clin Oncol* 1996; 15: 538.

25. Glaspy JA, Shpall EJ, LeMaistre CF et al, Peripheral blood progenitor cell mobilization using stem cell factor in combination with filgrastim in breast cancer patients. *Blood* 1997; 90: 2939–51.

26. Stiff PJ, Bayer RA, Kerger C et al, Autologous stem cell transplants for ovarian cancer: high rate of platelet engraftment delays related to poor stem cell mobilization. *Blood* 1996; 88 (Suppl 1): 678a.

27. Dreger P, Klass M, Petersen B et al, Autologous progenitor cell transplantation: prior exposure to stem cell-toxic drugs determines yield and engraftment of peripheral blood progenitor cells but not of bone marrow grafts. *Blood* 1995; 86: 3970–8.

28. Oostendorp RA, Dormer P, VLA-4-mediated interactions between normal human hematopoietic progenitors and stromal cells. *Leuk Lymphoma* 1997; 24: 423–35.

29. Waller CF, Bertz R, Wenger MK et al, Mobilization of peripheral blood progenitor cells for allogeneic transplanta-

tion: efficacy and toxicity of a high dose rhG-CSF regimen. *Bone Marrow Transplant* 1996; **18**: 279–83.

30. Zellner W, VonSteiglity J, Dominka T et al, Mobilization of blood stem cells using G-CSF without preceding chemotherapy. *Beitr Infusion Ther* 1993; **31**: 118–23.

31. Grigg AP, Roberts AW, Raunow H et al, Optimizing dose and scheduling of filgrastim (granulocyte colony-stimulating factor) for mobilization and collection of peripheral blood progenitor cells in normal volunteers. *Blood* 1995; **15**: 4437–45.

32. Kroger N, Zeller W, Hassan HT et al, Stem cell mobilization with G-CSF alone in breast cancer patients: higher progenitor cell yield by delivering divided doses ($2 \times 5$ µg/kg) compared to a single dose ($1 \times 10$ µg/kg). *Bone Marrow Transplant* 1999; **23**: 125–9.

33. Stiff PJ, Management strategies for the hard to mobilize patient. *Bone Marrow Transplant* 1999; **23**(Suppl 2): 529–33.

34. Watts MJ, Sullivan AM, Leveott D et al, Back-up bone marrow is frequently ineffective in patients with poor peripheral blood progenitor cell mobilization. *Blood* 1997; **90**(Suppl 1): 213a.

35. Stiff P, Gingrich R, Luger S et al, A randomized phase 2 study of PBPC mobilization by stem cell factor and filgrastim in heavily pretreated patients with Hodgkin's disease or non-Hodgkin's lymphoma. *Bone Marrow Transplant* 2000; in press.

36. Weaver Ch, Tauer K, Zhen B et al, Second attempts at mobilization of peripheral blood stem cells in patients with initial low CD34+ cell yields. *J Hematother* 1998; **7**: 241–9.

37. Hogge DE, Cashman JD, Humphries RK, Eaves CJ, Differential and synergistic effects of human granulocyte–macrophage colony stimulating factor and human granulocyte colony-stimulating factor on hematopoiesis in human long-term marrow cultures. *Blood* 1991; **77**: 493–9.

38. Winter JN, Lazarus HM, Rademaker A et al, Phase I/II study of combined granulocyte colony-stimulatory factor and granulocyte–macrophage colony-stimulating factor administration for the mobilization of hematopoietic progenitor cells. *J Clin Oncol* 1996; **14**: 277–86.

39. Armitage JO, Emerging applications of recombinant human granulocyte-macrophage colony-stimulating factor. *Blood* 1998; **92**: 4491–508.

40. Lane TA, Law P, Maruyana M et al, Harvesting and enrichment of hematopoietic progenitor cells mobilized into the peripheral blood of normal donors by granulocyte–macrophage colony-stimulating factor (GM-CSF) or G-CSF: potential role in allogeneic marrow transplantation *Blood* 1995; **85**: 275–82.

41. Socinski MA, Cannistra SA, Elias A et al, Granulocyte–macrophage colony stimulatory factor expands the circulating hematopoietic progenitor cell compartment in man. *Lancet* 1988; **28**: 1194–8.

42. Sienna S, Bregini M, Brando B et al, Circulation of CD34+ hematopoietic stem cells in the peripheral blood of high-dose cyclophosphamide-treated patients: enhancement by intravenous human granulocyte–macrophage colony stimulatory factor. *Blood* 1989; **74**: 1905–14.

43. Rowlings PA, Bagly JL, Rowling CM et al, A comparison of peripheral blood stem cell mobilization after chemotherapy and cyclophosphamide as a single agent in doses of $4 \text{ g/m}^2$ or $7 \text{ g/m}^2$ in patients with advanced cancer. *Aust NZ J Med* 1992; **22**: 660–4.

44. Lie AK, Rowling TP, Bayly JL, To LB, Progenitor cell yield in sequential blood stem cell mobilization in the same patients: insights into chemotherapy dose escalation and combination of hematopoietic growth factors and chemotherapy. *Br J Haematol* 1996; **95**: 39–44.

45. Gianni A, Sienna S, Bregni M et al, Granulocyte–macrophage colony stimulating factor to harvest circulating hematopoietic stem cells for autotransplantation. *Lancet* 1989; **ii**: 580–4.

46. Haas R, Ho A, Bredthauer U et al, Successful autologous transplantation of blood stem cells mobilized with recombinant human granulocyte–macrophage colony-stimulating factor. *Exp Hematol* 1990; **18**: 94–8.

47. Schwartzberg LS, Weaver CH, Birch R et al, A randomized trial of two doses of cyclophosphamide with etoposide and G-CSF for mobilization of peripheral blood stem cells in 318 patients with stage II–III breast cancer. *J Hematother* 1998; **7**: 141–50.

48. Demirer T, Buckner CD, Storer B et al, Effect of different chemotherapy regimens on peripheral blood stem cell collections in patients with breast cancer receiving granulocyte colony-stimulating factor. *J Clin Oncol* 1997; **15**: 684–90.

49. Weaver CH, Schwartzberg LS, Birch R et al, Collection of peripheral blood stem cells following administration of paclitaxel, cyclophosphamide and filgrastim in patients with breast and ovarian cancer. *Biol Blood Marrow Transplant* 1997; **3**: 83–90.

50. Perez-Simon JA, Caballero MD, Corral M et al, Minimal number of circulating CD34+ cells to ensure successful leukapheresis and engraftment in autologous peripheral blood progenitor cell transplantation. *Transfusion* 1998; **38**: 385–91.

51. Gandhi MK, Jestice K, Scott MA et al, The minimum CD34 threshold depends on prior chemotherapy in autologous peripheral blood stem cell recipients. *Bone Marrow Transplant* 1999; **23**: 9–13.

52. Bensinger W, Appelbaum F, Rowley S et al, Factors that influence collection and engraftment of autologous peripheral-blood stem cells. *J Clin Oncol* 1995; **13**: 2547–55.

53. Demirer T, Buckner CD, Bensinger WI, Optimization of peripheral blood stem cell mobilization. *Stem Cells* 1996; **14**: 106–16.

54. Tricot G, Jagannath S, Vesole D et al, Peripheral blood stem cell transplants for multiple myeloma: identification of favorable risk factors for rapid engraftment in 225 patients. *Blood* 1995; **85**: 588–96.

55. Haas R, Mohle R, Fruhauf S et al, Patient characteristics associated with successful mobilizing and autografting of peripheral blood progenitor cells in malignant lymphoma. *Blood* 1994; **23**: 3783–94.

56. Moskowitz CH, Glassman JR, Wuest D et al, Factors affecting mobilization of peripheral blood progenitor cells in patients with lymphoma. *Clin Cancer Res* 1998; **4**: 311–16.

57. Pecora AL, Preti. RA, Gleam GO et al, CD34+CD33− cells influence days to engraftment and transfusion requirements in autologous blood stem-cell recipients. *J Clin Oncol* 1998; **16**: 2093–104.

58. Demirer T, Buckner CD, Gooyel T et al, Factors influencing collection of peripheral blood stem cells in patients with multiple myeloma. *Bone Marrow Transplant* 1996; **17**: 937–41.

59. Parthasarathy M, Stiff P, Oldenberg D et al, Re-mobilization with high dose G-CSF is successful for autologous transplant candidates who mobilize poorly with standard G-CSF. *Abstracts First Combined ABMTR/IBMTR/ASBMT Meeting, 1999.*

60. Stiff P, LeMaistre CF, Luger S et al, Resource utilization following initial PBPC mobilization failure. *Proc Am Soc Clin Oncol* 1998; **17**: 83a.

61. Stiff P, Malhotra D, Bayer R et al, High dose G-CSF improves stem cell mobilization and collection in patients with ovarian cancer which leads to a decrease in delayed platelet engraftment following stem cell transplants *Blood* 1997; **90**(Suppl): 591a.

62. Weaver CH, Birch R, Gecco FA, Mobilization and harvesting of peripheral blood stem cells: randomized evaluations of different doses of filgrastim. *Br J Haematol* 1998; **100**: 338–47.

63. Moskovitz C, Stiff P, Gordon MS et al, Recombinant methionyl human stem cell factor (r-met-HuSCF) and filgrastim

for PBPC mobilization and transplantation in non-Hodgkin's lymphoma patients. Results of a phase I/II trial. *Blood* 1998; **89**: 3136–47.

64. Andrews RG, Briddel RA, Knitler GH et al, In vivo synergy between recombinant human stem cell factor and recombinant human granulocyte colony-stimulatory factor in baboons. Enhanced circulation of progenitor cells. *Blood* 1994; **84**: 800–10.

65. Shpall EJ, Wheeler CA, Turner SA et al, A randomized phase 3 study of peripheral blood progenitor cell mobilization by stem cell factor and filgrastim in high risk breast cancer patients. *Blood* 1998; **93**: 2491–501.

66. Lyman SD, James L, VandenBos T et al, Molecular cloning of a ligand for the flt3/flk-2 tyrosine kinase receptor: a proliferative factor for primitive hematopoietic cells. *Cell* 1993; **75**: 1157–67.

67. Lyman SD, Williams DE, Biology and potential clinical applications of flt3 ligand. *Curr Opin Hematol* 1995; **2**: 177–81.

68. Lyman SD. Biologic effects and potential clinical applications of Flt3 ligand. *Curr Opin Hematol* 1998; **5**: 192–6.

69. Shurin MR, Esche C, Lotze MT, FLT3 receptor and ligand. Biology and potential clinical applications. *Cytokine Growth Factor Rev* 1998; **9**: 37–48.

70. Lyman SD, Brasel K, Rousseau AM, Williams DE, The flt3 ligand: a hematopoietic stem cell factor whose activities are distinct from steel factor. *Stem Cells (Dayt)* 1994; **12**(Suppl 1): 99–107.

71. Lyman SD, Jacobsen SEW, C-kit ligand and Flt3 ligand: stem/progenitor cell factors with overlapping but distinct activities. *Blood* 1998; **91**: 1101–34.

72. Hjertson M, Sundstrom C, Lyman SD et al, Stem cell factor, but not flt3 ligand induces differentiation and activation of human mast cells. *Exp Hematol* 1996; **24**: 748–54.

73. Brasel K, McKenna HJ, Morrissey PJ et al, Hematologic effects of flt3 ligand in vivo in mice. *Blood* 1996; **88**: 2004–12.

74. Ashihara E, Shimazaki C, Sudo Y et al, FLT-3 ligand mobilizes hematopoietic primitive and committed progenitor cells into blood in mice. *Eur J Hematol* 1998; **60**: 86–92.

75. Molineux G, McCrea C, Yan QX et al, Flt3 ligand synergizes with granulocyte colony-stimulating factor to increase neutrophil numbers and to mobilize peripheral blood stem cells with long-term repopulating potential. *Blood* 1997; **89**: 3998.

76. Neipp M, Zarina T, Domenick MA et al, Effect of FLT3 ligand and granulocyte-stimulating factor on expansion and mobilization of facilitating cells and hematopoietic stem cells in mice: kinetics and repopulating potential. *Blood* 1998; **92**: 3177–88.

77. Winton EF, Bucur SZ, Bond LD et al, Recombinant human (rh) FLT3 ligand plus rh-GM-CSF or G-CSF causes a marked CD34+ cell mobilization to blood in rhesus monkeys. *Blood* 1996; **88**: 642a.

78. Lynch DH, Andreasen A, Maraskovsky E et al, Flt3 ligand induces tumor progression and anti-tumor immune responses in vivo. *Nature Med* 1997; **3**: 625–31.

79. Chem K, Braun SE, Lyman SD et al, Soluble and membrane bound isoforms of Flt3-ligand induced antitumor immunity in vivo. *Blood* 1996; **88**(Suppl 1): 274a.

80. Winton EF, Bucur SZ, Bray RA et al, The hematopoietic effects of recombinant human (rh) FLT3 ligand administered to non-human primates. *Blood* 1995; **86**(Suppl 1): 424a.

81. Lebsack ME, McKenna HJ, Hoek JA et al, Safety of FLT3 ligand in healthy volunteers. *Blood* 1997; **90**(Suppl 1): 170a.

82. Maraskovsky E, Roux E, Tepe M et al, Flt3 ligand increases peripheral blood dendritic cells in healthy volunteers. *Blood* 1997; **90**(Suppl 1): 581a.

83. Lebsack ME, Maraskovsky E, Roux E et al, Increased circulating dendritic cells in healthy human volunteers following administration of FLT3 ligand alone or in

combination with GM-CSF or G-CSF. *Blood* 1998; **92**(Suppl 1): 581a.

84. Chao N, Litzow MR, Geller RB et al, Randomized phase II study of FLT3 ligand (Mobist™) in combination with GM-CSF or G-CSF for mobilization of peripheral blood progenitor cells in patients with breast cancer. *Blood* 1999; **94**: 666a.

85. Stiff PJ, Beveridge RA, Vose J et al, Randomized phase II study of FLT 3 ligand (Mobist™) in combination with GM-CSF or G-CSF for mobilization of peripheral blood progenitor cells in patients with lymphoma or ovarian cancer. *Blood* 1999; **94**: 666a.

# 3
# Matched unrelated marrow transplantation: The true indications

Ann E Woolfrey, Effie W Petersdorf, Claudio Anasetti, Paul J Martin, Joachim Deeg, William Bensinger, Jean E Sanders, John A Hansen

## PRINCIPLES OF UNRELATED MARROW TRANSPLANTATION

Genetic disparities associated with unrelated marrow grafts increase the immunologic barriers that must be overcome to ensure engraftment and achieve tolerance. While graft rejection and graft-versus-host (GvH) reactions must be controlled for successful outcome, there is an associated graft-versus-leukemia (GvL) response that plays an important role in the success of allogeneic marrow transplantation for treatment of hematologic malignancies. The GvL reaction appears to be more significant in unrelated donor grafts, such that negative effects resulting from strengthened graft rejection and GvH reactions are counterbalanced by this favorable allogeneic response.

### Engraftment

Differences in histocompatibility antigens associated with unrelated donor grafts, including HLA as well as minor histocompatibility antigen, disparities, promote a stronger host alloimmune response, thereby increasing the risk of graft rejection. Graft rejection can be found in 2–7% of unrelated marrow recipients, either as failure of primary engraftment or as secondary graft loss.[1–5] The risk of graft failure for patients with HLA phenotypically identical unrelated marrow grafts is significantly lower than for those who receive HLA-mismatched grafts. Other factors that determine risk of graft failure include pretransplant diagnosis, intensity of the conditioning regimen, and the number of both marrow cells and T cells in the graft. Intensity of the conditioning regimen and pretransplant diagnosis, which may reflect the extent of previous chemotherapy and subsequent host immunity, are important factors that determine the magnitude of residual host T or NK cells capable of causing graft rejection. Donor T cells play a primary role in establishing a marrow graft; thus there is an increased risk of graft rejection following transplantation of

T-cell-depleted marrow.[3] High marrow cell dose also appears to have a favorable affect on engraftment.[4]

## Graft-versus-host disease

Recipients of unrelated marrow grafts have a higher probability of developing acute graft-versus-host disease (GvHD) compared with recipients of HLA-matched sibling grafts, presumably owing to differences in major or minor histocompatibility antigens. Grade II–IV acute GvHD occurs in 49–83% of HLA-A, -B, -DRB1 matched and in 67–98% of HLA-mismatched transplants (Table 3.1).[2,6–9] Severe GvHD (grade III–IV) occurs in approximately 25% of matched and 35% of mismatched transplants, respectively. Significant factors associated with the development of acute GvHD include HLA disparity, female donor, and older patient age, while T-cell depletion significantly decreases the risk for acute GvHD.[2,3,10] Compared with recipients of HLA-identical related grafts, recipients of unrelated marrow have a higher probability of developing extensive chronic GvHD (Table 3.1).[2,3,9] Furthermore, the duration of GvHD and length of treatment is prolonged (median 3.2 years).[11] Significant factors associated with the development of chronic GvHD include HLA disparity, female donor for a male recipient, and patient age.[9,12] Quality of life for patients who survive two years after transplantation is not significantly different for unrelated marrow recipients compared with other groups of long-term survivors, despite prolonged therapy for chronic GvHD.[9,11]

## Relapse and GvL

The capacity of donor immune cells to generate antileukemic reactivity appears to be increased in unrelated marrow grafts, presumably induced by

## Table 3.1 GvHD after unmodified unrelated marrow transplantation

| Ref. | No. of patients | Grade II–IV acute (%) | | Grade III–IV acute (%) | | Extensive chronic (%) | |
|------|------|-------|-----------|-------|-----------|-------|-----------|
| | | Match | Mismatch[a] | Match | Mismatch[a] | Match | Mismatch[a] |
| 13 | 196 | 77 | >88 | 35 | 37–50 | 67[b] | |
| 2 | 88 | 83 | 98 | 37 | 62 | 37 | |
| 7 | 112 | 78 | 94 | 36 | 51 | 61 | 74 |
| 6 | 50 | 49 | 67 | 23 | 30 | 50 | 57 |
| 3[c] | 462 | 64[b] | | 47[b] | | 35[b] | |

[a]HLA match or mismatch defined by serologic typing for HLA-A, -B, and -DRB1 allele typing.
[b]Includes both HLA-matched and -mismatched marrow grafts.
[c]Includes T-cell-depleted marrow grafts.

disparities in histocompatibility antigens. Enhancement of the GvL effect is supported by observations that recipients of unrelated marrow have a lower risk of relapse compared with recipients of genetically HLA-identical marrow.[4,10] Patients who receive HLA-mismatched unrelated grafts or those who develop GvHD also have a lower risk of relapse.[2,4,7] These studies suggest that there is enhanced donor reactivity to antigens found on residual host leukemic cells when there is no familial relationship between donor and host. It remains to be established whether the GvL reaction is directed primarily toward disparate histocompatibility antigens, as a manifestation of the global GvH response, or whether leukemic-specific antigens may be identified, allowing separation of GvL from GvH responses.

# FACTORS ASSOCIATED WITH IMPROVED OUTCOME OF UNRELATED MARROW GRAFTS

## Histocompatibility

Conventional methods for histocompatibility testing used serologic and cellular assays to determine phenotypic HLA type. With these methods, genetic identity between donor and recipient could not be determined, except through family study and segregation analysis. These latter methods cannot be used to determine genetic HLA compatibility among unrelated persons. The advent of DNA-based HLA typing methods has made it evident that many serologically determined antigens are polymorphic. These polymorphic alleles may contribute to undetected HLA mismatch among unrelated donor–recipient pairs.[13,14] Petersdorf et al[13] studied the extent of polymorphism among 300 phenotypically HLA-A, -B, -DR matched donor–recipient pairs using DNA sequencing-based methods. Previously undetected allele-level polymorphisms were found in 159 pairs (53%), while only 142 donor–recipient pairs were HLA-A, -B, -C, -DRB1, -DQB1 identical at the allele level (47%) (Table 3.2). Among the 159 pairs mismatched for one or more alleles, HLA-C mismatch

### Table 3.2  HLA-A, -B, -C, -DRB1, -DQB1 matching among 300 donor–recipient pairs

| Donor disparity | No. of pairs (% of total) |
| --- | --- |
| Allele-matched | 146 (49) |
| Mismatch at a single class I allele | 58 (19) |
| Mismatch at multiple class I alleles | 31 (10) |
| Mismatch at a single class II allele | 25 (8) |
| Mismatch at multiple class II alleles | 6 (2) |
| Mismatch at both class I and class II alleles | 39 (13) |

was found in 87, HLA-B mismatch in 58, HLA-A mismatch in 50, HLA-DQB1 mismatch in 48, and HLA-DRB1 mismatch in 36 pairs. Multiple mismatches were found in 70 (23%) of phenotypically HLA-A, -B, -DR matched donor–recipient pairs. The importance of these undetected mismatches is suggested by observations of increased incidence of graft rejection and GvHD after transplantation of HLA-A, -B, -DR phenotypically identical marrow compared with HLA-genetically identical marrow. Graft rejection occurs in 2% of patients after HLA-A, -B, -DR phenotypically identical marrow transplants, compared with less than 1% after HLA-A, -B, -DR genotypically identical marrow.[1,3,7] Similarly, grade II–IV acute GvHD occurs in 70–80% of patients after HLA-A, -B, -DR phenotypically identical marrow, compared with 30–40% after HLA-A, -B, -DR genotypically identical marrow. Based on these observations, we have studied the relationship of HLA allelic mismatch to survival, and risk of graft rejection or GvHD.

Advances in DNA typing technologies were first used to discriminate HLA class II alleles. Initial studies of patient–donor pairs serologically matched at HLA-A and -B found that DRB1 or DQB1 disparity increased the risk for grades III–IV GvHD and decreased survival, but the extent of molecular polymorphisms within serologically defined class I antigens was not analyzed.[8,15] A recent study of 300 donor–recipient pairs using molecular techniques to identify allele disparities at HLA-A, -B, -C, -DRB1, and -DQB1 found that disparity of DRB1 or DQB1 alleles increased the risk of grades III–IV GvHD (relative risk, RR = 1.8; 95% confidence interval, CI = 1.0–3.4; $p = 0.06$) (Figure 3.1).[13] The effect of DRB1 or DQB1 disparity was most significant when found in combination with disparity at one or more class I loci. When class II alleles are matched, disparity for class I alleles does not appear to confer an increased risk for severe GvHD, even if more than one disparity is detected.

In contrast to GvHD, graft rejection appears to be more closely associated with disparities of class I HLA. This was suggested initially by studies using sequence-based typing methods that evaluated the extent of allele mismatch in 21 patients with graft failure. Molecular typing of donor–recipient pairs detected a statistically significant increase in allelic disparity for HLA-C alone, or in combination with HLA-A or -B disparities, compared with case-matched unrelated marrow controls without graft failure.[5] These results have recently been confirmed in a cohort of 300 patients with chronic myelogenous leukemia transplanted with unrelated marrow during chronic phase. An increased risk of graft failure was associated with mismatching for two or more class I alleles, but not with mismatching for class II DRB1 or DQB1 alleles, as shown in Table 3.3.[13] Increased risk of rejection was also observed with DRB1 or DQB1 mismatch when associated with a class I mismatch. These studies indicate that graft failure is associated primarily with HLA-class I disparity, particularly in the presence of two or more disparate class I alleles.

These studies underline the importance of detecting HLA-allele disparities to improve survival following unrelated marrow transplantation. Patients who receive unrelated marrow grafts that are incompatible for more than one allele

## Table 3.3  Graft failure according to donor HLA disparity among 292 donor–recipient pairs

| Donor disparity | No. of pairs | No. of graft failures (% of total) |
|---|---|---|
| No disparity (allele match) | 146 | 3  (2) |
| Single class I | 50 | 1  (2) |
| Multiple class I | 31 | 9 (29) |
| Class I and class II | 35 | 4 (11) |
| Single class II | 24 | 0 |
| Multiple class II | 6 | 0 |

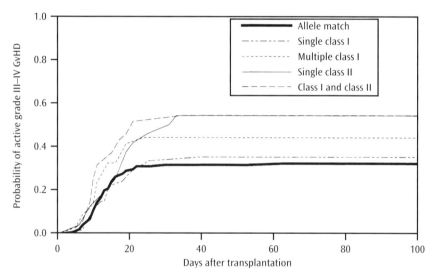

Figure 3.1

Probability of grade III–IV acute GvHD according to recipient disparity for class I HLA-A, -B, -C and class II HLA-DRB1, -DQB1 alleles. Unmodified marrow infusions were given to 292 patients with chronic myelogenous leukemia in chronic phase following a total-body irradiation-containing conditioning regimen.

have a significantly increased risk of mortality (Figure 3.2). The risk of death is 3.5 times greater for patients mismatched for multiple class I alleles ($p < 0.001$) and 3 times greater for patients mismatched for class I and class II alleles together ($p < 0.001$).[13] A single allelic disparity for HLA class I or class II does not appear to be associated with a significant increase in mortality. Results of these and similar studies[16] indicate that comprehensive matching of HLA class I and class II alleles should improve outcome for recipients of unrelated marrow grafts.

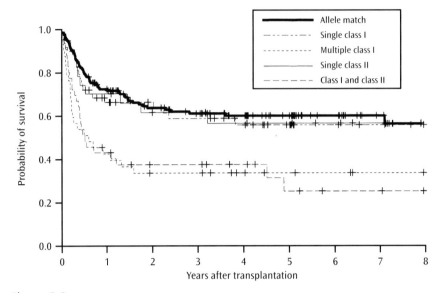

**Figure 3.2**

Probability of survival according to donor or recipient disparity for class I HLA-A, -B, -C and class II HLA-DRB1, -DQB1 alleles. Unmodified marrow infusions were given to 292 patients with chronic myelogenous leukemia in chronic phase following a total-body irradiation-containing conditioning regimen. Methotrexate and cyclosporine were given as GvHD prophylaxis. Tic marks represent patients alive at the time of last contact.

## Stem cell dose

Optimization of stem cell dose improves outcome of unrelated marrow transplantation, particularly for patients with acute leukemia. In a multivariate analysis of 204 patients with acute leukemia transplanted from unrelated donors, marrow cell dose greater than the median dose ($>3.65 \times 10^8$/kg) was associated with significantly better leukemia-free survival (LFS) ($p = 0.01$).[4] High marrow cell dose was associated with improved graft recovery, including faster recovery of peripheral blood granulocytes ($p = 0.01$), lymphocytes ($p = 0.002$), and platelets ($p < 0.001$). Higher marrow cell dose also was associated with a lower incidence of grade III–IV GvHD (36% versus 51–68%; $p = 0.01$) and non-leukemic mortality (64% versus 54% for patients less than 18 years old and 63% versus 24% for those 18 years or older; $p < 0.001$). Mortality from infection was lower in patients with higher marrow cell dose, particularly for those transplanted in remission (32% versus 3%; $p = 0.006$), and marrow cell dose was the only variable associated with improved LFS for remission patients (RR = 0.3; 95% CI = 0.2–0.6, $p = 0.0009$). Among patients less than 18 years old, the LFS rate was 46% for those with high marrow dose, compared with 30% with lower cell dose, and for patients 18 years or older, the LFS rate with high or low cell dose was 52% versus 17%, respectively.

A recent prospective study of 121 patients with hematologic malignancies evaluated dose effect of CD34, CD14, CD3, CD4, CD8, CD56, and CD19 subsets in unrelated marrow grafts.[17] Only CD34$^+$ cell dose was found to be associated with outcome. The median CD34$^+$ cell dose in this study was $2.6 \times 10^6$/kg (range $(0.02–19.8) \times 10^6$/kg). Patients who received CD34$^+$ cell doses of $2.5 \times 10^6$/kg or more had fewer episodes of delayed neutropenia ($p = 0.008$), improved platelet recovery ($p = 0.007$), and improved one-year survival (70% versus 48%; $p = 0.008$) compared with those with lower CD34$^+$ cell dose. The risk of mortality was threefold higher for patients with low CD34$^+$ cell dose, primarily because of higher non-relapse mortality (40% versus 18%).

# UNRELATED MARROW TRANSPLANTATION FOR TREATMENT OF HEMATOLOGIC MALIGNANCIES

## Chronic myelogenous leukemia

Allogeneic marrow transplantation from an HLA-matched sibling donor has been established as the best treatment for patients with chronic myelogenous leukemia (CML). Younger patients can expect a four-year event-free survival (EFS) rate of 75% if transplant is carried out within one year of diagnosis.[18] In contrast, only 25% of patients survive five years with conventional therapy.[19] Advances in the treatment of CML with interferon-alpha (IFN-α), given alone or in combination with chemotherapy, has prolonged the time to disease progression and has improved survival in a significant portion of patients.[20–22] However, treatment with IFN-α is not curative for most patients, and survival is inferior when compared with marrow transplantation (seven-year EFS rate: 32% versus 58%).[23]

The use of unrelated marrow increases the opportunity for CML patients to receive curative therapy, and large studies have demonstrated that outcome with unrelated donors approaches the outcome with HLA-matched related donors.[12,24–26] Analysis of 196 patients with chronic-phase CML at the Fred Hutchinson Cancer Research Center showed a 57% five-year survival rate.[12] Transplant-related mortality accounted for most deaths, and the cumulative incidence of relapse was 10% at five years. Factors associated with improved survival included HLA matching, transplantation within one year of diagnosis, age less than 50 years, and use of prophylaxis against fungus and cytomegalovirus (CMV). Patients less than 50 years of age who received an HLA-A, -B, and -DRB1 matched unrelated marrow transplant within one year after diagnosis had a 74% probability of surviving five years (Figure 3.3), comparable to results for patients transplanted with HLA-matched related marrow.[12,18] Other studies also show that younger age, HLA compatibility, and shorter time from diagnosis to treatment, as well as high marrow cell dose, are associated with favorable survival.[11,12,24] Encouragingly, patients transplanted in recent years have improved survival, possibly reflecting better methods of supportive care, such as prophylaxis for fungal and viral disease.[11,26] Based

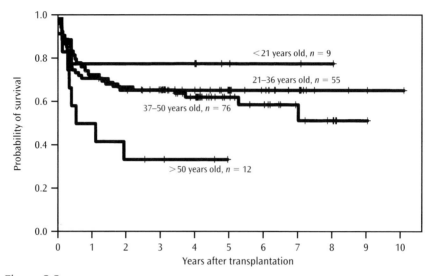

Figure 3.3

Probability of survival according to age for 152 patients with CML in chronic phase. Patients received unmodified marrow from an HLA-A, -B, -DRB1 matched donor following conditioning with cyclophosphamide and fractionated total body irradiation. Methotrexate and cyclosporine were given as GvHD prophylaxis. Tic marks represent patients alive at the time of last contact.

upon these studies, marrow transplantation should be considered the optimal treatment for younger patients who have an HLA-A, -B, -DRB1 identical related or unrelated donor.[27]

Factors that affect outcome need to be considered in determining when to initiate unrelated marrow transplantation. Outcome is improved if transplantation is done within one year of diagnosis.[12,24] Patients treated with IFN-α for more than six months have a greater incidence of grade III–IV acute GvHD (55% versus 34%; $p = 0.01$) and non-relapse mortality (56% versus 38%; $p = 0.05$) compared with those treated for less than six months before transplantation.[11,28] These findings indicate that patients with suitable unrelated donors should not receive prolonged treatment with IFN-α and should be transplanted within one year of diagnosis, if possible. This strategy must be modified, however, to take into account the benefit of an optimally matched unrelated donor, a procedure that remains time-consuming.

The value of optimizing the HLA match between the donor and recipient by use of advanced DNA-typing technology appears to be particularly important for chronic-phase CML patients because survival is determined primarily by complications of GvHD.[12,13] Our studies have shown that compatibility for HLA alleles improves survival for chronic-phase CML patients. The risks of graft rejection, severe acute GvHD, and mortality are increased significantly for patients mismatched at HLA class I and class II alleles. Likewise, recipients of unrelated grafts with multiple HLA class I allele disparities have a significantly increased incidence of graft failure and mortality.

Overall survival rates for patients transplanted in accelerated phase, blast crisis, or second chronic phase have been estimated at 27–60%, 0–20%, and 22–40%, respectively, with either related or unrelated donors.[10,24] Outcomes for patients with advanced-phase CML transplanted using marrow from unrelated donors appear comparable to those for HLA-matched related donors.

## Myelodysplastic and myeloproliferative syndromes

Myelodysplastic syndrome (MDS) patients with poor-risk cytogenetics, higher percentage of marrow blasts, or progressive cytopenias have high risk of progression to acute leukemia.[29,30] Like other stem cell disorders, MDS responds poorly to conventional chemotherapy, particularly when therapy is initiated before leukemic transformation.[31] MDS patients treated with marrow transplantation alone have a four-year EFS rate of 40–45%.[32,33] Factors associated with favorable outcome include younger age and transplantation during early disease phase.

The use of unrelated marrow donors does not appear to compromise survival. Anderson et al[34] studied outcome for 52 MDS patients (median age 33 years) transplanted from unrelated donors. The two-year EFS rate was 38%, and there was a trend for improved survival in patients transplanted with early-phase disease (i.e. refractory anemia (RA)/refractory anemia with excess blasts (RAEB)) compared with advanced-phase (i.e. refractory anemia with excess blasts in transformation (RAEB-t)/acute myelogenous leukemia) (47% versus 26%; $p = 0.14$). Patients less than 20 years of age had a 53% EFS rate. Other investigators have also reported that younger age and early-phase disease are associated with improved outcome.[35] Evidence for a GvL effect has been suggested in several studies.[33–35] In a European Blood and Marrow Transplantation Group (EBMT) study of 118 patients, the probability of relapse was 26% for patients with grade II–IV acute GvHD, compared with 42% for those with less than grade II GvHD.[35]

Marrow transplantation has shown promising results for children with MDS.[36–38] Marrow transplantation for 47 patients less than 18 years old resulted in a two-year EFS rate of 59% for RA patients, 56% for RAEB and 14% for RAEB-t or chronic myelomonocytic leukemia (CMML).[36] Seventeen patients received unrelated marrow grafts, with survival similar to those with closely matched related donors, although the risk of severe GvHD was significantly higher (24% versus 12%; $p = 0.001$). Marrow transplantation plays an important role in the treatment of juvenile CML (J-CML), a lethal myeloproliferative/myelodysplastic stem cell disorder characterized by hepatosplenomegaly, lymphadenopathy, eczematous rash, leukocytosis, thrombocytopenia, and hypercellular, dysplastic marrow. Although some cases respond to therapy with isotretinoin, marrow transplantation has been the only treatment reported to be curative.[39] In several small series of patients, 40–50% EFS rates were observed at two years after marrow transplantation.[39–41] In these studies, outcome with unrelated donors appeared comparable to outcome with closely matched related donors.

## Marrow transplantation for acute leukemia

Despite the observations that unrelated marrow transplantation is associated with increased risks of rejection, GvHD, and transplant-related mortality, the use of unrelated donors as source of stem cells for patients with acute leukemia does not appear to compromise outcome. While the risks of graft rejection and acute and chronic GvHD are higher in unrelated marrow recipients, the risk of relapse is lower, and EFS is not significantly different.[2,4] In patients with acute leukemia, primary engraftment occurs in 96–99% who receive unmanipulated marrow grafts, although the incidence of late graft failure is 6–8%. Neutrophil recovery occurs at a median of 21 days, 50% of patients achieve platelet counts of more than 50 000 by day 100, and 50% of patients no longer require platelet transfusions after day 25. Factors that are significantly associated with improved neutrophil and platelet engraftment include a high marrow cell dose ($>3.6 \times 10^8$ cells/kg) and transplantation in complete remission. Acute GvHD grade II–IV occurs in 82% and severe (grade III–IV) GvHD occurs in 47% of patients who receive unmanipulated marrow. Higher marrow cell dose is significantly associated with a lower incidence of severe GvHD, as is younger patient age and T-cell depletion.[3,4] Chronic GvHD occurs in 52% of surviving patients who receive unmanipulated marrow, and occurs more frequently in recipients of HLA-disparate grafts, those with an antecedent history of severe acute GvHD, and in older patients, and less frequently in patients with T-cell-depleted grafts.[3,4]

Phase of leukemia at time of transplant is highly predictive for the risks of leukemic relapse and death from non-relapse causes. In particular, patients transplanted in relapse with over 30% circulating blasts have very poor survival following unrelated transplantation.[4] Death from causes other than relapse occurs in approximately 40% of unrelated marrow recipients, and most deaths occur within the first 100 days. Marrow cell dose has been shown to be inversely correlated with non-relapse mortality, presumably due to more rapid engraftment and lower incidence of fatal infections in those receiving high cell doses, in addition to the association with lower risk of GvHD. Several studies have found that T-cell depletion may reduce the risk of early non-relapse mortality, although outcome is similar to that for non-T-cell-depleted grafts.[3,42]

Relapse is the major cause of death following transplantation for acute leukemia. Factors found to be significantly associated with risk of relapse include phase of disease at time of transplant and HLA-mismatch. We have shown a two- to fivefold reduction in risk of relapse for patients transplanted in remission compared with those in relapse ($p = 0.0001$).[2,4] Among patients transplanted in relapse, patients with over 30% leukemic blasts in the marrow have the highest risk of relapse (cumulative incidence $>70\%$ versus $<50\%$; $p = 0.01$). Recipients of HLA-A, -B, or -DRB1 mismatched marrow have a lower

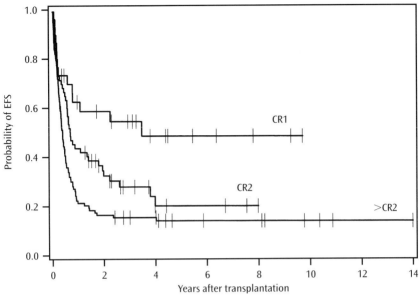

Figure 3.4

Probability of event-free survival (EFS) for patients with acute leukemia according to phase of disease at time of transplantation. Patients receive unmodified marrow from donors matched for HLA-A, -B, -DRB1 or mismatched for a single antigen following cyclophosphamide and fractionated total-body irradiation. Patients were in first remission (CR1, *n* = 31), second remission (CR2, *n* = 60) or had persistent disease or relapse (*n* = 109) at time of transplant. Tic marks represent patients alive at the time of last contact.

risk of relapse ($p = 0.01$), consistent with a GvL effect, but EFS is not different from that for recipients of HLA-matched grafts because of an increase in transplant-related mortality. The EFS rate is approximately 50% for patients in remission at the time of transplant, compared with less than 15% for those with more advanced disease, and this outcome appears to be similar for patients with acute lymphoblastic leukemia (ALL) and those with acute myelogenous leukemia (AML) (Figure 3.4).[2,4] Factors that favor leukemia-free survival include transplantation during complete remission, higher marrow cell dose, and CMV-negative recipient, younger age, and HLA-A, -B, -DRB1 match.[2–4]

### Acute lymphoblastic leukemia

The majority of children with ALL will be cured with conventional chemotherapy.[43] Cooperative group studies have defined groups of high-risk patients with long-term survival rates of less than 30% following conventional chemotherapy, including those with the clonal cytogenetic abnormalities t(9;22) and t(4;11) and those who have poor response to induction therapy (Table 3.4).[43–45] Marrow transplantation has been studied as a means to

**Table 3.4 Features associated with acute leukemia that predict outcome after conventional chemotherapy**

|  | ALL | AML |
|---|---|---|
| **Unfavorable outcome** | | |
| Clinical features | Time to CR >4 weeks<br>Induction failure | Secondary AML |
| Cytogenetics | t(4;11)<br>t(9;22) | 5q−<br>Monosomy 7<br>Translocations involving 11q23<br>Complex abnormalities |
| **Favorable outcome** | | |
| Clinical features | Age 1–9 years<br>WBC <10 000 | Down syndrome<br>FAB-M3 |
| Cytogenetics | Hyperdiploidy (>50)<br>t(12;21) | t(8;21)<br>inv(16)<br>t(15;17) |

provide higher intensity therapy for high-risk ALL patients once remission is achieved. A conditioning regimen containing total-body irradiation followed by transplantation from matched sibling donors in first complete remission (CR1) appears to provide a survival advantage, with reports of 45–84% three-year EFS rates.[45–47] Marrow transplantation may improve survival for infants considered to have very poor outcome with standard chemotherapy; in our experience 64% of high-risk infants transplanted during first remission survive without recurrent disease (JE Sanders, unpublished data). Unrelated marrow transplants have been performed for high-risk ALL patients who do not have suitably matched related donors. Studies in patients with Philadelphia-chromosome-positive ALL have shown a two-year EFS rate of 37–45% for those transplanted in first remission, approaching that found with matched sibling donors.[48,49] These studies suggest that unrelated marrow transplantation offers a significant survival advantage over conventional chemotherapy when an HLA-identical related donor is not available, but prospective studies should be performed to confirm these promising results.

Prognosis for children who develop first marrow relapse depends on the duration of first remission. Patients with late relapse (more than 2 years from diagnosis) may have relatively good outcome with conventional chemotherapy alone, although some studies continue to show potential for late second relapse.[50] In contrast, children who relapse in the marrow within two years of diagnosis have poor outcome, primarily due to treatment failure.[50,51] Marrow transplantation appears to improve survival, and 40–50% EFS rates have been reported for patients in second complete remission (CR2) transplanted from

HLA-identical related donors.[52,53] It has been difficult to compare outcomes of patients treated with chemotherapy or marrow transplantation, since patient populations are not necessarily equivalent. Patients with aggressive disease die earlier and may not be included in studies of marrow transplantation, resulting in selection bias.[54] To address this question, matched-pair analyses have been performed for CR2 patients treated with chemotherapy or HLA-identical related marrow transplants.[55,56] Particularly for those patients with early first relapse, marrow transplant resulted in significantly better EFS rates at five years compared with chemotherapy alone (40% versus 17%; $p < 0.001$).[55] Marrow transplantation was associated with a reduced risk of relapse that was not negated by increased treatment-related deaths.

While these and other studies support the use of HLA-identical sibling marrow transplantation for treatment of ALL in CR2, particularly for those with early marrow relapse, the role of unrelated marrow transplantation has not been directly addressed. We have observed a 45% disease-free survival rate at 3 years after unrelated marrow transplantation for children in CR2 (Figure 3.5),

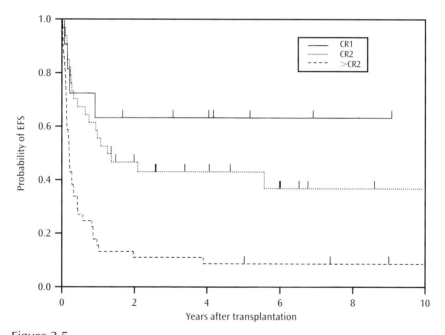

Figure 3.5

Probability of event-free survival (EFS) for children with ALL according to phase of disease at time of transplant. Patients received unmodified marrow from donors matched for HLA-A, -B, -DRB1 or mismatched for a single antigen following cyclophosphamide and fractionated total-body irradiation. At time of transplant, patients were in first remission (CR1, $n = 11$) or in second remission (CR2, $n = 35$), or were in third or greater remission, relapse, or had refractory disease (>CR2, $n = 44$). Tic marks represent patients alive at the time of last contact.

comparable to earlier reports of matched sibling marrow transplants.[52,57] Other studies report EFS rates with unrelated marrow grafts of 42–53%.[42,58,59] These studies suggest that unrelated marrow provides similar results to matched related marrow for treatment of ALL in CR2, although direct comparative trials are needed to avoid selection bias.

The role of marrow transplantation in the treatment of patients with isolated extramedullary relapse has not been determined, since many patients can achieve prolonged survival with chemotherapy alone. In these cases, unrelated marrow transplantation should be undertaken only on an established research protocol. On the other hand, patients who have refractory relapse and those who relapse after second remission have extremely poor outcome despite further treatment with conventional chemotherapy. Although allogeneic marrow transplantation might provide these patients with a survival advantage, the true impact on EFS is difficult to assess because of selection bias. EFS rates in the range of 10–30% at two to three years after transplantation has been reported in multiple small series that include advanced-stage ALL patients, and source of marrow (matched related versus unrelated) did not appear to affect outcome.[4,59,60] Importantly, for patients with advanced leukemia, disease burden is associated with outcome: survival is significantly worse for patients with over 30% marrow blasts, and particularly poor for those with circulating blasts.[4]

### Acute myelogenous leukemia

Despite intensive chemotherapy, less than half of all patients with AML will survive in the long term.[61–63] Allogeneic marrow transplantation using HLA-matched related donors appears to improve survival for young adults and children when used as post-remission therapy. Collaborative group studies of young adults have shown 43–55% disease-free survival at four years with marrow transplantation compared with 30–43% for patients receiving consolidation chemotherapy alone.[64–66] Marrow transplant patients were found to have lower risk of relapse, but this advantage was offset by greater treatment-related mortality compared with chemotherapy alone. The benefit of allogeneic transplantation is more apparent for pediatric AML patients. Several prospective cooperative group trials have shown 50–60% EFS rates after allogeneic marrow transplantation, compared with 30–40% after autologous transplants or chemotherapy alone.[67,68] Currently, allogeneic marrow transplantation should be considered for young patients with HLA-identical related donors, particularly for those with poor-risk cytogenetics or other poor-risk features.

Unrelated marrow transplantation has not been demonstrated to improve outcome for patients in first remission. Outcome has improved for patients treated with chemotherapy alone: younger AML patients in first remission currently have a 50–60% EFS rate.[67–69] Marrow transplantation in early first relapse or second remission results in 30–40% EFS rates at two years after transplantation.[70] Thus far, it is not apparent that the majority of AML patients would benefit from unrelated marrow transplantation in CR1 (unpublished data). Unrelated marrow transplantation in first remission might be considered for patients with high-risk features (Table 3.4), such as extramedullary disease or poor-prognosis cytogenetics, but transplantation should be undertaken only on an established research protocol. Specifically, infants with high-risk features might benefit from unrelated marrow transplantation in CR1, since the transplant-related mortality rate is 10% or less and the EFS rate is 55%, regardless of donor source.[71]

Marrow transplantation has an important role in the treatment of relapsed AML because outcome is poor with chemotherapy alone. Marrow transplantation in early first untreated relapse or CR2 results in a two-year EFS rate of 30–40%.[72,73] Analyses that attempt to compare outcome based on treatment have shown a survival advantage for patients who receive marrow transplants compared with chemotherapy alone, particularly for younger patients and for those with longer first remission.[74] Results of unrelated marrow transplantation have been similar to those of matched related marrow transplantation for treatment of advanced-stage AML. While unrelated marrow transplants are associated with an increased risk of transplant-related mortality, the risk of relapse is lower, and the two-year EFS rate is 30–40%.[4,75] The use of high marrow cell doses can reduce the risk of transplant-related mortality.[4] Transplantation during second remission is associated with favorable survival compared with transplantation during more advanced phases of disease.[2,4] Unrelated marrow transplantation may provide long-term survival for patients with AML in relapse, particularly those in early untreated first relapse, but patients transplanted with over 30% marrow blasts or circulating peripheral blasts have extremely poor outcome.[4]

## Unrelated marrow transplantation for treatment of non-malignant disorders

### Severe aplastic anemia

Marrow transplantation using an HLA-matched related donor is the treatment of choice for severe aplastic anemia (SAA), resulting in long-term survival rates of over 90%.[76] When an HLA-compatible family donor is not available, most patients are treated with high-dose immunosuppression, using antithymocyte globulin (ATG) plus cyclosporine, with or without granulocyte colony-stimulating factor (G-CSF). Approximately 70–80% of patients respond to immunosuppression, although the actuarial 10-year survival rate is about 40%.[77–80] Marrow transplantation from unrelated donors has generally been reserved for those patients who do not respond to or who relapse after immunosuppressive therapy.

In the 1980s, studies reported poor survival rates after unrelated marrow transplantation, but results of more recent studies are encouraging. Margolis et al[81] reported their single-institution experience with 28 children and young adults (median age 8.5 years), all but one of whom had relapsed after immunosuppressive therapy. The one-year survival rate after HLA-A, -B, -DRB1 matched ($n = 9$) or mismatched ($n = 19$) was 54%. A recent study of 141 SAA patients transplanted with unrelated marrow also shows improved survival, particularly for young patients transplanted within three years of diagnosis using HLA-matched donors (62% three-year probability of survival).[82] All patients in this study had received one or more cycles of immunosuppressive therapy prior to transplantation, with a median of 13 months between diagnosis and transplantation. Donors were phenotypically HLA-matched (74%) or mismatched for one antigen (26%). Graft failure occurred in 11% of patients, and was associated with HLA-mismatched donors (7% versus 24%; $p = 0.01$), T-cell depletion (6% versus 21%; $p = 0.01$), and low marrow cell dose (3% versus 10–16%; $p = 0.23$). Acute GvHD grade II–IV and grade III–IV occurred in 52% and 37% of evaluable patients, respectively, and extensive chronic GvHD occurred in 31%. The Kaplan–Meier estimate of probability of survival was 0.34 at five years. Factors that improved survival according to multivariate analysis were transplant within three years of diagnosis and use of HLA-A, -B, -DR matched donor.

This study demonstrated the importance of detecting allele-level HLA mismatch. DRB1 allele typing found mismatch to occur in 26 of 81 evaluable serologically HLA-A, -B, and -DR matched patient–donor pairs.[82] The survival rate for patients with serologically HLA-A, -B, and -DRB1 allele-matched marrow grafts was 56% at two or three years, compared with 15% for those with HLA-mismatched marrow.

### Immunodeficiency syndromes

Bone marrow transplantation cures life-threatening immunodeficiency disorders by providing immune-competent donor cells. Unrelated and mismatched related marrow grafts have been used successfully when HLA-matched related donors are not available. Compared with haploidentical marrow grafts, which generally are depleted of T cells, infusion of unmanipulated unrelated marrow results in improved immune reconstitution, and consequently decreased incidence of opportunistic infections or Epstein–Barr virus (EBV) lymphoproliferative disorders, although overall survival is similar.[83,84] Filipovich[85] reported outcomes of 27 children with immunodeficiency diseases transplanted with unrelated donor marrow, including patients with severe combined immunodeficiency (SCID). The overall survival rate was estimated to be 61%. Donor engraftment was documented in 22 patients, with the majority of survivors achieving stable mixed hematopoietic chimerism and resolution of clinical immunodeficiency. No post-transplant EBV lymphoproliferative disorders were reported for this group of unrelated donor patients. Improved outcome was observed for patients without severe pretransplant complications, such as pneumonitis, GvHD, or other life-threatening illness. For patients with Wiskott–Aldrich syndrome, younger age was associated with better outcome.

There are multiple reports of successful unrelated marrow transplants for the treatment of life-threatening non-malignant conditions, including Hurler syndrome and other storage diseases,[86–88] familial erythrophagocytosis,[86,89] thalassemia,[86] and congenital bone marrow failure syndromes.[86,90–92] In the National Marrow Donor Program (NMDP) database, 438 patients have been transplanted for a variety of non-malignant conditions, with reported 43% four-year survival rate.[93] In our institution, 14 children with rare life-threatening non-malignant conditions have received unrelated marrow grafts after con-

ditioning with busulfan, cyclophosphamide and ATG (Table 3.5). Seven survive without disease recurrence at a median follow-up of 6.4 years (range 0.6
–8.1 years). We have observed an association between lower serum levels of
busulfan and graft failure, establishing the importance of adjusting busulfan
dose to achieve the targeted steady-state concentration of over 600 ng/ml in
recipients of unrelated marrow grafts.[94]

# FUTURE DIRECTIONS

## Optimizing donor selection: DNA-based HLA typing

Our studies indicate the value of optimal HLA matching to improve survival
and decrease the risks of graft rejection and GvHD. Matching for HLA-A, -B,
-C, -DRB1, and -DQB1 alleles using DNA-based typing technology is particularly important for chronic-phase CML patients. The importance of allele
matching for patients with other diagnoses is currently being studied. Matching other HLA loci may also be important in determining outcome. Currently
the role of DP matching is being studied in our institution. In the future, large
databases with donor–recipient allele typing may allow evaluation of the relative impact of certain mismatches on outcome – for example, certain combinations of allele mismatches may be more tolerable than other combinations.
Determination of acceptable and unacceptable mismatches may one day
increase the number of acceptable donors for each patient.

## Table 3.5  Unrelated marrow transplantation for the treatment of 14 children with lethal congenital disorders

| Diagnosis | Age (years) | Sex | Survival (days) | Cause of death |
|---|---|---|---|---|
| Hurler syndrome | 1.2 | M | >2925 | |
| Hurler syndrome | 1.6 | M | 736 | Multiorgan failure |
| Metachromatic leukodystrophy | 3.1 | M | >2511 | |
| Metachromatic leukodystrophy | 5.4 | F | 177 | Disseminated CMV |
| Hurler syndrome | 2.3 | F | >2596 | |
| Combined immunodeficiency | 3.8 | M | 29 | Veno-occlusive disease |
| Severe combined immunodeficiency | 0.9 | F | >2292 | |
| Chédiak–Higashi syndrome | 5.2 | F | 328 | Chronic GvHD |
| Wiskott–Aldrich syndrome | 3.3 | M | >1371 | |
| Bare lymphocyte syndrome | 2.2 | M | 327 | Late graft rejection |
| Niemann–Pick disease | 1.6 | M | 24 | Graft rejection |
| Severe combined immunodeficiency | 0.7 | F | 37 | Pneumonitis |
| Severe combined immunodeficiency | 0.7 | M | >403 | |
| Wiskott–Aldrich syndrome | 4.2 | M | >180 | |

## Peripheral blood stem cell transplantation: increasing cell dose

High marrow cell and CD34$^+$ cell dose confers survival benefit for unrelated marrow recipients, particularly for patients with acute leukemia. Attainment of high marrow cell dose is limited by the quantity of marrow that can be harvested safely. One method to increase hematopoietic stem cell dose is through collection of mobilized peripheral blood stem cells (PBSC). The benefit of increased cell dose has been shown in recent studies of allogeneic PBSC transplants using HLA-identical related donors. Results of a randomized study of allogeneic PBSC versus marrow, just completed in our institution, show significantly improved survival for patients receiving PBSC compared with marrow (70% versus 45%; $p = 0.02$) There was no significant difference in the incidence of acute or chronic GvHD, but patients with marrow grafts had a twofold increase in risk of relapse ($p = 0.07$). Among patients with acute leukemia, the risk of mortality was increased twofold for those with marrow grafts compared with PBSC ($p = 0.02$).[95] While there is limited experience with unrelated PBSC transplantation, it has been used successfully in a number of European and North American centers. The NMDP has just opened a study to evaluate the use of unrelated PBSC in large numbers of patients.

## CONCLUSIONS

Unrelated marrow transplantation provides an important therapy in the management of hematologic malignancies and other life-threatening disorders. Suitably matched unrelated donors are acceptable alternatives in the majority of instances in which marrow transplantation is indicated and HLA-matched or closely matched related donors are not available. Outcome after unrelated marrow transplantation has improved over time with the development of better methods for supportive care and improved appreciation for the importance of HLA allele compatibility and hematopoietic cell dose. The availability of unrelated marrow transplantation for the treatment of life-threatening diseases should increase as donor registries grow and increase recruitment of minority donors.

## ACKNOWLEDGMENTS

This work is supported by National Institutes of Health Grants CA18029, AI33484, CA15704, and DK02431.

# REFERENCES

1. Hansen JA, Petersdorf EW, Unrelated donor hematopoietic cell transplantation. In: *Hematopoietic Cell Transplantation*, Vol II (Forman S, Blume K, Thomas ED, eds). Blackwell Science: Cambridge, MA, 1998: 915–28.

2. Balduzzi A, Gooley T, Anasetti C et al, Unrelated donor marrow transplantation in children. *Blood* 1995; **86**: 3247–56.

3. Kernan NA, Bartsch G, Ash RC et al, Analysis of 462 transplantations from unrelated donors facilitated by the National Marrow Donor Program. *N Engl J Med* 1993; **328**: 593–602.

4. Sierra J, Storer B, Hansen JA et al, Transplantation of marrow cells from unrelated donors for treatment of high-risk acute leukemia: the effect of leukemic burden, donor HLA-matching, and marrow cell dose. *Blood* 1997; **89**: 4226–35.

5. Petersdorf EW, Longton GM, Anasetti C et al, Association of HLA-C disparity with graft failure after marrow transplantation from unrelated donors. *Blood* 1997; **89**: 1818–23.

6. Davies SM, Shu XO, Blazar BR et al, Unrelated donor bone marrow transplantation: influence of HLA A and B incompatibility on outcome. *Blood* 1995; **86**: 1636–42.

7. Beatty PG, Anasetti C, Hansen JA et al, Marrow transplantation from unrelated donors for treatment of hematologic malignancies: effect of mismatching for one HLA locus. *Blood* 1993; **81**: 249–53.

8. Petersdorf EW, Longton GM, Anasetti C et al, The significance of HLA-DRB1 matching on clinical outcome after HLA-A, -B, -DR identical unrelated donor marrow transplantation. *Blood* 1995; **86**: 1606–13.

9. Morton AJ, Anasetti C, Gooley T et al, Chronic graft versus host disease (GVHD) following unrelated donor transplantation. *Blood* 1997; **90**: 590a.

10. Beatty PG, Hansen JA, Longton GM et al, Marrow transplantation from HLA-matched unrelated donors for treatment of hematologic malignancies. *Transplantation* 1991; **51**: 443–7.

11. Morton AJ, Gooley T, Hansen JA et al, Association between pretransplant interferon-alpha and outcome after unrelated donor marrow transplantation for chronic myelogenous leukemia in chronic phase. *Blood* 1998; **92**: 394–401.

12. Hansen JA, Gooley TA, Martin PJ et al, Bone marrow transplants from unrelated donors for patients with chronic myeloid leukemia. *N Engl J Med* 1998; **338**: 962–68.

13. Petersdorf EW, Gooley TA, Anasetti C et al, Optimizing outcome after unrelated marrow transplantation by comprehensive matching of HLA class I and II alleles in the donor and recipient. *Blood* 1998; **92**: 3515–20.

14. Santamaria P, Reinsmoen NL, Lindstom AL et al, Frequent HLA class I and DP sequence mismatches in serologically (HLA-A, HLA-B, HLA-DR) and molecularly (HLA-DRB1, HLA-DQA1, HLA-DQB1) HLA-identical unrelated bone marrow transplant pairs. *Blood* 1994; **83**: 280–7.

15. Petersdorf EW, Longton GM, Anasetti C et al, Definition of HLA-DQ as a transplantation antigen. *Proc Natl Acad Sci USA* 1996; **93**: 15 358–63.

16. Sasazuki T, Juji T, Morishima Y et al, Effect of matching of class I HLA alleles on clinical outcome after transplantation of hematopoietic stem cells from an unrelated donor. *N Engl J Med* 1998; **339**: 1177–85.

17. Anasetti C, Heimfeld S, Rowley S et al, Higher CD34 cell dose is associated with improved survival after marrow transplantation from unrelated donors. *Blood* 1999; **93**: 561a.

18. Clift RA, Buckner CD, Thomas ED et al, Marrow transplantation for chronic myeloid leukemia: a randomized study comparing cyclophosphamide and total body irradiation with busulfan and cyclophosphamide. *Blood* 1994; **84**: 2036–43.

19. Italian Cooperative Study Group on Chronic Myeloid Leukaemia. Evaluating survival after allogeneic bone marrow transplant for chronic myeloid leukaemia in chronic phase: a comparison of transplant versus no-transplant in a cohort of 258 patients first seen in Italy between 1984 and 1986. *Br J Haematol* 1993; **85**: 292–9.

20. Italian Cooperative Study Group on Chronic Myeloid Leukemia. Interferon alfa-2a as compared with conventional chemotherapy for the treatment of chronic myeloid leukemia. *N Engl J Med* 1994; **330**: 820–5.

21. Italian Cooperative Study Group on Chronic Myeloid Leukemia. Long-term follow-up of the Italian trial of interferon-alpha versus conventional chemotherapy in chronic myeloid leukemia. *Blood* 1998; **92**: 1541–8.

22. Chronic Myeloid Leukemia Trialists' Collaborative Group, Interferon alfa versus chemotherapy for chronic myeloid leukemia: a meta-analysis of seven randomized trials. *J Natl Cancer Institute* 1997; **89**: 1616–20.

23. Gale RP, Hehlmann R, Zhang MJ et al, Survival with bone marrow transplantation versus hydroxyurea or interferon for chronic myelogenous leukemia. The German CML Study Group. *Blood* 1998; **91**: 1810–19.

24. McGlave P, Bartsch G, Anasetti C et al, Unrelated donor marrow transplantation therapy for chronic myelogenous leukemia: initial experience of the National Marrow Donor Program. *Blood* 1993; **81**: 543–50.

25. Marks DI, Cullis JO, Ward KN et al, Allogeneic bone marrow transplantation for chronic myeloid leukemia using sibling and volunteer unrelated donors. A comparison of complications in the first 2 years. *Ann Intern Med* 1993; **119**: 207–14.

26. Dini G, Lamparelli T, Rondelli R et al, Unrelated donor marrow transplantation for chronic myelogenous leukaemia. *Br J Haematol* 1998; **102**: 544–52.

27. Lee SJ, Kuntz KM, Horowtiz MM et al, Unrelated donor bone marrow transplantation for chronic myelogenous leukemia: a decision analysis. *Ann Intern Med* 1997; **127**: 1080–8.

28. Beelen DW, Graeven U, Elmaagacli AH et al, Prolonged administration of interferon-alpha in patients with chronic-phase Philadelphia chromosome-positive chronic myelogenous leukemia before allogeneic bone marrow transplantation may adversely affect transplant outcome. *Blood* 1995; **85**: 2981–90.

29. Greenberg P, Cox C, LeBeau MM et al, International scoring system for valuating prognosis in myelodysplastic syndromes. *Blood* 1997; **89**: 2079–88.

30. Passmore SJ, Hann IM, Stiller CA et al, Pediatric myelodysplasia: a study of 68 children and a new prognostic scoring system. *Blood* 1995; **85**: 1742–50.

31. Hasle H, Kerndrup G, Yssing M et al, Intensive chemotherapy in childhood myelodysplastic syndrome. A comparison with results in acute myeloid leukemia. *Leukemia* 1996; **10**: 1269–73.

32. Appelbaum FR, Storb R, Ramberg RE, Allogeneic marrow transplantation in the treatment of preleukemia. *Ann Intern Med* 1984; **100**: 689–93.

33. Anderson JE, Appelbaum FR, Fisher LD et al, Allogeneic bone marrow transplantation for 93 patients with myelodysplastic syndrome. *Blood* 1993; **82**: 677–81.

34. Anderson JE, Anasetti C, Appelbaum FR et al, Unrelated donor marrow transplantation for myelodysplasia (MDS) and MDS-related acute myeloid leukaemia. *Br J Haematol* 1996; **93**: 59–67.

35. Arnold R, deWitte T, vanBiezen A et al, Unrelated bone marrow transplantation in patients with myelodysplastic syndromes and secondary acute myeloid leukemia: an EBMT survey. European Blood and Marrow Transplantation Group. *Bone Marrow Transplant* 1998; **21**: 1213–16.

36. Frangoul HA, Gooley TA, Sander JE et al, Allogeneic bone marrow transplantation (BMT) in children with de novo myelodysplastic syndrome (MDS). *Blood* 1998; **92**: 687a.

37. Guinan EC, Tarbell NJ, Tantravahi R, Weinstein HJ, Bone marrow transplantation for children with myelodysplastic syndromes. *Blood* 1989; **73**: 619.

38. Davies SM, Wagner JE, Defor T et al, Unrelated donor bone marrow transplantation for children and adolescents with aplastic anaemia or myelodysplasia. *Br J Haematol* 1997; **96**: 749–56.

39. Sanders JE, Buckner CD, Thomas ED et al, Allogeneic marrow transplantation for children with juvenile chronic myelogenous leukemia. *Blood* 1988; **71**: 1144–6.

40. Chown SR, Potter MN, Cornish J et al, Matched and mismatched unrelated donor bone marrow transplantation for juvenile chronic myeloid leukaemia. *Br J Haematol* 1996; **93**: 674–6.

41. Locatelli F, Pession A, Comoli P et al, Role of allogeneic bone marrow transplantation from an HLA-identical sibling or a matched unrelated donor in the treatment of children with juvenile chronic myeloid leukaemia. *Br J Haematol* 1996; **92**: 49–54.

42. Oakhill A, Pamphilon DH, Potter MN et al, Unrelated donor bone marrow transplantation for children with relapsed acute lymphoblastic leukaemia in second complete remission. *Br J Haematol* 1996; **94**: 574–8.

43. Rivera GK, Pinkel D, Simone JV et al, Treatment of acute lymphoblastic leukemia. 30 years experience at St. Jude Children's Research Hospital. *N Engl J Med* 1993; **329**: 1343–4.

44. Ortega JJ, Olive T, Haematopoietic progenitor cell transplant in acute leukaemias in children: indications, results and controversies. *Bone Marrow Transplant* 1998; **21**(Suppl 2): S11–16.

45. Bordigoni P, Vernant JP, Souillet G et al, Allogeneic bone marrow transplantation for children with acute lymphoblastic leukemia in first remission: a cooperative study of the Groupe d'Etude de la Greffe de Moelle Osseuse. *J Clin Oncol* 1989; **7**: 747–53.

46. Stockschlader M, Hegewisch-Becker S, Kruger W et al, Bone marrow transplantation for Philadelphia-chromosome-positive acute lymphoblastic leukemia. *Bone Marrow Transplant* 1995; **16**: 663–7.

47. Snyder DS, Chao NJ, Amylon MD et al, Fractionated total body irradiation and high-dose etoposide as a preparatory regimen for bone marrow transplantation for 99 patients with acute leukemia in first complete remission. *Blood* 1993; **82**: 2920–8.

48. Sierra J, Radich J, Hansen JA et al, Marrow transplants from unrelated donors for treatment of Philadelphia chromosome-positive acute lymphoblastic leukemia. *Blood* 1997; **90**: 1410–14.

49. Marks DI, Bird JM, Cornish JM et al, Unrelated donor bone marrow transplantation for children and adolescents with Philadelphia-positive acute lymphoblastic leukemia. *J Clin Oncol* 1998; **16**: 931–6.

50. Chessels JM, Leiper AD, Richards SM, A second course of treatment for childhood acute lymphoblastic leukaemia: long-term follow-up is needed to assess results. *Br J Haematol* 1994; **86**: 48–54.

51. Henze G, Fengler R, Hartmann R et al, BFM group treatment results in relapsed childhood acute lymphoblastic leukemia. *Hämatologie Bluttransfusion* 1990; **33**: 619–26.

52. Sanders JE, Flournoy N, Thomas ED. Marrow transplant experience in children with acute lymphoblastic leukemia: an analysis of factors associated with survival, relapse and graft-versus-host disease. *Med Pediatr Oncol* 1985; **13**: 165–72.

53. Brochstein JA, Kernan NA, Groshen S et al, Allogeneic bone marrow transplantation after hyperfractionated total-body irradiation and cyclophosphamide in children with acute leukemia. *N Engl J Med* 1987; **317**: 1618.

54. Pinkel D. Bone marrow transplantation in children. *J Pediatr* 1993; **122**: 331–41.

55. Barrett AJ, Horowitz MM, Pollock BH et al, Bone marrow transplants from

HLA-identical siblings as compared with chemotherapy for children with acute lymphoblastic leukemia in a second remission. *N Engl J Med* 1994; **331**: 1253–8.

56. Wheeler K, Richards S, Bailey C, Chessells J, Comparison of bone marrow transplant and chemotherapy for relapsed childhood acute lymphoblastic leukaemia: the MRC UKALL X experience. Medical Research Council Working Party on Childhood Leukaemia. *Br J Haematol* 1998; **101**: 94–103.

57. Woolfrey AE, Frangoul H, Anasetti C et al, Unrelated marrow transplants for children with acute lymphocytic leukemia (ALL). *Blood* 1999; **93**: 712a.

58. Weisdorf DJ, Billett AL, Hannan P et al, Autologous versus unrelated donor allogeneic marrow transplantation for acute lymphoblastic leukemia. *Blood* 1997; **90**: 2962–8.

59. Hongeng S, Krance RA, Bowman LC et al, Outcomes of transplantation with matched-sibling and unrelated-donor bone marrow in children with leukaemia. *Lancet* 1997; **350**: 767–71.

60. Greinix HT, Reiter E, Keil F et al, Leukemia-free survival and mortality in patients with refractory or relapsed acute leukemia given marrow transplants from sibling and unrelated donors. *Bone Marrow Transplant* 1998; **21**: 673–8.

61. Bennet JM, Young ML, Andersen JW et al, Long-term survival in acute myeloid leukemia. *Cancer* 1997; **8**: 2205.

62. Wells RJ, Woods WG, Buckley JD et al, Treatment of newly diagnosed children and adolescents with acute myeloid leukemia: a Childrens Cancer Group study. *J Clin Oncol* 1994; **12**: 2367.

63. Woods WG, Kobrinsky N, Buckley J et al, Intensively timed induction therapy followed by autologous or allogeneic bone marrow transplantation for children with acute myeloid leukemia or myelodysplastic syndrome: a Childrens Cancer Group pilot study. *J Clin Oncol* 1993; **11**: 1448.

64. Zittoun RA, Mandelli F, Willemze R et al, Autologous or allogeneic bone mar-

row transplantation compared with intensive chemotherapy in acute myeloid leukemia. *N Engl J Med* 1995; **332**: 217–23.

65. Harousseau JL, Cahn JY, Pignon B et al, Comparison of autologous bone marrow transplantation and intensive chemotherapy as postremission therapy in adult acute myeloid leukemia. *Blood* 1997; **90**: 2978–86.

66. Cassileth PA, Harrington DP, Appelbaum FR et al, Chemotherapy compared with autologous or allogeneic bone marrow transplantation in the management of acute myeloid leukemia in first remission. *N Engl J Med* 1998; **339**: 1649–56.

67. Woods WG, Kobrinsky N, Buckley J et al, Timed-sequential induction therapy improves postremission outcome in acute myeloid leukemia: a report from the Children's Cancer Group. *Blood* 1996; **87**: 4979.

68. Amadori S, Testi AM, Arico M et al, Prospective comparative study of bone marrow transplantation and post-remission chemotherapy for childhood acute myelogenous leukemia. *J Clin Oncol* 1993; **11**: 1046.

69. Stevens RF, Hann IM, Wheatley K, Gray RG, Marked improvements in outcome with chemotherapy alone in pediatric acute myeloid leukaemia: results of the United Kingdom Medical Research Council's 10th AML trial. MRC Childhood Leukaemia Working Party. *Br J Haematol* 1998; **101**: 130–40.

70. Clift RA, Buckner CD, Appelbaum FR et al, Allogeneic marrow transplantation during untreated first relapse of acute myeloid leukemia. *J Clin Oncol* 1992; **10**: 1723.

71. Woolfrey AW, Gooley T, Milner L et al, Bone marrow transplantation for children less than 2 years of age with acute myelogenous leukemia or myelodysplastic syndrome. *Blood* 1998; **92**: 3546–56.

72. Appelbaum FR, Clift RA, Buckner CD et al, Allogeneic marrow transplantation for acute nonlymphoblastic leukemia after first relapse. *Blood* 1983; **61**: 949–53.

73. Chown SR, Marks DE, Cornish JM et al, Unrelated donor bone marrow transplantation in children and young adults with acute myeloid leukaemia in remission. *Br J Haematol* 1997; **99**: 36–40.

74. Gale RP, Horowitz MM, Rees JK et al, Chemotherapy versus transplants for acute myelogenous leukemia in second remission. *Leukemia* 1996; **10**: 13–19.

75. Ash RC, Casper JT, Chitambar CR et al, Successful allogeneic transplantation of T cell-depleted bone marrow from closely HLA-matched unrelated donors. *N Engl J Med* 1990; **322**: 485–94.

76. Storb R, Etzioni R, Anasetti C et al, Cyclophosphamide combined with antithymocyte globulin in preparation for allogeneic marrow transplants in patients with aplastic anemia. *Blood* 1994; **84**: 941.

77. Doney K, Pepe M, Storb R et al, Immunosuppressive therapy of aplastic anemia: Results of a prospective randomized trial of antithymocyte globulin (ATG), methylprednisolone and oxymetholone to ATG, very high-dose methylprednisolone and oxymetholone. *Blood* 1992; **79**: 2566.

78. Doney K, Leisenring W, Storb, R, Appelbaum FR, for the Seattle Bone Marrow Transplant Team, Primary treatment of acquired aplastic anemia: outcomes with bone marrow transplantation and immunosuppressive therapy. *Ann Intern Med* 1997; **126**: 107.

79. Bacigalupo A, Hows J, Gluckman E et al, Bone marrow transplantation (BMT) versus immunosuppression for the treatment of severe aplastic anaemia (SAA): a report of the EBMT SAA Working Party. *Br J Haematol* 1988; **70**: 177.

80. Frickhofen N, Kaltwasser JP, Schrezenmeier H et al, Treatment of aplastic anemia with antilymphocyte globulin and methylprednisolone with or without cyclosporine. *N Engl J Med* 1991; **324**: 1297.

81. Margolis D, Camitta B, Pietryga D et al, Unrelated donor bone marrow transplantation to treat sever aplastic anaemia in children and young adults. *Br J Haematol* 1996; **94**: 65–72.

82. Deeg HJ, Schoch G, Ramsey N et al, Marrow transplantation from unrelated donors for patients with aplastic anemia (AA) who failed immunosuppressive therapy. *Blood* 1997; **90**: 397a.

83. Filipovich AH, Shapiro RS, Ramsay NK et al, Unrelated donor bone marrow transplantation for correction of lethal congenital immunodeficiencies. *Blood* 1992; **80**: 270–6.

84. Buckley RH, Schiff SE, Schiff RI et al, Haploidentical bone marrow stem cell transplantation in human severe combined immunodeficiency. *Semin Hematol* 1993; **30**: 92–104.

85. Filipovich AH, Stem cell transplantation from unrelated donors for correction of primary immunodeficiencies. *Immunol Allergy Clin North Am* 1996; **16**: 377–92.

86. Miano M, Porta F, Locatelli F et al, Unrelated donor marrow transplantation for inborn errors. *Bone Marrow Transplant* 1998; **21**: S37–41.

87. Peters C, Balthazor M, Shapiro EG et al, Outcome of unrelated donor bone marrow transplantation in 40 children with Hurler syndrome. *Blood* 1996; **87**: 4894–902.

88. Ringden O, Groth CG, Erikson A et al, Ten years' experience of bone marrow transplantation for Gaucher disease. *Transplantation* 1995; **59**: 864–70.

89. Baker KS, DeLaat CA, Steinbuch M et al, Successful correction of hemophagocytic lymphohistiocytosis with related or unrelated bone marrow transplantation. *Blood* 1997; **89**: 3857–63.

90. Gluckman E, Auerbach AD, Horowitz MM et al, Bone marrow transplantation for Fanconi anemia. *Blood* 1995; **86**: 2856–62.

91. Smith OP, Chan MY, Evans J, Veys P, Shwachman–Diamond syndrome and matched unrelated donor BMT. *Bone Marrow Transplant* 1995; **16**: 717–18.

92. Langston AA, Sanders JE, Deeg HJ et al, Allogeneic marrow transplantation for aplastic anaemia associated with dyskeratosis congenita. *Br J Haematol* 1996; **92**: 758–65.

93. National Marrow Donor Program (http://www.marrow.org).

94. Slattery JT, Sanders JE, Buckner CD, Graft-rejection and toxicity following bone marrow transplantation in relation to busulfan pharmacokinetics. *Bone Marrow Transplant* 1995; **16**: 31–42.

95. Bensinger W, Martin P, Clift R et al, A prospective randomized trial of peripheral blood stem cells (PBSC) or marrow (BM) for patients undergoing allogeneic transplantation for hematologic malignancies. *Blood* 1999; **93**: 368a.

# 4

# Novel preparative regimens I: Tagged antibodies

James E Butrynski, Dana C Matthews

## INTRODUCTION

Beginning with the first human marrow transplants in the 1960s, developments in all aspects of transplantation have benefited patients with otherwise fatal hematological malignancies. However, despite more aggressive preparative regimens and improved supportive care, relapse of disease and regimen-related toxicities continue to be the main causes of failure. New therapies that selectively target tumor cells are being developed with the goal of decreasing both relapse rates and toxicity. Monoclonal antibodies reactive with hematopoietic antigens have impacted hematopoietic stem cell (HSC) transplantation (HSCT) in several ways. These include the use of unmodified antibodies to purge or enrich stem cell products, and the use of antibodies labeled with toxic moieties such as drugs or radioactive isotopes to increase antitumor effects. This chapter will focus on the history, advances, and controversies regarding radiolabeled antibodies used in preparative regimens for HSCT.

## BACKGROUND

Lymphohematopoetic malignancies are radiation-sensitive, and thus the majority of stem cell transplantation regimens have used total-body irradiation (TBI) as part of the preparative regimen.[1] However, despite high-dose TBI, relapse continues to be a major cause of failure, particularly for patients transplanted at an advanced disease stage. Efforts to reduce relapse have included increasing the dose of TBI, as examined in two randomized trials investigating the effect of TBI dose escalation on relapse rates. In these trials, TBI was delivered as 12 gray (Gy) in six fractions or 15.75 Gy in seven fractions, and was combined with standard high-dose cyclophosphamide (Cy) for patients receiving matched related bone marrow transplants for myeloid leukemias. In patients with acute myelogenous leukemia (AML) in first remission, the relapse rate was 12% after 15.75 Gy, compared with 35% after 12 Gy.[2] In patients with chronic myelogenous leukemia (CML) in chronic phase, the relapse rate was 0% after 15.75 Gy and 25% after 12 Gy.[3] However, in both studies, the transplant-related mortality was higher following 15.75 Gy TBI, and thus there was no difference in the long-term disease-free survival between the two radiation doses.

These and other trials confirmed the radiosensitivity of lymphohematopoetic tumors, but also demonstrated that the escalation of radiation dose delivered as TBI is limited by normal organ tolerance. However, these studies suggest that the ability to target radiation to the malignant cell and spare normal tissues, thus allowing the delivery of higher radiation doses to the tumor without excessive toxicity, has the potential to improve the outcome of HSCT. The availability of monoclonal antibodies reactive with hematopoietic antigens provides a means of delivering targeted radiation by coupling a radioisotope to an antibody to produce a radioimmunoconjugate (RIC). In contrast to unlabeled monoclonal antibodies, the tumor cell killing effects of RIC do not require host effector mechanisms such as antibody-dependent cellular cytotoxicity (ADCC) to kill cells, nor do they require internalization to be effective as is required by drug–antibody conjugates or immunotoxins. Additionally, beta-particle emissions are capable of killing cells over a distance of several cell diameters, resulting in potential cell kill of both antigen-positive and -negative tumor cells.[4] The 'cross-fire' created by the RIC is also advantageous in situations of heterogeneous distribution of RIC in large tumor masses.

## COMPONENTS OF TAGGED ANTIBODY THERAPY

### Antigen

The target antigen plays a critical role in the outcome of tagged antibody therapy. Target antigen variables that affect the biodistribution of RIC include the pattern of expression in tissues, the number of antigenic sites per cell, and the fate of the antigen–antibody complex after binding, i.e. whether the complex internalizes into the cell (Table 4.1).

Truly 'tumor-specific' antigens are uncommon, with the best example being antibody reactive with the immunoglobulin idiotype expressed by non-Hodgkin's lymphoma cells, an approach that has been impractical given the need to generate unique antibodies for individual patients.[5] Most trials have targeted antigens expressed by tumor cells and a subset of normal non-clonogenic lymphoid or myeloid cells. The targeting of antigen expressed by both tumor and normal cells at sites of tumor cell residence may be advantageous in that the maximum radiation to a tissue such as bone marrow may occur if the majority of cells in that tissue are bound by antibody.

A large copy number of target antigens per cell is desirable to provide maximum binding sites and thus optimize the local concentration of radioisotope.[6] When antigen expression is very limited, in terms of both numbers of antigen-positive cells and the copy number per cell, only a small amount of antibody

**Table 4.1 Components of tagged antibody therapy**

| Component | Important properties |
|---|---|
| Antigen | Expression in target and non-target tissues<br>Target sites per cell<br>Fate of antigen–antibody complex |
| Antibody | Avidity<br>Immunogenicity<br>Size<br>Ease of labeling |
| Isotope | Type of emission<br>Energy of emission<br>Half-life<br>Stability of label |
| Toxin | Protein synthesis disruption or DNA damage<br>Immunogenicity<br>Internalization required |

can be administered without saturating all of the binding sites. There may be a limit to the amount of radioisotope with which a small amount of protein can be labeled, thus limiting the radiation dose that can be delivered. However, when cell death requires only a small number of toxic moieties per cell, as with high-energy alpha particles or some drug or toxin conjugates, relatively low antigen expression per cell may be sufficient.

The characteristics of the target antigen prior to and following antibody binding may also affect antibody biodistribution. Antigens that are shed from the cell surface and thus circulate in appreciable quantities can bind antibody in circulation, decreasing the amount available to bind to target tissue. Following antibody binding to the target antigen, the complex may remain on the cell surface or may internalize into the cell. Antigen–antibody complexes remaining at the cell surface are optimal for unlabeled antibodies requiring ADCC for effect.[7,8] Conventionally iodinated antibodies may undergo rapid metabolism if internalized, and be dehalogenated in lysosomes, with subsequent rapid excretion of small iodine-containing moieties.[9,10] Thus the radioiodine will be retained best at the target site if the antigen remains stable on the cell surface or if the method for coupling iodine to antibody is resistant to intracellular degradation, as has been shown with tyramine cellobiose labeling.[11] Internalization of RIC not prone to intracellular metabolism, such as those labeled with radiometals (e.g. yttrium-90) or radioiodinated using such alternative conjugation methods, may improve the accumulation of isotope at the target site. Finally, internalized antigens are not available to bind antibody until they are resynthesized by the cell, which may require several days.

## Antibody

Antibody characteristics that may affect both the biodistribution of RIC and practical treatment options include avidity, immunogenicity, size, and the ease of radiolabeling. Furthermore, the dose of antibody administered may affect biodistribution and the ratio of radiation delivered to the tumor as compared with non-target organs by impacting the degree of antigen saturation and the half-life of antibody in circulation.

Antibody avidity for target antigen will affect both 'on' and 'off' rates for antibody binding to target antigen. In addition, although high avidity of antibody for antigen may enhance retention after binding, very high avidity may result in heterogeneity of antibody distribution within a tumor mass as described by Weinstein and colleagues in their model of the 'binding site barrier'.[12–14] This model predicts that diffusion of antibody into a tumor may be hampered by its avid binding at the first site of entry in perivascular regions.

The use of murine monoclonal antibodies often results in the production of human anti-mouse antibody (HAMA), usually within one to two months post exposure. The presence of HAMA generally precludes further treatment with murine antibody, or changes the biodistribution of subsequent antibody administered. Even patients with severe immunosuppression associated with their underlying disease can mount a HAMA response.[15] Chimeric antibodies of mostly human origin have been engineered in an effort to decrease the immune response to antibody.[16,17] These chimeric proteins generally retain the murine variable region for epitope recognition but are placed into a human immunoglobulin backbone. The absence of an immune response to these constructs allows repeat dosing.[18]

Ideally, antibodies must have access to tumor cells in every disease location. Antibody penetration into a tumor may be limited by poor vascularity at the tumor site, poor capillary permeability, and high interstitial pressure within the tumor.[19–21] Intact antibodies penetrate tumors less homogeneously than smaller antibody fragments (Fab′, single-chain Fv (scFv)).[21,22] However, antibody fragments, because of their small size, are cleared more rapidly from the circulation, resulting in decreased serum concentration and a diminished serum-to-tumor gradient. Dimeric and trimeric Fab′ have had better tumor uptake than scFv in some studies, and novel genetically engineered antibody constructs, including $C_H2$ domain deletions and 'minibodies' composed of scFv fused to the $C_H3$ domain, may potentially improve tumor targeting.[23–25]

The dose and dosing schedule for optimal biodistribution must be determined for each antibody construct. As the antibody dose is increased above its optimal level, non-specifically circulating antibody delivers radiation to all sites, with the potential to increase toxicity. However, large doses of antibody may be required to saturate antigen-positive cells in sites such as the spleen and maintain a serum concentration high enough to allow the antibody to permeate tumor masses.

Finally, the antibody must retain its immunoreactivity when labeled with radioisotope. In situations where the specific activity (amount of radioactivity in millicuries per amount of antibody in milligrams, denoted mCi/mg) that can be achieved without adversely affecting antibody binding is relatively low, schemes that incorporate repeat dosing may be used in order to deliver the desired amount of radioactivity.

## Isotope

Several radioisotopes have been used for clinical radiolabeled antibody therapy (Table 4.2). Most trials to date have used beta-emitting isotopes, such as iodine-131 ($^{131}$I) and yttrium-90 ($^{90}$Y), although a recent trial has employed bismuth-213 ($^{213}$Bi), an alpha-emitter. Important characteristics of the radioisotope include particle energy, half-life, availability, and ease of conjugation to antibody.

Beta particles, which are electrons, are approximately 1/7300 the mass of alpha particles, which are helium nuclei (composed of two protons and two neutrons).[26] Because of their low mass, beta particles have a much greater penetrating power and a longer range through tissue than alpha particles, with a mean path length ranging from 0.3 to 5.3 mm for commonly used isotopes.

The primary mode of energy loss by alpha particles passing through tissue is

## Table 4.2  Radioisotopes for radiolabeled antibody therapy

| Radionuclide | Mean path (mm) | Particle energy (MeV) | Half-life | Comments |
|---|---|---|---|---|
| *Beta-emitters* | | | | |
| Iodine-131 ($^{131}$I) | 0.8 | 0.6 | 8.0 days | Readily available, high-energy gamma requires patient radiation isolation |
| Yttrium-90 ($^{90}$Y) | 5.3 | 2.3 | 2.8 days | Every beta component high; lack of gamma component requires imaging with Indium-111 ($^{111}$I) |
| Rhenium-186 ($^{186}$Re) | 0.9 | 1.1 | 3.8 days | Gamma acceptable for imaging |
| Rhenium-188 ($^{188}$Re) | 4.4 | 2.1 | 17 hours | Gamma acceptable for imaging |
| Lutetium-177 ($^{177}$Lu) | 0.3 | 0.5 | 67 days | Gamma acceptable for imaging |
| Copper-67 ($^{67}$Cu) | 0.3 | 0.6 | 2.6 days | Gamma acceptable for imaging |
| Holmium-166 ($^{166}$Ho) | 4.0 | 1.9 | 1.1 days | Gamma acceptable for imaging |
| Samarium-153 ($^{153}$Sm) | 0.9 | 0.7 | 1.9 days | Gamma acceptable for imaging |
| *Alpha-emitters* | | | | |
| Bismuth-213 ($^{213}$Bi) | 0.06 | 6.1 | 1 hour | High-energy particle, short half-life |
| Astatine-211 ($^{211}$At) | 0.06 | 5.9 | 7.2 hours | High-energy particle, short half-life |

by inelastic collision with atomic electrons. Their range of energy deposition in tissues is in the range of micrometres, and alpha particles are capable of significant damage as they dissipate their energy, with lethal damage resulting from as few as two or three particles per cell.[27,28]

Gamma rays are a form of electromagnetic radiation (photons), and penetrate tissue easily, with little interaction with matter. The main advantage of gamma emissions is the ability to perform planar imaging for estimation of radiation absorbed dose calculations. This longer range energy also has the potential to deliver a 'TBI' component from the circulating radiolabeled antibody. However this may increase the non-specific organ toxicity of the RIC. Furthermore, gamma emissions represent a radiation hazard to the patient's family and staff, necessitating treatment in radiation isolation.

[131]I is readily available and its coupling chemistry is well established. Dehalogenation reactions, which can uncouple monoiodotyrosine from antibody, occur when internalized iodinated antibodies have been labeled by standard chloramine T or Iodo-Gen (Pierce Chemical Co) methods.[9] Coupling chemistry utilizing a tyramine cellobiose or 5-iodo-3-pyridinecarboxylate bridge to incorporate radioiodine with antibody is an alternative labeling approach that is resistant to dehalogenation.[11,29]

[90]Y has a greater path length of energy deposition as compared with [131]I (5.3 mm versus 0.8 mm), and thus may produce more homogeneous radiation in a tumor mass. In addition, [90]Y has no significant gamma emissions. When coupled to internalizing antibodies [90]Y-metabolites are retained intracellularly. The coupling between [90]Y (as well as other non-halogen radionuclides such as rhenium-186 ([186]Re) and copper-67 ([67]Cu)) and antibody relies upon chelation chemistry, and may be prone to dechelation and release of free isotope. Although this may lead to localization of free [90]Y in bone or liver, recently developed chelates appear to be more stable.[30] The absence of gamma emissions requires labeling of the antibody with an alternative radioisotope, usually indium-111 ([111]In), for imaging. The ability to extrapolate from the biodistribution of [111]In to estimated radiation doses delivered by the same antibody labeled with [90]Y depends upon the assumption that the localization of the two isotopes is identical, which requires that both isotopes be stably bound to the antibody by the chelate.

Alpha emitters have recently been used in human trials in leukemia.[31] Their short range of action and high-energy deposition may result in more specific and effective cell kill. However, their short half-lives complicate their clinical use. Although these short half-lives as well as the limited path length, makes alpha-particle RIC less practical for mass lesions, leukemia may represent an ideal target, given the rapid access of RIC to malignant cells in the highly vascular marrow and spleen.

## Toxin

Toxins that have been coupled to antibodies include diphtheria toxin, ricin, maytansinoids, gelonin, *Pseudomonas* exotoxin, and a novel drug, calicheamicin.[32–39] These agents are highly potent, and many act by disrupting protein synthesis or causing DNA damage. Most require internalization following antibody–antigen binding to reach the cytosol or nucleus in order to achieve their effect. No trials of toxin-tagged antibodies have been performed in the context of preparative regimens prior to HSCT. However, in a recent dose-escalation trial of the novel drug–antibody conjugate CMA-676 (calicheamicin conjugated to anti-CD33 antibody) in patients with relapsed or refractory AML, 8 of 39 patients (21%) had elimination of leukemic blasts from blood and marrow with minimal toxicity.[40] In a phase II study, 17 of 45 patients (38%) with AML in untreated first relapse achieved a remission with this agent.[41] This drug–antibody conjugate may play a role in a preparative regimen in the future, or could be used to reduce tumor burden either before, or as consolidation, after HSCT.

## BIODISTRIBUTION AND RADIATION ABSORBED DOSE ESTIMATES OF RADIOLABELED ANTIBODIES

Ideally, radiolabeled antibody therapy includes determination of RIC biodistribution and estimation of radiation absorbed doses delivered to target and normal tissues. Accurate estimation of radiation absorbed doses in tissues of interest (measured as centigray (cGy) delivered to tissue per millicurie of isotope administered) allows individualized determination of the dose delivered both to sites of tumor, for correlation of estimated dose with antitumor effect, and to normal organs, for correlation of estimated dose with toxicity. The dosimetric calculations are based on information derived from serial blood (or tissue) sampling and serial quantitative external gamma-camera scanning following the infusion of a given dose of antibody labeled with a trace amount of isotope. Time–activity curves of the concentration of radioisotope in organs and tumor over time are generated and used to estimate radiation absorbed doses to each tissue using methods developed by the Medical Internal Radiation Dose Committee of the Society of Nuclear Medicine.[42–44] These calculations include the contribution of radiation from isotope bound directly in the tissue of interest, as well as any contribution from adjacent organs. These methods provide estimates that allow the determination of whether a favorable biodistribution (i.e. more radiation delivered to target as compared with non-target organs) was achieved with a given dose of antibody, comparison of radiation dose ratios achieved with different antibody doses or RIC, and individualization of radiation doses delivered to critical normal organs. Other clinical trials have administered isotope based on a predetermined number of millicuries per square meter or weight in kilograms.

## CLINICAL TRIALS

Clinical trials of HSCT preparative regimens employing tagged antibodies have been performed in leukemia, non-Hodgkin's lymphoma, and Hodgkin's disease. In each trial performed to date, the antibodies have been labeled with radioisotopes. In multiple myeloma, targeted radiation delivered to bone marrow by radioisotope-containing chelates that bind directly to bone has been incorporated into the conditioning regimens. In addition, in neuroblastoma, $^{131}$I-metaiodobenzylguanidine (MIBG), a molecule that specifically targets neuroblastoma cells, has been used in combination with autologous bone marrow support. The use of antibodies to deliver non-radioactive toxins or to purge hematopoietic stem cell products will not be discussed here.

## LEUKEMIA/MYELODYSPLASTIC SYNDROME

Most studies using radiolabeled antibodies as part of HSCT preparative regimens for leukemia or myelodyslastic syndrome (MDS) have targeted the hematopoietic antigens CD33 and CD45. A recent study used rhenium-188 ($^{188}$Re)-labeled antibody reactive with the granulocytic antigen CD66c.

### CD33 antigen

CD33 is a cell surface protein present on normal maturing myeloid precursors and on AML cells but not on normal hematopoietic stem cells or non-hematopoietic tissues.[45–48] AML blast cells from 90% of patients express this antigen. The exact function of CD33 is unknown, but its structural and binding characteristics identify it as a member of the sialoadhesin family of proteins. Antigen expression ranges from 10 000 copies per cell on normal precursors to more than 10-fold higher levels on some leukemic cells. The antigen–antibody complex is internalized after binding by antibody.[9]

The Memorial Sloan-Kettering group has used radiolabeled anti-CD33 murine monoclonal antibody (M195) as part of conditioning prior to HSCT. In the initial non-transplant pilot trial examining the biodistribution of trace-labeled M195 antibody, 10 patients with relapsed AML ($n = 3$), refractory AML ($n = 6$), or chronic myelomonocytic leukemia (CMML) ($n = 1$) were treated with multiple doses of unlabeled antibody, with the first dose trace-labeled with $^{131}$I (5 mCi).[49] The acute infusional toxicity was minimal. HAMA responses were documented in 4 of 6 evaluable patients. Visualization of the $^{131}$I-M195 antibody biodistribution using whole-body imaging demonstrated rapid specific bone marrow targeting at the lowest dose of antibody and saturation of available binding sites at antibody doses of 5 mg/m$^2$. Radiation absorbed dose estimates to liver and marrow were 1.1–6.1 cGy/mCi and 1.7–33.5 cGy/mCi, respectively, with the highest percentage of injected dose per gram of bone marrow seen at the 5 mg/m$^2$ antibody dose level. Two patients had a transient drop in peripheral blast counts after unlabeled antibody. There were no significant tumor responses with saturating doses of M195 antibody, but this study demonstrated that radiolabeled M195 antibody could deliver more radiation to marrow and spleen than to other organs in the majority of patients.

A follow-up study examined the bone marrow suppression and toxicities of escalating doses of $^{131}$I delivered by M195 antibody in 24 patients with relapsed or refractory AML ($n = 16$), blast-phase MDS ($n = 5$), secondary AML ($n = 2$), and blastic CML ($n = 1$).[50] Patients received 50–210 mCi/m$^2$ of $^{131}$I-M195 antibody in divided doses. The dosing regimen was chosen to allow re-expression of the CD33 antigen on the surface of the target cells between infusions. Twenty-two patients were able to receive all planned doses. Toxicity during the infusions was minimal and non-hematological toxicities were manageable. Seven of 19 patients developed HAMA, and the two patients retreated after development of HAMA had abrogated targeting and leukemic cell killing.

The 22 patients demonstrated marked uptake of tagged antibody into all areas of bone marrow, as well as variable blood pooling, as determined by whole-body gamma imaging. Seventeen of 19 patients demonstrated decreases in the absolute number of blasts per millimeter of bone marrow biopsy, with a direct correlation between $^{131}$I dose level and mean blast kill. Eight patients had sufficient marrow cytoreduction to require infusion of previously stored autologous stem cells. Three of these achieved complete remissions (CR), while no CR were achieved at the non-myeloablative dose levels. A maximum tolerated dose was not reached in this study. This clinical trial demonstrated leukemic cytoreduction using radiolabeled antibody as a single agent even in patients with chemotherapy-refractory leukemias.

In an attempt to increase leukemic cell kill, a subsequent trial combined $^{131}$I-M195 antibody with standard busulfan (Bu) and Cy, followed by allogeneic bone marrow transplant (BMT) in 19 patients.[50] Ten patients had relapsed ($n = 2$) or refractory ($n = 8$) AML, and five patients had CML in accelerated phase ($n = 2$) or blast crisis ($n = 3$). Four additional patients received a second BMT for either relapsed chronic-phase ($n = 1$) or accelerated ($n = 3$) CML. Doses of $^{131}$I ranged from 120 to 230 mCi/m$^2$ delivered in two to four divided doses of 3 mg/m$^2$ M195 antibody per dose. Patients then received Bu (16 mg/kg) and Cy (120 mg/kg for first BMT and 90 mg/kg for second BMT) followed by infusion of unprocessed HLA-matched allogeneic bone marrow. Cyclosporine (CSP) and corticosteroids were given as prophylaxis against graft-versus host-disease (GvHD).

No significant infusional toxicity following $^{131}$I-M195 antibody was reported. The 4 patients undergoing second BMT died in complete remission of transplant-related complications and 6 of 15 patients undergoing first transplant died in CR of GvHD or infection. Acute GvHD was observed in 7 patients and included grade I ($n = 2$), grade II ($n = 3$), and grade IV ($n = 2$). Chronic GvHD was seen in 2 patients. HAMA developed in 6 of 16 evaluable patients. All patients engrafted, with a median time to neutrophil recovery of 14 days and a median time to platelet recovery of 27 days. Fourteen of the 15 patients undergoing their first BMT achieved a CR. At the time of report, three remained in CR at 18, 26, and 29 months after BMT, and six patients had relapsed 3–36 months following BMT. [131]I-M195 antibody added to this preparative regimen did not appear to increase toxicity or negatively influence engraftment.

In an effort to decrease immunogenicity and to mediate ADCC against a leukemic target, a humanized version of M195 antibody (HuM195) was developed. In the initial non-transplant trial to evaluate the biodistribution of trace-labeled HuM195 antibody, 13 patients with relapsed ($n = 7$) or refractory ($n = 6$) AML were treated with 0.5–10.0 mg/m$^2$ per dose of HuM195 antibody.[51] At least six doses per patient were given over 18 days. The first administered dose was trace-labeled with [131]I. The optimal biodistribution occurred at 3 mg/m$^2$ as determined by the extent of saturation of available sites and specific bone marrow localization at this dose. Toxicity at 3.0 and 10 mg/m$^2$ was manageable, and no patients developed HAMA. No CR were observed, but tumor responses were seen in two patients. HuM195 antibody has also been delivered at supersaturating doses of up to 36 mg/m$^2$/dose for eight doses over 18 days.[52] Although unlabeled HuM195 antibody has not been incorporated into HSCT preparative regimens, it has been studied in the setting of minimal residual disease in patients with acute promyelocytic leukemia (APL).[53]

Appelbaum and colleagues[54] examined the biodistribution of an alternative murine anti-CD33 antibody, p67. This phase I study combined [131]I-p67 antibody with standard Cy and 12 Gy TBI. Nine patients with AML in second remission ($n = 5$) or in relapse ($n = 4$) received biodistribution infusions of trace-labeled [131]I-p67 antibody at doses of 0.05–0.5 mg/kg. Although there was initial uptake of [131]I-p67 antibody in the marrow in most patients, marrow retention of [131]I-p67 antibody was short ($t_{1/2} = 21.4$ hours), presumably because of rapid internalization and dehalogenation of the radiolabeled antibody. As a consequence of this short half-life, the average radiation absorbed dose to marrow was low (1.6 cGy/mCi). The average dose to liver was 1.5 cGy/mCi. Favorable biodistribution (marrow and spleen estimated to receive a higher dose of radiation than any normal organ) was seen in four of nine patients.

These four patients received therapy doses of antibody labeled with the amount of [131]I-p67 antibody (110–330 mCi) estimated to deliver 1.75 Gy to the normal organ receiving the highest dose (lung or liver), followed by Cy, TBI, and HSCT. All patients engrafted normally and no grade III or IV toxicity (life-threatening or fatal, respectively) was seen.[55] Three of the four treated patients relapsed after transplant, while one patient survives disease-free more than seven years later. This study showed that modest radiation doses delivered by [131]I-p67 antibody could be combined with a standard conditioning regimen without significant toxicity. However, the use of [131]I-p67 antibody was limited by the short marrow half-life and the low antibody doses that would saturate CD33. These two factors limited the dose of radiation deliverable to the leukemic cells.

Recently, HuM195 antibody labeled with alternate radioisotopes, $^{90}$Y and $^{213}$Bi, has been evaluated in patients with advanced myeloid leukemias.[56,57] In a phase I dose escalation trial of $^{90}$Y-HuM195 antibody, 15 patients with relapsed or refractory AML were treated with antibody labeled with 0.1–0.3 mCi/kg of $^{90}$Y as a single dose in the outpatient department[56] (JG Jurcic, personal communication). A tracer dose of $^{111}$In-HuM195 antibody was used to determine the biodistribution. Localization of $^{111}$In-HuM195 antibody in the bone marrow, liver, and spleen occurred within one hour of infusion, with retention at these sites for at least three days following treatment. Infusional toxicity was mild, and myelosuppression was proportional to the amount of $^{90}$Y administered. Although most patients receiving 0.22–0.3 mCi/kg had transient elimination of leukemia in the marrow two to four weeks after treatment, the AML recurred with marrow recovery in all of these patients with refractory leukemia. Although HSCT was not used in this phase I study, the delivery of significant radiation to marrow with $^{90}$Y-HuM195 antibody suggests its potential utility as part of a preparative regimen for HSCT.

In a phase I study, HuM195 antibody labeled with the alpha-emitting isotope $^{213}$Bi, in escalating doses of 0.28 to 1 mCi/kg, was infused in three to six fractions over two to four days in 17 patients with relapsed ($n = 13$) or refractory ($n = 3$) AML or CMML ($n = 1$).[57] No acute toxicity was observed, but myelosuppression lasted up to 34 days. Bone marrow, liver, and spleen uptake of radioisotope occurred within 10 minutes after infusion, and was maintained throughout the half-life of the isotope. The estimates of $^{213}$Bi-HuM195 antibody radiation dose delivered to marrow, liver, spleen, and blood were 656–4676 cSv, 242–2752 cSv, 290–4399 cSv, and 108–673 cSv, respectively (the sievert (Sv) is a radiological unit of human dose equivalent, and relates the absorbed dose in human tissue to the effective biological damage of the radiation). These estimates were many-fold higher than to the whole body. No CR have been seen, but 10 of 12 evaluable patients had reductions in peripheral blood leukemia cells and 12 of 17 patients had decreases in the percentage of bone marrow blasts. Thus, in this first human study using an alpha-emitting isotope, $^{213}$Bi-HuM195 antibody appears safe and possesses antileukemic activity. Incorporation into a preparative regimen may lead to an additive effect on tumor cell death while not adding appreciably to toxicity.

In summary, radiolabeled anti-CD33 antibody has antileukemic activity alone in a heavily pretreated cohort, and, when used as part of a preparative regimen, does not appear to add significant toxicity. The achievable specific activities and relatively short retention in marrow when using $^{131}$I may limit the role of this isotope, but $^{213}$Bi and $^{90}$Y, with higher linear energy transfer properties, may obviate the need for such high specific activities.

## CD45 antigen

CD45 is a cell surface tyrosine phosphatase that is expressed by all circulating leukocytes and lymphocytes but not by erythrocytes or platelets.[58–60] Approximately 70% of nucleated cells in the marrow and all leukocytes in lymph nodes and spleen express CD45, as do 85–90% of AML cells and the majority of acute lymphoblastic leukemia (ALL) cells. CD45 antigen expression is relatively high (on average 200 000 sites per cell), and the antigen–antibody complex remains on the cell surface.[9] CD45 antigen offers several advantages as a target for tagged antibody therapy. Because this antigen is expressed by both malignant cells of myeloid and lymphoid lineage, and non-malignant cells in bone marrow, spleen, and lymphoid tissue, anti-CD45 antibody will bind to the majority of cells in these tissues whether patients are in remission or relapse.

Preclinical studies of [131]I anti-CD45 antibody in mice demonstrated relative specific delivery of radiation to tissues of hematopoietic and lymphoid origin.[61] In these experiments, estimates of radiation absorbed dose to the marrow and lymph nodes were two- to threefold and three- to eightfold, respectively, greater than to the lung, the normal tissue with the highest radiation absorbed dose. In the macaque model, estimates of radiation absorbed dose demonstrated that two different [131]I-anti-CD45 antibodies could deliver up to 5 times more radiation to lymph nodes and up to 2.6 times more to bone marrow than to lung or liver.[62]

Based on these preclinical results, a phase I trial examining the biodistribution of [131]I-labeled murine anti-CD45 antibody (BC8) and determining the maximum tolerated dose of radiation delivered by [131]I-BC8 antibody when combined with Cy, 12 Gy TBI, and HSCT was initiated.[63,64] Antibody biodistribution was determined in 44 patients with AML, ALL, or MDS (Figure 4.1). Thirty-one patients had AML in second or third remission ($n = 9$) or relapsed or refractory disease ($n = 22$), 10 patients had ALL in second remission ($n = 5$) or relapsed or refractory disease ($n = 5$), and 3 patients had MDS (refractory anemia with excess blasts (RAEB) ($n = 2$) or refractory anemia with excess blasts in transformation (RAEB-t) ($n = 1$). Favorable biodistribution of trace-labeled [131]I-BC8 antibody was observed in 37 patients (84%). The average estimated radiation absorbed doses (cGy/mCi [131]I ± SEM) in this study were bone marrow 6.5 ± 0.5, spleen 13.5 ± 1.3, liver 2.8 ± 0.2, lung 1.8 ± 0.1, kidney 0.6 ± 0.04, and total body 0.4 ± 0.02. The normal organ that received the highest estimated radiation absorbed dose was the liver in all but one patient.

Thirty-four patients were treated with a therapeutic dose of [131]I-BC8 antibody labeled with the amount of [131]I estimated to deliver from dose level 1 (3.5 Gy) to level 6 (12.25 Gy) to the normal organ receiving the highest dose. This dose was administered on day −14, followed by Cy 60 mg/kg on days −8 and −7 and TBI as daily 2 Gy fractions on days −6 to −1 (to a total dose of 12 Gy). HSC (allogeneic or autologous marrow or peripheral blood) were infused on day 0. CSP and methotrexate (MTX) were given to allogeneic recipients as GvHD prophylaxis.

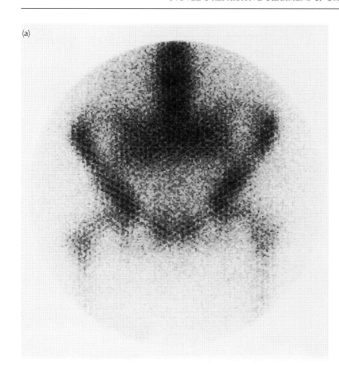

(a)

## Figure 4.1

[131]I-anti-CD45 antibody (BC8) localization in a patient immediately following (a) and 17 hours following (b) infusion of trace-labeled BC8 antibody. This anterior gamma-camera image shows accumulation and retention of [131]I in marrow in the lower lumbar vertebral bodies and the pelvic axial skeleton.

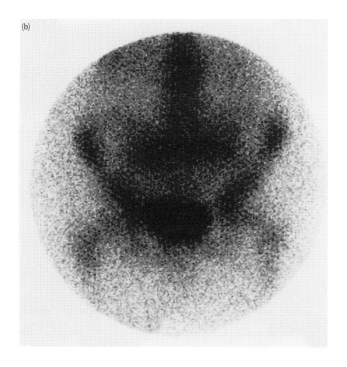

(b)

Toxicities during or following infusion of [131]I-BC8 antibody included chills, fever, malaise, throat tightness, nausea, vomiting, and diarrhea in two-thirds of the patients. A minority of patients were hospitalized for one to two days because of mild persistent hypotension or fever related to the infusion. Limiting the antibody infusion rate to 7.5 mg/hour decreased, but did not eliminate, these infusion-related side-effects.

Grade III/IV regimen-related toxicity (mucositis) developed in both patients treated at dose level 6, 12.25 Gy to liver, and in one of six patients treated at level 5, 10.5 Gy to liver (grade III veno-occlusive disease (VOD) of the liver). Thus the maximum tolerated dose (MTD) was estimated to be 10.5 Gy to liver, which based on the average estimates of radiation absorbed dose on this study, would allow delivery of an average of 24 Gy supplemental radiation to marrow and 50 Gy to spleen in addition to Cy and 12 Gy TBI. Of note, one patient received an estimated radiation absorbed dose of 31 Gy to the marrow from [131]I-BC8 antibody and failed to engraft by the time of her death at day 30 post treatment. Three subsequent patients had their dose of [131]I-BC8 antibody limited to the amount that would deliver no more than 28 Gy to the marrow, and engrafted normally.

Of the 25 patients with AML or MDS, seven survive disease-free 26–100 months (median 76 months) post-transplant. Thirteen patients relapsed 2–77 months post-transplant and 5 died of infectious complications. Of the 9 patients with ALL, 3 survive disease-free 34, 70, and 82 months post-transplant. Four patients relapsed 0.5–11 months post-transplant and 2 died of infection.

In summary, this clinical study demonstrated that specific targeting of radiation to spleen and marrow as compared with non-target organs can be achieved using [131]I-BC8 antibody as part of a preparative regimen. An estimated absorbed dose of 10.5 Gy to the liver delivered by [131]I-BC8 antibody was well tolerated when given with Cy/TBI and HSCT. Ongoing phase II studies of this preparative regimen for patients with advanced leukemia have been expanded to include unrelated donors.

In a second, ongoing phase I/II study for patients with less advanced AML, [131]I-BC8 antibody has been combined with Bu 16 mg/kg, Cy 120 mg/kg, and matched related allogeneic BMT.[65] Forty-eight patients in first remission ($n = 32$), untreated first relapse ($n = 7$) and second remission ($n = 9$) have received a biodistribution dose of antibody, with favorable biodistribution in 42 patients (88%).

Thirty-six patients have received a therapeutic dose of BC8 antibody labeled with the amount of [131]I calculated to deliver 3.5 Gy ($n = 4$) to 5.25 Gy ($n = 32$) to the liver (100–260 mCi) on day $-14$ followed by Bu (to achieve ≤900 ng/ml steady-state serum concentration) on days $-8$ to $-5$, Cy on days $-3$ and $-2$, and marrow infusion on day 0. GvHD prophylaxis consisted of CSP and MTX.

The overall toxicity was acceptable. Two of the 32 patients treated at dose level II (5.25 Gy to the liver) developed grade III mucositis. One patient, who died on day 38 of a sepsis syndrome, was considered to have grade IV regimen-related toxicity, and one died of VOD on day 22.

The estimated radiation absorbed doses ranged from 6 to 16 Gy to marrow and 14 to 62 Gy to spleen. Eighteen of 24 patients transplanted in first remission are alive and disease-free at a median of 45 months (13–66 months) following transplant. The remaining six patients have either relapsed ($n = 2$) or died of transplant-related causes ($n = 4$). Three of seven patients transplanted in second remission are disease-free three to nine months following transplant. The remaining four have died ($n = 2$) or relapsed ($n = 1$), or are too early to evaluate ($n = 1$). Three of the five patients transplanted in untreated relapse have relapsed. Overall, for patients with less advanced AML, this regimen was tolerable and has resulted in an impressive disease-free survival for patients transplanted in first remission. The study is continuing accrual of patients in first remission.

## Other targets

In a recently reported trial using an antibody reactive with the non-specific cross-reacting granulocytic antigen specific for early myelopoiesis, Bunjes and colleagues[66] intensified conditioning with [188]Re-labelled anti-CD66c in patients with high-risk hematological malignancies. Thirty-seven patients with acute or chronic leukemias at high risk of relapse after standard induction were treated. All demonstrated favorable biodistribution, and were treated with a median dose of 289 mCi [188]Re-labeled anti-CD66c antibody in two to four fractions. This resulted in a median red marrow dose of 13 Gy. Further conditioning consisted of 12 Gy TBI and Cy 120 mg/kg in 27 patients, Bu/Cy in 5 patients, and 12 Gy TBI/Cy and thiotepa 10 mg/kg in 5 patients. Thirty patients received T-cell-depleted allogeneic peripheral HSC, 4 patients received T-cell-depleted allogeneic bone marrow, and 3 patients received unpurged autologous HSC. Toxicity included mild acute GvHD ($n = 13$), chronic GvHD ($n = 7$), and VOD ($n = 1$), and 5 patients died of transplant-related complications (infectious and cerebral hemorrhage). At a median follow-up of six months, 28 patients (76%) are alive and 27 are disease-free. This approach appears to offer a safe and possibly effective means to intensify the preparative regimen.

## NON-HODGKIN'S LYMPHOMA

Non-Hodgkin's lymphoma (NHL) is a radiosensitive disease and thus a suitable setting for the use of radiolabeled monoclonal antibodies. Several groups have used antibodies reactive with B-cell antigens to deliver radiation at dose levels that have not been myeloablative and have not required hematopoietic stem cell rescue.[67–76] A variety of different antigens have been targeted, but the majority of clinical trials have used anti-CD20 antibodies. CD20 antigen is a B-lymphocyte-specific cell surface marker expressed on mature B cells (normal and malignant) but not on precursor B cells or stem cells.[77] It is a non-glycosylated surface membrane phosphoprotein, involved in B-cell activation and progression through the cell cycle. Upon binding of antibodies directed at its extracellular domain, CD20 antigen is not shed from the cell surface or appreciably internalized.

Several investigators have used HSCT to allow escalation of the radiation dose beyond that which is myeloablative, with the goal of taking maximum advantage of the dose response of lymphoma to radiation. The first such clinical study using [131]I-labeled anti-B-cell antibodies was a phase I dose-escalation study determining the effect of antibody dose on biodistribution, and, for patients with favorable biodistribution, the maximum tolerated dose of radiation delivered to the normal organ receiving the highest dose in patients supported with autologous HSCT.[78,79] In this study, the biodistribution of three anti-B-cell antibodies was determined. Forty-three patients were administered sequential weekly infusions of 0.5, 2.5, and 10 mg/kg of anti-CD20 antibodies (B1 or IF5) or anti-CD37 antibodies (MB-1) trace-labeled with 5 to 10 mCi [131]I. Positive tumor imaging was noted in 36 patients, including 25 of 26 patients who received [131]I-B1 antibody. Favorable biodistribution – defined as greater estimated radiation absorbed doses to all tumor sites as compared with critical normal organs – was observed in 24 of 43 patients. The two factors most strongly influencing antibody biodistribution were tumor burden and the presence of splenomegaly. Favorable biodistribution was seen in 23 of 31 patients (74%) with tumor burdens of 500 ml or less, compared with 1 of 12 patients (8%) with tumor burdens exceeding 500 ml ($p < 0.001$). Five of five splenectomized patients (100%) had favorable biodistribution, compared with 17 of 23 patients (74%) with normal sized spleens and 2 of 15 patients (13%) with splenomegaly ($p < 0.001$). This study also suggested that the optimal antibody dose for anti-CD20 antibody was 2.5 mg/kg, which resulted in a higher rate of favorable biodistribution as compared with the optimal dose of anti-CD37 antibody, 10 mg/kg.

Of the 24 patients achieving a favorable biodistribution, 19 were treated with a therapeutic infusion of [131]I-anti-CD20 or anti-CD37 antibody. The therapy dose of antibody was labeled with the amount of [131]I estimated to deliver a predetermined dose (10–30.75 Gy) to the normal organ receiving the highest radiation dose.

Acute toxicities during the therapeutic infusion were mild. All patients developed myelosuppression, and 15 patients received purged autologous marrow reinfusion, with neutrophil recovery occurring a median of 22 days and platelet recovery a median of 20 days following marrow infusion. Treatable infections occurred in nine patients. Non-hematological toxicity included mild nausea (79%), fever (74%), elevated serum thyroid-stimulating hormone (TSH) (42%), mild alopecia (21%), hyperbilirubinemia (37%), and mild serum creatinine elevations associated with empiric amphotericin B therapy (33%). The severity of these toxicities correlated with the estimated radiation absorbed dose delivered to normal organs by [131]I-antibody. One of three patients receiving an estimated dose of 27.25 Gy to the lungs developed reversible hemorrhagic pneumonitis and congestive cardiomyopathy, and one patient receiving an estimated dose of 30.75 Gy to the lungs developed reversible grade II hypotension. Based on these toxicities, the dose of [131]I delivering 27.25 Gy to normal organs was estimated to be the MTD.

The tumor response rate was high, with a CR in 16 of 19 patients (84%), partial response (PR) in 2 (11%), and one minor response. At the time of reporting, the median duration of response exceeded 11 months for those receiving [131]I-B1 antibody. Myelosuppression was severe, but was manageable with autologous HSCT. This study demonstrated that large doses of [131]I that could be selectively targeted to CD20 or CD37, delivered an average of 10 times as much radiation to tumor compared with the whole body and 2–3 times as much compared with critical organs.

Based on the encouraging results of the phase I trial, Press and colleagues[80] conducted a phase II trial of [131]I-B1 antibody in patients with relapsed NHL. Twenty-five patients with follicular small cleaved cell ($n = 12$), follicular mixed ($n = 3$), follicular large cell ($n = 3$), mantle cell ($n = 3$), diffuse small cleaved ($n = 2$), and diffuse large cell ($n = 2$) lymphoma underwent a biodistribution infusion of trace-labeled [131]I-B1 antibody. Twenty-two of 25 patients (88%) achieved a favorable biodistribution. This high rate of favorable biodistribution reflects the fact that tumor volumes were less than 500 ml in 19 of 22 patients at the time of biodistribution studies. Three of the 22 patients converted from unfavorable to favorable biodistribution after chemotherapy cytoreduction reduced the volume of the tumor. Twenty-one patients received a therapeutic infusion of [131]I-B1 antibody labeled with 343–785 mCi of [131]I estimated to deliver 25–31 Gy to the normal organ receiving the greatest dose of radiation. Autologous marrow or peripheral blood HSC were reinfused when the neutrophil count fell below 200/μL for two consecutive days, provided the total-body activity of [131]I was less than 2 mR/h at 1 m.

Myelosuppression occurred in all patients following therapeutic infusion. Neutrophils recovered a median of 23 days following marrow infusion and 13–17 days following PBSC infusion. Platelet recovery occurred a median of 22 days, regardless of stem cell source. Two patients died before achieving neutrophil recovery, one from sepsis and the other from progression of high-grade lymphoma, but both had trilineage engraftment by marrow biopsy at autopsy. Three patients had serious infections. Non-hematologic toxicities included nausea (71%), mild mucositis (24%), elevated TSH (30%), reversible cardiomyopathy and interstitial pneumonitis in one patient, mild pericarditis in one, and transient hypotension in one. HAMA developed in four patients two to three weeks after exposure to [131]I-B1 antibody.

After a reported median follow-up of over 12 months, 19 of 21 patients (91%) remain alive and 17 (81%) remain progression-free. Pooling the patients from the phase I and II trials who received [131]I-B1 antibody, the projected overall and progression-free survival rates were 93% and 62% at a median follow-up of two years. Stratifying patients by dose level into those receiving greater or less than 20 Gy to dose-limiting normal organs, those receiving the higher dose levels had a progression-free survival rate of 70%, compared with 20% for those receiving the lower dose level. Interestingly, the CR rates between those receiving the higher dose and those receiving the lower dose were not different, suggesting that these radiosensitive malignancies respond readily to low doses of radiation and that the durability of the response is improved by higher radiation doses.

Recently, long-term follow-up of these patients treated with [131]I-B1 antibody and autologous HSCT noted estimated overall and progression-free survival rates of 68% and 42%, respectively, at a median follow-up of 42 months.[81] The most recent update is presented (Figure 4.2). Fourteen of 29 patients remain in unmaintained remissions 27–87 months after treatment, with a median time to treatment failure (TTF) of 37 months. Eleven of 19 patients with indolent lymphomas are still in remission 32–72 months after treatment. In contrast, patients with aggressive histologies fared less well, with 3 of 10 patients with aggressive lymphoma remaining free from progression. Twenty-one of the 29 patients (72%) experienced longer TTF following [131]I-B1 antibody therapy than with the last chemotherapy regimen prior to this trial. Among the 29 patients, the TTF following [131]I-B1 antibody therapy exceeded the TTF with the last chemotherapy regimen ($p < 0.001$), and exceeded the longest TTF with any prior therapeutic regimen ($p < 0.16$) (Figure 4.3).

Late toxicities included hypothyroidism in 60% of patients, as manifested by

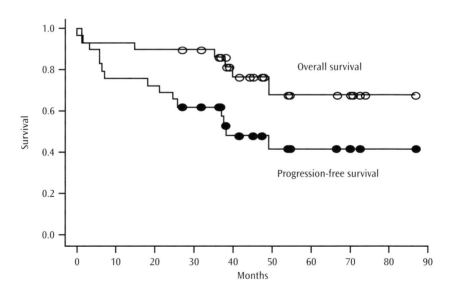

Figure 4.2

Progression-free and overall survival of 29 patients with B-cell non-Hodgkin's lymphoma treated with [131]I-B1 antibody plus autologous HSCT.

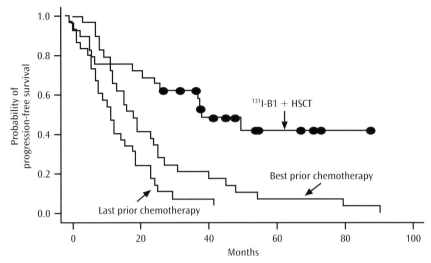

Figure 4.3

Progression-free survivals after [131]I-B1 antibody plus autologous HSCT, after longest remission with any prior therapy regimen, and after last prior chemotherapy.

an elevated TSH and the development of HAMA in 35% of patients. One patient developed functional cardiac impairment in the setting of previous doxorubicin-induced cardiomyopathy, and two patients developed functional pulmonary impairment in the setting of previous systemic lupus erythematosis and pre-existent restrictive lung disease. Two patients have developed solid tumors approximately three years after therapy. One developed stage I transitional cancer of the bladder in the setting of a heavy smoking history and prior treatment with Cy. The other patient developed colon carcinoma metastatic to the liver and died of complications from the colon cancer. Since the reported follow-up, two patients have developed MDS/leukemia. This rate is comparable to other reports of MDS/leukemia in autologous HSCT follow-up in NHL.[82,83]

This phase II study demonstrated impressive and often durable tumor responses with tolerable toxicities. To improve upon the results of the high-dose [131]I-B1 antibody plus HSCT, Press and colleagues[84] are conducting a phase I/II dose-finding study combining myeloablative doses of [131]I-B1 antibody with high-dose Cy and etoposide with HSCT. Cy, etoposide, and TBI is a standard HSCT preparative treatment for relapsed lymphoma, but relapse remains a problem for patients treated with that regimen. The goal of this study is to replace TBI with targeted radiotherapy in order to increase the radiation dose delivered to the tumor.

For this study, first Cy (100 mg/kg) and then etoposide (60 mg/kg) were added to [131]I-B1 antibody delivering 20 Gy (estimated radiation absorbed dose to the normal organ receiving the greatest dose of radiation). The dose of radiation delivered by antibody has subsequently been escalated in increments of 2 or 3 Gy to 27 Gy. To date, 47 patients have been treated. Thirty-two patients (68%) had low-grade lymphoma and 15 patients (32%) had intermediate- or high-grade lymphomas. Toxicities observed have been comparable to those with standard high-dose chemoradiotherapy with autologous HSCT, and have been higher than seen with [131]I-B1 antibody alone. After a median follow-up of two years, 40 (85%) patients are alive and 36 (77%) patients are progression-free (OW Press, personal communication). Longer follow-up will allow a more meaningful comparison with historical cohorts and the patients treated with [131]I-B1 antibody alone with autologous HSCT.

Two additional studies have used myeloablative doses of radiolabeled antibodies with autologous HSCT to treat NHL. Juweid and colleagues[85] evaluated [131]I-labeled anti-CD22 antibody (LL2). Non-myeloablative ($n = 21$) and myeloablative ($n = 3$) doses of [131]I-LL2 antibody were used to treat patients with relapsed NHL. Six of the 17 assessable patients receiving the non-myeloablative doses (range 24–130 mCi) had a CR ($n = 2$), PR ($n = 2$), minor response ($n = 1$), and mixed response ($n = 1$), and two of the three patients receiving myeloablative doses (range 145–183 mCi) followed by autologous BMT had partial responses. These investigators have suggested that repeated delivery of non-myeloablative doses of radiolabeled antibody may be attempted first, with consideration (if disease progression occurs) of myeloablative doses of radiolabeled antibody with HSCT.

Knox and colleagues[86] conducted a phase I/II study of [90]Y-anti-CD20 antibody, evaluating the effect of preinfusion of unlabeled antibody on the biodistribution of radiolabeled antibody and determining the maximum tolerated dose not requiring HSCT. Eighteen patients with relapsed NHL were treated with total doses ranging from 13.5 to 53.0 mCi [90]Y per patient. Doses of less than 40 mCi of [90]Y-anti-CD20 antibody were not myeloablative, while two of four patients at the 50 mCi dose level met criteria for autologous HSCT. The use of unlabeled antibody decreased splenic uptake and improved antibody biodistribution. The overall response rate was 72% and included six CR and seven PR, with freedom from progression of 3–29+ months. Fourteen of 18 patients had better or longer responses to the radiolabeled antibody than with their most recent therapy. Compared with doses of external-beam radiation required to achieve similar results, targeted therapy achieved tumor responses with lower average estimated delivered doses of radiation, raising the possibility that antibody-induced apoptosis or other factors may have contributed to the tumor responses. The investigators postulated that selection of patients with favorable responses or use of the higher doses of unlabeled pretreatment antibody may further improve this therapeutic approach.

# HODGKIN'S DISEASE

In Hodgkin's disease, lymph nodes involved with tumor are made up of a collection of multiple cell types, making the selection of a potential target antigen expressed by tumor cells difficult. To date, all studies using radiolabeled antibodies to target Hodgkin's disease have targeted ferritin. Ferritin, a tumor-associated protein found in Hodgkin's disease tissues, is synthesized and secreted by T cells, present in high numbers in many nodes involved with disease; thus there may be a higher concentration of ferritin in these tissues compared with normal tissues.[87–89]

Initial studies in advanced Hodgkin's disease utilized [131]I-polyclonal antiferritin antibodies at non-myeloablative doses.[90] Thirty-seven patients were treated with a single cycle of 30 mCi of [131]I-antiferritin antibody on day 0 and 20 mCi of [131]I-antiferritin antibody on day 5. The toxicities were primarily leukopenia and thrombocytopenia. Two patients had nadir white blood cell (WBC) counts below 1000/$\mu$L. No non-hematologic toxicity was seen. Forty percent of patients demonstrated an objective measurable response, including 1 CR and 14 PR. The majority of responses were seen in patients whose disease was confined to lymph nodes. The median survival of all patients was 53 weeks, with no difference between responsive and unresponsive disease.

Vriesendorp and colleagues explored the use of [90]Y-antiferritin antibody with and without high-dose chemotherapy and autologous HSCT in a series of clinical trials. In phase I and II studies, 45 patients with advanced-stage Hodgkin's disease received trace-labeled [111]In-antiferritin antibody to determine dechelation (as a surrogate measure of rapid degradation of the [90]Y-antiferritin antibody) and tumor targeting, and to estimate radiation absorbed doses to tumor, tissue surrounding tumor, and liver.[91,92] Patients were only treated with [90]Y-antiferritin antibody with or without subsequent HSCT if they showed tumor targeting (ratio between tumor and surrounding tissue greater than 3) and no evidence of dechelation. Thirty patients received at least one cycle of [90]Y-antiferritin antibody (20–50 mCi). Approximately half of the patients receiving 20 mCi and all receiving >20 mCi had marrow reinfused 18 days following therapeutic infusion. Forty patients (89%) showed tumor targeting. In patients with tumors larger than 2 cm (75% of patients), the estimated radiation absorbed doses to tumor ranged from 3 to 30 Gy, with a median of 9 Gy. The normal organ with the largest estimated delivered dose was the liver, receiving approximately 7 Gy.

Hematologic toxicity was observed in all patients. The pace of hematologic recovery after a 20 mCi dose was not affected by the administration of autologous marrow. In contrast, more profound nadirs of granulocytes and platelets were seen after 30 or 40 mCi [90]Y-antiferritin antibody, with earlier recovery (generally by 10 days) in patients receiving autologous marrow. However, three patients (two at 20 mCi and one at 50 mCi) had prolonged aplasia and died despite autologous marrow infusion. This study suggested that 40 mCi was the highest dose that could be administered as predominantly outpatient therapy, without excessive hospitalization resulting from marrow suppression. No significant non-hematologic toxicity was encountered.

Eighteen of 29 assessable patients (62%) had tumor responses, including nine patients achieving CR. The median duration of response was six months (range 2–26 months). Tumor responses were more common in patients with small disease volume and long disease histories. Six patients recurred in areas of previous bulk disease areas. Five patients recurred in new locations while remaining disease-free in previous bulk disease areas.

A follow-up report of this study noted an overall response rate of 51% of 39 assessable patients.[93] Ten CR and 10 PR were achieved, and the median overall survival was six months. Responses were more frequent in patients with a blood radioactivity level of 10 $\mu$Ci/ml or greater one hour following therapeutic infusion. The authors speculated that the lower blood radioactivity levels observed in the majority not responding may reflect a larger volume of distribution as a consequence of 'substances' released in patients with bulky Hodgkin's disease leading to increased capillary permeability. Immune responses to antiferritin antibodies were not detected.

Bierman and colleagues[94] studied $^{90}$Y-antiferritin antibody followed by high-dose chemotherapy and autologous BMT in 12 patients with poor-prognosis Hodgkin's disease. All patients exhibited tumor targeting as determined by scintigraphy with trace-labeled $^{111}$In-antiferritin antibody and were treated with 2–5 mg $^{90}$Y-antiferritin antibody (18–33 mCi) between days $-13$ and $-11$, followed by Cy (total dose 6 g/m$^2$), carmustine (total dose 300 mg/m$^2$), and etoposide (total dose 750 mg/m$^2$) on days $-6$ to $-3$, with autologous marrow infusion on day 0. The radiation dose to large tumor masses in five patients ranged between 5 and 10 Gy. Radiation absorbed dose estimates to bone marrow and liver were 0.18 and 0.3 Gy/mCi, respectively.

Five patients experienced early deaths due to diffuse alveolar damage ($n = 2$), upper airway bleeding ($n = 1$), and fungal infections ($n = 2$). Chest irradiation had been received previously by all patients who experienced early death. Engraftment occurred in the eight evaluable patients. Four patients were alive at the time of report 24–28 months following transplant, with three free of disease progression. The estimated one-year overall survival and progression-free survival rates were 36% and 21%, respectively. In contrast to the previous study,[91] all instances of tumor progression occurred at sites of prior involvement. The authors suggested that this combined approach was most likely to be effective, with acceptable toxicity, in patients with less advanced disease or earlier in their disease course.

## FUTURE DIRECTIONS

In two diseases, multiple myeloma and neuroblastoma, radioisotopes are being delivered to sites of disease using targeting approaches that do not employ antibodies, but which result in radiation doses to marrow high enough to require HSCT.

As resistance to standard therapy will ultimately develop in all patients with multiple myeloma, high-dose therapy with or without HSCT is being actively explored in this disease. Both regimen-related mortality and relapse rates have been high in this patient population, suggesting the need for better-tolerated, more effective preparative regimens. Because myeloma is largely confined to the bone and bone marrow, bone-seeking radiopharmaceuticals that accumulate in the skeleton are attractive because they target areas of active bone turnover and trabecular bone and thus will radiate sites of metastases and bone marrow, respectively.[95,96] Such a bone seeking reagent, holmium-166-DOTMP ([166]Ho-DOTMP), has been evaluated as a single agent or as part of a preparative regimen with HSCT.

In a phase I trial, six patients who failed conventional therapy were treated with a diagnostic dose of 30 mCi [166]Ho-DOTMP and three therapeutic doses (range 518–2066 mCi), followed by autologous HSCT.[97,98] All patients demonstrated marrow suppression, but had normal engraftment of infused stem cells. No other significant toxicities were observed. The total radiation absorbed dose delivered to bone marrow ranged from 7.9 to 41.1 Gy.

In two ongoing phase I/II trials, [166]Ho-DOTMP, in escalating doses, is being combined with melphalan 140 mg/m$^2$ or 200 mg/m$^2$ alone or melphalan 140 mg/m$^2$ combined with 8 Gy fractionated TBI, followed by autologous or syngeneic HSCT.[99] The [166]Ho-DOTMP dose to be delivered to the red bone marrow started at 20 Gy and has been escalated by 10 Gy increments. All 28 patients evaluable for safety at dose levels of 20, 30, and 40 Gy delivered by [166]Ho-DOTMP (with 140 mg/m$^2$ melphalan) engrafted neutrophils by day 17, and 26 patients engrafted platelets by day 19. All four patients evaluable for safety at 20 Gy delivered by [166]Ho-DOTMP (with 200 mg/m$^2$ melphalan) engrafted neutrophils by day 10 and platelets by day 20. Two patients receiving 30 Gy delivered by [166]Ho-DOTMP combined with melphalan and TBI had delayed platelet engraftment (days 28 and 44). No significant extramedullary toxicity (>grade II) or transplant-related mortality was observed. A CR rate of 53%, with an overall response rate of 65%, was observed in 17 patients evaluable for response (dose levels 20 and 30 Gy). These regimens have thus resulted in high response rates with minimal toxicity, and accrual continues.

In refractory neuroblastoma, targeted radiotherapy has been studied with and without autologous HSC rescue. [131]I-labeled MIBG, a guanethidine derivative with a structure analogous to norepinephrine (noradrenaline), is taken up specifically by neuroblastoma cells. Matthay and colleagues[100] have treated 30 patients with refractory neuroblastoma with [131]I-MIBG labeled with 3–18 mCi/kg. The main toxicity was hematologic, and six patients required HSCT at doses of 15 mCi/kg or more. Responses were seen in 37% of patients (1 CR and 10 PR). This encouraging response rate in refractory neuroblastoma suggests that this agent combined with a myeloablative preparative regimen and HSCT may improve outcome in this disease.

In addition, neuroblastoma cells are recognized by anti-disialoganglioside ($G_{D2}$) antibody (3F8). [131]I-3F8 antibody has been studied in phase I and II trials. In a phase I trial, doses of 6–28 mCi/kg of $^{131}$I-3F8 antibody were used to treat patients with refractory high-risk neuroblastoma. Responses were noted in bone marrow and soft tissue masses. Total-body and marrow absorbed radiation dose estimates following administration of 20–24 mCi/kg $^{131}$I-3F8 antibody were 500–700 cGy. A subsequent phase II trial investigated the efficacy of intensive chemotherapy and radiation to bulk disease delivered by external beam as induction followed by the administration of 20 mCi/kg $^{131}$I-3F8 antibody with autologous HSCT as consolidation.[101] $^{131}$I-3F8 antibody therapy was well tolerated, with minimal non-hematopoietic toxicity. Twenty of 24 patients (83%) were progression-free at a median follow-up of 12 months. Recurrence of the disease in the central nervous system has been noted in two patients, suggesting the importance of directing therapy to all sites of disease.

In the setting of allogeneic transplants for acute leukemia, studies to date have added targeted therapy to conventional preparative regimens. While this approach may decrease the risk of relapse, it has not decreased the regimen-related toxicities associated with the procedure. The inclusion of myeloablative doses of TBI or Bu ensures that the patient will be immunosuppressed and thus not reject the graft, but limits the potential dose escalation of the RIC. Recently, several investigators have developed non-myeloablative regimens that allow at least partial donor chimerism of granulocyte colony-stimulating factor (G-CSF)-mobilized peripheral blood HSC in patients who would not tolerate conventional preparative regimens.[102,103] In cases of mixed chimerism, the initial transplant may be followed by donor lymphocyte infusions (DLI) to optimize the potential graft versus leukemia (GvL) effect. In one such regimen, 2 Gy TBI is combined with the immunosuppressive agents CSP and mycophenolate mofetil, with partial or complete chimerism occurring in 80% of patients.[104] Thus the potential exists to use such non-myeloablative regimens to achieve engraftment when combined with radiolabeled antibody. Since the GvL effect previously achieved by DLI post-transplant has been most effective in minimal disease states, the combination of targeted hematopoietic irradiation delivered by $^{131}$I-anti-CD45 antibody and non-myeloablative regimens with HSCT is being studied in a phase I trial in Seattle. The goal of the addition of targeted radiolabeled antibody is to augment leukemia-cell kill without excessive toxicity. This approach is being examined in patients with relapsed or refractory AML who are between the ages of 55 and 70 years and thus would not tolerate conventional preparative regimens.

## CONCLUSIONS

The inclusion of tagged antibody therapy in HSCT preparative regimens offers the potential to decrease relapse rates and perhaps to decrease toxicity. Despite the promise of this approach, challenges remain. The exact role of antibody targeted therapy and the best time to employ this therapy in the course of a given disease are being evaluated at many centers. Improvements in this therapy may include optimization in targeting of the tagged antibody to tumor sites, retention of isotope by selected cells, the discovery of novel target antigens, methods to selectively upregulate target antigens, and novel ways to reduce the non-specific radiation that is delivered to normal tissues. Efforts are also underway to understand the relative biological effects of radiation delivered by RIC. While the ready vascular access and radiosensitivity of hematological malignancies make them a particularly attractive target for RIC, optimizing targeted therapy for hematologic malignancies may also lead to enhanced utility of this approach in solid tumors.

## ACKNOWLEDGMENT

This work was supported by US National Institutes of Health Grant CA44991. Dana C Matthews is a Clinical Scholar of the Leukemia and Lymphoma Society.

## REFERENCES

1. Uckun FM, Kim TH, Ramsay NC et al, Radiobiological heterogeneity of leukemic lymphocyte precursors from acute lymphoblastic leukemia patients. *Int J Radiat Biol* 1989; **56**: 611–15.

2. Clift RA, Buckner CD, Appelbaum FR et al, Allogeneic marrow transplantation in patients with acute myeloid leukemia in first remission: a randomized trial of two irradiation regimens. *Blood* 1990; **76**: 1867–71.

3. Clift RA, Buckner CD, Appelbaum FR et al, Allogeneic marrow transplantation in patients with chronic myeloid leukemia in the chronic phase: a randomized trial of two irradiation regimens. *Blood* 1991; **77**: 1660–5.

4. Nourigat C, Badger CC, Bernstein ID, Treatment of lymphoma with radiolabeled antibody: elimination of tumor cells lacking target antigen. *J Natl Cancer Inst* 1990; **82**: 47–50.

5. Miller RA, Maloney DG, Warnke R et al, Treatment of B-cell lymphoma with monoclonal anti-idiotype antibody. *N Engl J Med* 1982; **306**: 517–22.

6. Shockley TR, Lin K, Sung C et al, A quantitative analysis of tumor specific monoclonal antibody uptake by human melanoma xenografts: effects of antibody immunological properties and tumor antigen expression levels. *Cancer Res* 1992; **52**: 357–66.

7. Reff ME, Carner K, Chambers KS et al, Depletion of B cells in vivo by a chimeric mouse human monoclonal antibody to CD20. *Blood* 1994; **83**: 435–45.

8. Shan D, Ledbetter JA, Press OW, Apoptosis of malignant human B cells by ligation of CD20 with monoclonal antibodies. *Blood* 1998; **91**: 1644–52.

9. van der Jagt RH, Badger CC, Appelbaum FR et al, Localization of radiolabeled antimyeloid antibodies in a human acute leukemia xenograft tumor model. *Cancer Res* 1992; **52**: 89–94.

10. Press OW, Shan D, Howell-Clark J et al, Comparative metabolism and retention of iodine-125, yttrium-90, and indium-111 radioimmunoconjugates by cancer cells. *Cancer Res* 1996; **56**: 2123–9.

11. Ali SA, Warren SD, Richter KY et al, Improving the tumor retention of radiolabeled antibody: aryl carbohydrate adducts. *Cancer Res* 1990; **50**: 783s–88s.

12. Fujimori K, Covell DG, Fletcher JE et al, Modeling analysis of the global and microscopic distribution of immunoglobulin G, F(ab')2, and Fab in tumors. *Cancer Res* 1989; **49**: 5656–63.

13. Fujimori K, Covell DG, Fletcher JE et al, A modeling analysis of monoclonal antibody percolation through tumors: a binding-site barrier. *J Nucl Med* 1990; **31**: 1191–8.

14. Weinstein JN, van Osdol W, The macroscopic and microscopic pharmacology of monoclonal antibodies. *Int J Immunopharmacol* 1992; **14**: 457–63.

15. Grossbard ML, Gribben JG, Freedman AS et al, Adjuvant immunotoxin therapy with anti-B4-blocked ricin after autologous bone marrow transplantation for patients with B-cell non-Hodgkin's lymphoma. *Blood* 1993; **81**: 2263–71.

16. LoBuglio AF, Wheeler RH, Trang J et al, Mouse/human chimeric monoclonal antibody in man: kinetics and immune response. *Proc Natl Acad Sci USA* 1989; **86**: 4220–4.

17. Yarnold S, Fell HP, Chimerization of antitumor antibodies via homologous recombination conversion vectors. *Cancer Res* 1994; **54**: 506–12.

18. Caron PC, Co MS, Bull MK et al, Biological and immunological features of humanized M195 (anti-CD33) monoclonal antibodies. *Cancer Res* 1992; **52**: 6761–7.

19. Hagan PL, Halpern SE, Dillman RO et al, Tumor size: effect on monoclonal antibody uptake in tumor models. *J Nucl Med* 1986; **27**: 422–7.

20. Jain RK, Physiological barriers to delivery of monoclonal antibodies and other macromolecules in tumors. *Cancer Res* 1990; **50**: 814s–819s.

21. Yokota T, Milenic DE, Whitlow M et al, Rapid tumor penetration of a single-chain Fv and comparison with other immunoglobulin forms. *Cancer Res* 1992; **52**: 3402–8.

22. Buchegger F, Haskell CM, Schreyer M et al, Radiolabeled fragments of monoclonal antibodies against carcinoembryonic antigen for localization of human colon carcinoma grafted into nude mice. *J Exp Med* 1983; **158**: 413–27.

23. Adams GP, McCartney JE, Tai MS et al, Highly specific in vivo tumor targeting by monovalent and divalent forms of 741F8 anti-c-erbB-2 single-chain Fv. *Cancer Res* 1993; **53**: 4026–34.

24. King DJ, Turner A, Farnsworth AP et al, Improved tumor targeting with chemically cross-linked recombinant antibody fragments. *Cancer Res* 1994; **54**: 6176–85.

25. Hu S, Shively L, Raubitschek A et al, Minibody: a novel engineered anti-carcinoembryonic antigen antibody fragment (single-chain Fv-CH3) which exhibits rapid, high-level targeting of xenografts. *Cancer Res* 1996; **56**: 3055–61.

26. Wang CH, Willis DL, Loveland WD, *Radiotracer Methodology in the Biological, Environmental, and Physical Sciences.* Prentice-Hall: Englewood Cliffs, NJ, 1975.

27. Macklis RM, Lin JY, Beresford B et al, Cellular kinetics, dosimetry, and radiobiology of alpha-particle radioimmunotherapy: induction of apoptosis. *Radiat Res* 1992; **130**: 220–6.

28. Kennel SJ, Stabin M, Roeske JC et al, Radiotoxicity of bismuth-213 bound to membranes of monolayer and spheroid cultures of tumor cells. *Radiat Res* 1999; **151**: 244–56.

29. Reist CJ, Garg PK, Alston KL et al, Radioiodination of internalizing monoclonal antibodies using N-succinimidyl 5-iodo-3-pyridinecarboxylate. *Cancer Res* 1996; **56**: 4970–7.

30. Kukis DL, DeNardo SJ, DeNardo GL et al, Optimized conditions for chelation of yttrium-90-DOTA immunoconjugates. *J Nucl Med* 1998; **39**: 2105–10.

31. Jurcic JG, McDevitt MR, Sgouros G et al, Phase I trial of targeted alpha-particle therapy for myeloid leukemias with bismuth-213-HuM195 (anti-CD33). *Proc Am Soc Clin Oncol* 1999; **18**: 7a.

32. Collier RJ, Effect of diphtheria toxin on protein synthesis: inactivation of one of the transfer factors. *J Mol Biol* 1967; **25**: 83–98.

33. Endo Y, Tsurugi K, Mechanism of action of ricin and related toxic lectins on eukaryotic ribosomes. *Nucleic Acids Symp Ser* 1986; **17**: 187–90.

34. Vitetta ES, Fulton RJ, May RD et al, Redesigning nature's poisons to create

anti-tumor reagents. *Science* 1987; **238**: 1098–104.

35. Zein N, Sinha AM, McGahren WJ et al, Calicheamicin gamma 1I: an antitumor antibiotic that cleaves double-stranded DNA site specifically. *Science* 1988; **240**: 1198–201.

36. Olsnes S, Sandvig K, How protein toxins enter and kill cells. *Cancer Treat Res* 1988; **37**: 39–73.

37. FitzGerald D, Pastan I, Targeted toxin therapy for the treatment of cancer. *J Natl Cancer Inst* 1989; **81**: 1455–63.

38. Kreitman RJ, Chaudhary VK, Waldmann T et al, The recombinant immunotoxin anti-Tac(Fv)-*Pseudomonas* exotoxin 40 is cytotoxic toward peripheral blood malignant cells from patients with adult T-cell leukemia. *Proc Natl Acad Sci USA* 1990; **87**: 8291–5.

39. Lambert JM, Goldmacher VS, Collinson AR et al, An immunotoxin prepared with blocked ricin: a natural plant toxin adapted for therapeutic use. *Cancer Res* 1991; **51**: 6236–42.

40. Sievers EL, Appelbaum FR, Spielberger RT et al, Selective ablation of acute myeloid leukemia using antibody-targeted chemotherapy: a phase I study of an anti-CD33 calicheamicin immunoconjugate. *Blood* 1999; **93**: 3678–84.

41. Sievers E, Larson RA, Estey E et al, Preliminary results of the efficacy and safety of CMA-676 in patients with AML in first relapse. *Proc Am Soc Clin Oncol* 1999; **18**: 7a.

42. Christy M, Eckerman KF, *Specific Absorbed Fractions of Energy at Various Ages from Internal Photon Sources.* ORNL/TM-8381, Vol 1-7. Oak Ridge National Laboratory: Oak Ridge, TN, 1987.

43. Society of Nuclear Medicine, *MIRD Primer for Absorbed Dose Calculations.* Society of Nuclear Medicine: Washington, DC, 1988.

44. Fisher DR, Badger CC, Breitz H et al, Internal radiation dosimetry for clinical testing of radiolabeled monoclonal antibodies. *Antib Immunoconj Radiopharm* 1991; **4**: 655–64.

45. Griffin JD, Linch D, Sabbath K et al, A monoclonal antibody reactive with normal and leukemic human myeloid progenitor cells. *Leuk Res* 1984; **8**: 521–34.

46. Dinndorf PA, Andrews RG, Benjamin D et al, Expression of normal myeloid-associated antigens by acute leukemia cells. *Blood* 1986; **67**: 1048–53.

47. Andrews RG, Takahashi M, Segal GM et al, The L4F3 antigen is expressed by unipotent and multipotent colony-forming cells but not by their precursors. *Blood* 1986; **68**: 1030–5.

48. Andrews RG, Singer JW, Bernstein ID, Monoclonal antibody 12-8 recognizes a 115-kd molecule present on both unipotent and multipotent hematopoietic colony-forming cells and their precursors. *Blood* 1986; **67**: 842–5.

49. Scheinberg DA, Lovett D, Divgi CR et al, A phase I trial of monoclonal antibody M195 in acute myelogenous leukemia: specific bone marrow targeting and internalization of radionuclide. *J Clin Oncol* 1991; **9**: 478–90.

50. Schwartz MA, Lovett DR, Redner A et al, Dose-escalation trial of M195 labeled with iodine 131 for cytoreduction and marrow ablation in relapsed or refractory myeloid leukemias. *J Clin Oncol* 1993; **11**: 294–303.

51. Caron PC, Jurcic JG, Scott AM et al, A phase 1B trial of humanized monoclonal antibody M195 (anti-CD33) in myeloid leukemia: specific targeting without immunogenicity. *Blood* 1994; **83**: 1760–8.

52. Caron PC, Dumont L, Scheinberg DA, Supersaturating infusional humanized anti-CD33 monoclonal antibody HuM195 in myelogenous leukemia. *Clin Cancer Res* 1998; **4**: 1421–8.

53. Jurcic JG, Caron PC, DeBlasio A et al, Targeted therapy with humanized anti-CD33 monoclonal antibody (huM195) reduces residual disease in acute promyelocytic leukemia. *Blood* 1995; **86**: 517a.

54. Appelbaum FR, Matthews DC, Eary JF et al, The use of radiolabeled anti-

CD33 antibody to augment marrow irradiation prior to marrow transplantation for acute myelogenous leukemia. *Transplantation* 1992; **54**: 829–33.

55. Bearman SI, Appelbaum FR, Back A et al, Regimen-related toxicity and early posttransplant survival in patients undergoing marrow transplantation for lymphoma. *J Clin Oncol* 1989; **7**: 1288–94.

56. Jurcic JG, Divgi CR, McDivitt MR et al, Potential for myeloablation with yttrium-90-labeled HuM195 (anti-CD33): a phase I trial in advanced myeloid leukemias. *Blood* 1998; **92**: 613a.

57. Jurcic JG, McDevitt MR, Sgouros G et al, Phase I trial of targeted alpha-particle therapy for myeloid leukemias with bismuth-213-HuM195 (anti-CD33). *Proc Am Soc Clin Oncol* 1999; **18**: 7a.

58. Omary MB, Trowbridge IS, Battifora HA, Human homologue of murine T200 glycoprotein. *J Exp Med* 1980; **152**: 842–52.

59. Andres TL, Kadin ME, Immunologic markers in the differential diagnosis of small round cell tumors from lymphocytic lymphoma and leukemia. *Am J Clin Pathol* 1983; **79**: 546–52.

60. Caldwell CW, Patterson WP, Hakami N, Alterations of HLe-1 (T200) fluorescence intensity on acute lymphoblastic leukemia cells may relate to therapeutic outcome. *Leuk Res* 1987; **11**: 103–6.

61. Matthews DC, Badger CC, Fisher DR et al, Selective radiation of hematolymphoid tissue delivered by anti-CD45 antibody. *Cancer Res* 1992; **52**: 1228–34.

62. Matthews DC, Appelbaum FR, Eary JF et al, Radiolabeled anti-CD45 monoclonal antibodies target lymphohematopoietic tissue in the macaque. *Blood* 1991; **78**: 1864–74.

63. Matthews DC, Appelbaum FR, Eary JF et al, Development of a marrow transplant regimen for acute leukemia using targeted hematopoietic irradiation delivered by [131]I-labeled anti-CD45 antibody, combined with cyclophosphamide and total body irradiation. *Blood* 1995; **85**: 1122–31.

64. Matthews DC, Appelbaum FR, Eary JF et al, Phase I study of [131]I-anti-CD45 antibody plus cyclophosphamide and total body irradiation for advanced acute leukemia and myelodysplastic syndrome. *Blood* 1999; **94**: 1237–47.

65. Matthews DC, Appelbaum FR, Eary JF et al, [131]I-anti-CD45 antibody plus busulfan/cyclophosphamide in matched related transplants for AML in first remission. *Blood* 1996; **88**: 142a.

66. Bunjes D, Seitz U, Duncker C et al, Results of a phase I–II study of radioimmunotherapy for the intensification of conditioning prior to stem cell transplantation for patients with high-risk haematological malignancies. *Blood* 1999; **94**: 711a.

67. Goldenberg DM, Horowitz JA, Sharkey RM et al, Targeting, dosimetry, and radioimmunotherapy of B-cell lymphomas with iodine-131-labeled LL2 monoclonal antibody. *J Clin Oncol* 1991; **9**: 548–64.

68. Kaminski MS, Fig LM, Zasadny KR et al, Imaging, dosimetry, and radioimmunotherapy with iodine 131-labeled anti-CD37 antibody in B-cell lymphoma. *J Clin Oncol* 1992; **10**: 1696–711.

69. Kaminski MS, Zasadny KR, Francis IR et al, Radioimmunotherapy of B-cell lymphoma with [131I]anti-B1 (anti-CD20) antibody. *N Engl J Med* 1993; **329**: 459–65.

70. Czuczman MS, Straus DJ, Divgi CR et al, Phase I dose-escalation trial of iodine 131-labeled monoclonal antibody OKB7 in patients with non-Hodgkin's lymphoma. *J Clin Oncol* 1993; **11**: 2021–9.

71. Waldmann TA, White JD, Carrasquillo JA et al, Radioimmunotherapy of interleukin-2R alpha-expressing adult T-cell leukemia with yttrium-90-labeled anti-Tac. *Blood* 1995; **86**: 4063–75.

72. Lewis JP, Denardo GL, Denardo SJ, Radioimmunotherapy of lymphoma: a UC Davis experience. *Hybridoma* 1995; **14**: 115–20.

73. Kaminski MS, Zasadny KR, Francis IR et al, Iodine-131-anti-B1 radioim-

munotherapy for B-cell lymphoma. *J Clin Oncol* 1996; **14**: 1974–81.

74. White CA, Halpern SE, Parker BA et al, Radioimmunotherapy of relapsed B-cell lymphoma with yttrium 90 anti-idiotype monoclonal antibodies. *Blood* 1996; **87**: 3640–9.

75. DeNardo GL, Lamborn KR, Goldstein DS et al, Increased survival associated with radiolabeled Lym-1 therapy for non-Hodgkin's lymphoma and chronic lymphocytic leukemia. *Cancer* 1997; **80**: 2706–11.

76. DeNardo GL, DeNardo SJ, Goldstein DS et al, Maximum-tolerated dose, toxicity, and efficacy of (131)I-Lym-1 antibody for fractionated radioimmunotherapy of non-Hodgkin's lymphoma. *J Clin Oncol* 1998; **16**: 3246–56.

77. Anderson KC, Bates MP, Slaughenhoupt BL et al, Expression of human B cell-associated antigens on leukemias and lymphomas: a model of human B cell differentiation. *Blood* 1984; **63**: 1424–33.

78. Press OW, Eary JF, Badger CC et al, Treatment of refractory non-Hodgkin's lymphoma with radiolabeled MB-1 (anti-CD37) antibody. *J Clin Oncol* 1989; **7**: 1027–38.

79. Press OW, Eary JF, Appelbaum FR et al, Radiolabeled-antibody therapy of B-cell lymphoma with autologous bone marrow support. *N Engl J Med* 1993; **329**: 1219–24.

80. Press OW, Eary JF, Appelbaum FR et al, Phase II trial of 131I-B1 (anti-CD20) antibody therapy with autologous stem cell transplantation for relapsed B cell lymphomas. *Lancet* 1995; **346**: 336–40.

81. Liu SY, Eary JF, Petersdorf SH et al, Follow-up of relapsed B-cell lymphoma patients treated with iodine-131-labeled anti-CD20 antibody and autologous stem-cell rescue. *J Clin Oncol* 1998; **16**: 3270–8.

82. Darrington DL, Vose JM, Anderson JR et al, Incidence and characterization of secondary myelodysplastic syndrome and acute myelogenous leukemia following high-dose chemoradiotherapy and autologous stem-cell transplantation for

lymphoid malignancies. *J Clin Oncol* 1994; **12**: 2527–34.

83. Stone RM, Neuberg D, Soiffer R et al, Myelodysplastic syndrome as a late complication following autologous bone marrow transplantation for non-Hodgkin's lymphoma. *J Clin Oncol* 1994; **12**: 2535–42.

84. Press O, Eary J, Liu S et al, A phase I/II trial of high dose iodine-131-anti-B1 (anti-CD20) monoclonal antibody, etoposide, cyclophosphamide, and autologous stem cell transplantation for patients with relapsed B cell lymphomas. *Proc Am Soc Clin Oncol* 1998; **17**: 3a.

85. Juweid M, Sharkey RM, Markowitz A et al, Treatment of non-Hodgkin's lymphoma with radiolabeled murine, chimeric, or humanized LL2, an anti-CD22 monoclonal antibody. *Cancer Res* 1995; **55**: 5899s–907s.

86. Knox SJ, Goris ML, Trisler K et al, Yttrium-90-labeled anti-CD20 monoclonal antibody therapy of recurrent B-cell lymphoma. *Clin Cancer Res* 1996; **2**: 457–70.

87. Order SE, Porter M, Hellman S, Hodgkin's disease: evidence for a tumor-associated antigen. *N Engl J Med* 1971; **285**: 471–4.

88. Katz DH, Order SE, Graves M et al, Purification of Hodgkin's disease tumor-associated antigens. *Proc Natl Acad Sci USA* 1973; **70**: 396–400.

89. Eshhar Z, Order SE, Katz DH, Ferritin, a Hodgkin's disease associated antigen. *Proc Natl Acad Sci USA* 1974; **71**: 3956–60.

90. Lenhard RE Jr, Order SE, Spunberg JJ et al, Isotopic immunoglobulin: a new systemic therapy for advanced Hodgkin's disease. *J Clin Oncol* 1985; **3**: 1296–300.

91. Vriesendorp HM, Herpst JM, Germack MA et al, Phase I–II studies of yttrium-labeled antiferritin treatment for end-stage Hodgkin's disease, including Radiation Therapy Oncology Group 87–01. *J Clin Oncol* 1991; **9**: 918–28 [erratum **9**: 1516].

92. Vriesendorp HM, Herpst JM, Leichner PK et al, Polyclonal [90]yttrium labeled

antiferritin for refractory Hodgkin's disease. *Int J Radiat Oncol Biol Phys* 1989; 17: 815–21.

93. Herpst JM, Klein JL, Leichner PK et al, Survival of patients with resistant Hodgkin's disease after polyclonal yttrium 90-labeled antiferritin treatment. *J Clin Oncol* 1995; **13**: 2394–400.

94. Bierman PJ, Vose JM, Leichner PK et al, Yttrium 90-labeled antiferritin followed by high-dose chemotherapy and autologous bone marrow transplantation for poor-prognosis Hodgkin's disease. *J Clin Oncol* 1993; **11**: 698–703.

95. Appelbaum FR, Sandmaier B, Brown PA et al, Myelosuppression and mechanism of recovery following administration of [153]samarium-EDTMP. *Antibod Immunoconj Radiopharm* 1988; **1**: 263–70.

96. Parks NJ, Kawakami TG, Avila MJ et al, Bone marrow transplantation in dogs after radio-ablation with a new Ho-166 amino phosphonic acid bone-seeking agent (DOTMP). *Blood* 1993; **82**: 318–25.

97. Bayouth JE, Macey DJ, Boyer AL et al, Radiation dose distribution within the bone marrow of patients receiving holmium-166-labeled-phosphonate for marrow ablation. *Med Phys* 1995; **22**: 743–53.

98. Bayouth JE, Macey DJ, Kasi LP et al, Pharmacokinetics, dosimetry and toxicity of holmium-166-DOTMP for bone marrow ablation in multiple myeloma. *J Nucl Med* 1995; **36**: 730–7.

99. Champlin R, Giralt S, Eary J et al, [166]Holmium-DOTMP in combination with melphalan with or without total body irradiation as a preparative regimen for autologous stem cell transplant (ASCT) for patients with multiple myeloma (MM). *Blood* 1999; **94**: 709a.

100. Matthay KK, DeSantes K, Hasegawa B et al, Phase I dose escalation of [131]I-metaiodobenzylguanidine with autologous bone marrow support in refractory neuroblastoma. *J Clin Oncol* 1998; **16**: 229–36.

101. Cheung NK, Kushner B, LaQuaglia M et al, N7: combination chemotherapy, radioimmunotherapy and adjuvant antibody therapy for high-risk neuroblastoma (NB). *Proc Am Soc Clin Oncol* 1998; **17**: 438a.

102. Giralt S, Estey E, Albitar M et al, Engraftment of allogeneic hematopoietic progenitor cells with purine analog-containing chemotherapy: harnessing graft-versus-leukemia without myeloablative therapy. *Blood* 1997; **89**: 4531–6.

103. Storb R, Yu C, Wagner JL et al, Stable mixed hematopoietic chimerism in DLA-identical littermate dogs given sublethal total body irradiation before and pharmacological immunosuppression after marrow transplantation. *Blood* 1997; **89**: 3048–54.

104. McSweeney PA, Wagner JL, Maloney DG et al, Outpatient PBSC allografts using immunosuppression with low-dose TBI before, and cyclosporine (CSP) and mycophenolate mofetil (MMF) after transplant. *Blood* 1998; **92**: 519a.

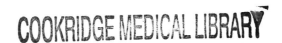

# 5
# Novel preparative regimens
# II: Non-myeloablative regimens

Angelo M Carella, Sergio Giralt

## INTRODUCTION

Traditionally, conditioning for allografting has relied on a combination of mye-loablative and immunosuppressive therapies, which result in substantial morbidity and mortality. In contrast, high-dose therapy followed by autografting has less-threatening toxicity. To circumvent the problems inherent to the toxicity and treatment-related deaths associated with allografting, it has recently been demonstrated that it is possible to achieve engraftment of donor hematopoietic stem cells (HSC) after immunosuppressive therapy combined with myelosuppressive but non-myeloablative therapy.[1,2] The observation that non-myeloablative regimens, based on fludarabine, have resulted in the engraftment of allogeneic cells in hematological malignancies raises the possibility that such conditioning might even be useful in achieving a graft-versus-tumor effect. In this chapter we shall discuss the general concepts regarding pilot clinical data. At the end, we shall also report on the Genoa experience with autografting followed by mini-allograft.

## GENERAL CONCEPTS

It is well known that the graft-versus-leukemia (GvL) effect is important to prevent relapse after allografting. Chronic myelogenous leukemia (CML) is the disease entity for which this immunologically mediated effect is most significant, although graft-versus-malignancy effects have also been demonstrated in other hematological neoplasia and in breast cancer.[3–9] The concept of a GvL effect is supported by the observation that patients with chronic-phase CML, who relapse after allografting, can achieve a complete cytogenetic and molecular remission by simple infusion of donor lymphocytes (DLI).[5,7,10] This occurs because, after relapse, leukemia recurs in host-derived cells but residual normal hematopoiesis and immunity remains largely donor-derived.[11] The infused donor lymphocytes are therefore not subject to rejection, but acute graft-versus-host (GvH) disease (GvHD) has developed in up to 80% of cases. After

DLI, responding patients may suddenly become hypoplastic, followed by recovery from donor-derived HSC and a return to complete chimerism. This long interval from DLI to clinical response is presumably related to the time required for proliferation of relevant alloreactive cells,[12] to reach a critical mass sufficient to eradicate the malignant cells. Considering that older and resistant patients represent the group with the worst prognosis following conventional myeloablative therapy, novel therapeutic options need to be explored. The success of DLI in inducing remission in patients with CML relapsing post transplant suggests that alternative approaches must be explored. A new perspective could come from the combination of an immunosuppressive non-myeloablative regimen followed by allogeneic HSC transplantation to achieve engraftment. DLI could then be given to induce complete remissions in patients with resistant disease. It has also been suggested that all these patients should receive autografting beforehand in order to reduce the neoplastic burden.[13] Fludarabine is the crucial drug for this non-myeloablative allografting. It has significant antileukemic properties and is an exceedingly effective immunosuppressive agent, as has been established at the MD Anderson Cancer Center.[1,14] It has been demonstrated that non-myeloablative chemotherapy using fludarabine combinations is sufficiently immunosuppressive to allow engraftment of allogeneic blood progenitor cells.[15]

This has led several groups of investigators to develop less toxic allotransplantation regimens that rely on a GvH effect rather than chemoradiation therapy for complete eradication of malignant cells. These non-myeloablative approaches can be roughly divided into three categories:

- myelosuppressive but non-myeloablative cytotoxic regimens;
- pretransplantation host immunosuppression combined with post-transplantation immunosuppression directed at both host and donor immune cells;
- high-intensity autotransplantation followed by immunosuppressive non-myelosuppressive/non-myeloablative regimens alone.

In all of these settings, allotransplantation is the platform for subsequent adoptive immunotherapy of the underlying malignancies using donor lymphocytes.

## MYELOSUPPRESSIVE NON-MYELOABLATIVE REGIMENS

Investigators at the MD Anderson Cancer Center used fludarabine-containing regimens in high-risk patients with hematological malignancies.[1] A total of 25 patients (22 acute myelogenous leukemia (AML) and 3 myelodysplastic syndrome (MDS)) were recently updated. The median age of the group was 61 years (range 24–74 years). Most patients were refractory or beyond first salvage therapy, with only six receiving transplants in first remission, or untreated first relapse. The median number of prior therapies was 2 (range 1–5), and the median percentage of bone marrow blasts was 10%. Fourteen patients received fludarabine, idarubicin and cytarabine, while 11 received a

## Table 5.1 Dose and treatment schedules for the FLAG-Ida and 2CDA/Ara-C regimens

| | Day | | | | |
|---|---|---|---|---|---|
| | $-5$ | $-4$ | $-3$ | $-2$ | $-1$ | 0 |
| FLAG-Ida | | | | | |
| Fludarabine (mg/m²) | 30 | 30 | 30 | 30 | |
| Ara-C (g/m²) | 2 | 2 | 2 | 2 | |
| Idarubicin (mg/m²) | 12 | 12 | 12 | | |
| 2CDA/Ara-C | | | | | |
| 2CDA (mg/m²) CI[a] | 12 | 12 | 12 | 12 | 12 |
| Ara-C (g/m²) | 1 | 1 | 1 | 1 | 1 |

[a] CI, continuous infusion.

combination of 2-chloroadenosine (2CDA) and cytarabine (Ara-C) in doses and schedules as presented in Table 5.1. Other patient and treatment characteristics are summarized in Table 5.2.

Among the 25 patients there was only one instance of regimen-related toxicity from pulmonary hemorrhage and multiorgan failure. Twenty patients recovered neutrophil counts of over $0.5 \times 10^9$/l at a median of 11 days post transplant (range 9–21 days), and 17 achieved platelet transfusion independence at a median of 15 days (range 8–78 days). Fifteen patients achieved complete remission (defined as less than 5% bone marrow blasts, with neutrophil and platelet recovery) after transplantation. Chimerism analysis in patients achieving a complete remission (CR) revealed that on day 30, 12 of the 15 patients had over 80% donor cells, either by cytogenetics or restriction fragment length polymorphism (RFLP) techniques. At 90 days, of the 10 patients remaining in CR, six had over 80% donor cells. At one year, of the three patients in CR, two had over 80% donor cells. Nine patients failed to respond to therapy and one patient died of graft failure.

Five patients developed grade II or more GvHD, with two having grades III–IV and one dying from this complication. The overall survival rate at one year for these very poor-risk patients was 28%. No significant differences were seen in survival among patients receiving either the fludarabine or 2CDA regimen (Figure 5.1), but, as one would expect, patients without peripheral blood blasts or those with less than 10% bone marrow blasts did significantly better (Figure 5.2).

Nine patients with CML have also received a non-myeloablative regimen with fludarabine. Patient and treatment characteristics are summarized in Table 5.3. All patients had neutrophil and platelet recovery, and only one patient died from transplant-related complications (grade IV GvHD). The seven recipients of cells from related donors had evidence of donor cell

**Table 5.2  Patient and treatment characteristics of MD Anderson Cancer Center patients with AML or MDS receiving FLAG-Ida or 2CDA/Ara-C**

| | |
|---|---|
| Number of patients | 25 |
| Age | 61 years (range 27–74 years) |
| Time to transplant | 361 days (range 77–1807 days) |
| Diagnosis: | |
|   AML | 22 |
|   MDS | 3 |
| Stage at transplantation:[a] | |
|   CR1 or 1st untreated relapse | 6 |
|   >1st untreated relapse or refractory | 19 |
| Number of prior radiotherapy treatments | 2 (range 1–5) |
| % BM blasts[b] | 10 (range 1–95) |
| % PB blasts[b] | 4 (range 0–98) |
| Preparative regimen:[c] | |
|   FLAG-Ida | 15 |
|   2CDA/AraC | 12 |
| GvHD prophylaxis:[d] | |
|   CSP/MP | 13 |
|   FK/MTX | 11 |
|   None | 1 |
| Donor type: | |
|   5/6 sibling | 6 |
|   6/6 sibling | 18 |
|   Syngeneic | 1 |
| Stem cell source:[b] | |
|   BM | 23 |
|   PB | 2 |

[a] CR1, 1st complete remission.
[b] BM, bone marrow; PB, peripheral blood.
[c] See Table 5.1.
[d] CSP, cyclosporine; MP, methylprednisolone; FK, tacrolimus (FK506); MTX, methotrexate.

engraftment at the time of initial engraftment, while the two patients who received cells from unrelated donors had autologous reconstitution without ever having evidence of donor cell engraftment. All four patients transplanted in advanced phase relapsed and have failed to respond to salvage therapy with immunosuppression withdrawal, interferon, donor lymphocyte infusions, or second transplantation. Two of the four patients in chronic phase who had evidence of donor cell engraftment are alive in complete cytogenetic remission at 12 and 18 months post transplant, one with and one without donor lymphocyte infusions.

This initial experience with FLAG-Ida and 2CDA/Ara-C in patients with myeloid malignancies revealed that engraftment of allogeneic progenitor cells could be achieved with non-myeloablative purine-analog-containing regimens;

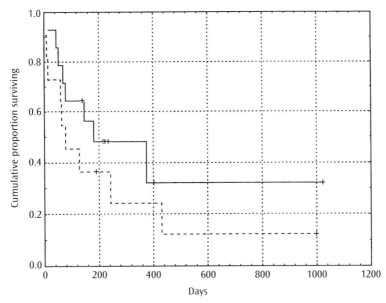

**Figure 5.1**

Survival according to preparative regimen, showing no difference (full line, FLAG-Ida; dashed line, 2CDA/Ara-C).

### Table 5.3  Patient and treatment characteristics of CML patients receiving FLAG-Ida and allogeneic progenitor cell transplantation

| | |
|---|---|
| Number of patients | 9 |
| Age | 55 years (range 42–67 years) |
| Time to transplant | 866 days (range 400–1249 days) |
| Stage at transplantation: | |
|     Late chronic phase | 5 |
|     Transformed phase | 4 |
| Prior interferon | 9 |
| Donor type:[a] | |
|     6/6 sibling | 7 |
|     6/6 MUD | 2 |
| Stem cell source:[b] | |
|     BM | 3 |
|     PB | 6 |
| GvHD prophylaxis:[c] | |
|     CS | 2 |
|     CSP/MP | 4 |
|     FK/MTX | 3 |

[a] MUD, matched unrelated donor.
[b] BM, bone marrow; PB, peripheral blood.
[c] CSP, cyclosporine; MP, methylprednisolone; FK, tacrolimus (FK 506); MTX, methotrexate.

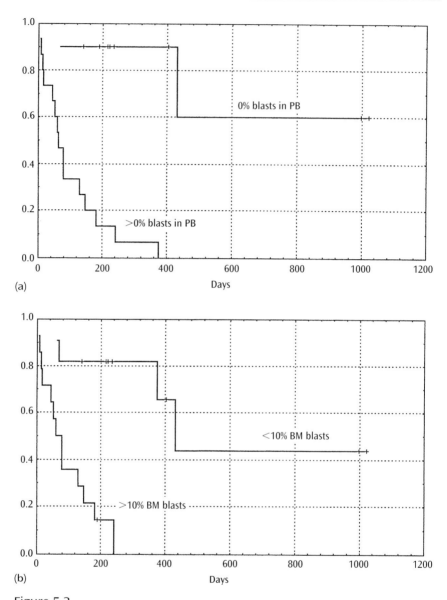

**Figure 5.2**

Survival according to tumor burden at time of transplant: (a) according to blasts in peripheral blood; (b) according to blasts in bone marrow.

however, long-term disease control was only achieved in patients with relatively low tumor burden who were transplanted early in the course of their disease. Likewise, these regimens may not be sufficiently immunosuppressive to allow engraftment of unrelated donor cells in the setting of CML. Therefore other novel non-myeloablative regimens needed to be developed. The combination of melphalan with purine analogs has been used at the MD Anderson Cancer Center as a more intense, but still non-myeloablative, regimen for patients considered as poor candidates for conventional myeloablative regimens. Eighty-six patients with a variety of hematologic malignancies have received one of three melphalan/purine-analog-containing preparative regimens. Patient and treatment characteristics are summarized in Table 5.4.

Seventy-seven patients had neutrophil recovery at a median of 14 days (range 9–35 days), and 55 patients recovered platelet-transfusion independence at a median of 21 days (range 9–118 days). All but one engrafting patients had documentation of over 80% donor cell engraftment by day 30, with one instance of autologous reconstitution and one of secondary graft failure. In this group of very poor-prognosis patients ineligible for conventional transplantation, the 100-day treatment-related mortality rate was 42% (36/86), with four out of eight patients in the 2CDA/melphalan arm dying from multiorgan failure, leading us to close this treatment arm. The overall survival rate for all patients was 29% at two years, and the disease-free survival rate was 23%. Patients transplanted in first CR/first chronic phase (CR1/CP1) or untreated first relapse (good- and intermediate-risk groups) did significantly better than patients with more advanced disease, with no difference seen among recipients of related or unrelated donor cells (Figure 5.3). Therefore fludarabine/melphalan combinations can allow engraftment of allogeneic progenitor cells, including cells obtained from matched unrelated donors. This strategy can produce long-term disease control in patients with hematologic malignancies early in the course of their disease with acceptable risk and toxicity in patients ineligible for conventional myeloablative transplant therapies. Treatment-related mortality from GvHD and disease recurrence remain the most common causes of treatment failure in this patient population.

## Minitransplants for lymphoid malignancies

The use of allogeneic transplantation is limited in patients with lymphoid malignancies such as chronic lymphocytic leukemia (CLL) or lymphomas because they typically affect older patients. Khouri and collaborators at the MD Anderson Cancer Center have evaluated the induction of a GvL effect as primary therapy for patients with lymphoid malignancies who are considered poor candidates for conventional transplant techniques.[16] Nine patients have been treated, eight of whom were more than 50 years old. All patients with advanced CLL ($n = 5$) or transformed lymphoma ($n = 4$), received one of two preparative regimens (fludarabine/cyclophosphamide or fludarabine/Ara-c/cisplatin). Mixed chimerism was observed in six of the nine patients, with the percentage of donor cells ranging from 50% to 100% one month post transplant. No regimen-related deaths were observed, and four patients achieved CR1 after DLI.

Investigators in Jerusalem reported on 26 allografts after a preparative

## Table 5.4 Patient and treatment characteristics of patients receiving melphalan/purine analog combinations

| | |
|---|---|
| Number of patients | 86 |
| Age | 52 years (range 22–70 years) |
| Sex: | |
|   Male | 52 |
|   Female | 34 |
| Diagnosis: | |
|   AML/MDS | 34/9 |
|   CML | 27 |
|   ALL/lymphoma | 3/13 |
| Status at transplantation:[a] | |
|   Early leukemia (CR1/CP1) | 1/6 |
|   1st untreated relapse | 10 |
|   ≥CR2 | 6 |
|   Transformed | 21 |
|   Refractory or >1st relapse | 42 |
| Number of prior therapies | 3 (range 0–8) |
| Prior BMT | 24 |
| Comorbid conditions:[b] | |
|   Age > 50 years | 48 |
|   MUGA < 50% | 5 |
|   PFTs < 50% | 4 |
|   GPT > 120 | 11 |
|   Prior BMT/or >3 Rx | 24/21 |
|   PS = 2/infection | 14/10 |
| Time to transplant | 547 days (range 27–6626 days) |
| Donor type:[c] | |
|   6/6 related | 39 |
|   5/6 related | 7 |
|   6/6 MUD | 40 |
| Stem cell source[d] | |
|   BM | 52 |
|   PB | 34 |
| CMV status[e] | |
|   (Neg/Neg) | 6 |
| Preparative regimen:[f] | |
|   FM 180 | 66 |
|   FM 140 | 12 |
|   2CDA/M 180 | 8 |
| GvHD prophylaxis:[g] | |
|   CSP/MP | 3 |
|   FK/MP | 2 |
|   FK/MTX | 81 |

[a] CR, complete remission; CP, chronic phase.
[b] MUGA, cardiac ejection factor; PFTs, pulmonary function tests; GPT, alanine aminotransferase; Rx, radiotherapy; PS, performance status.
[c] MUD, matched unrelated donor.
[d] BM, bone marrow; PB, peripheral blood.
[e] CMV, cytomegalovirus.
[f] FM 180, fludarabine–melphalan (180 mg); FM 140, fludarabine–melphalan (140 mg); 2CDA/M 180, 2-chloroadenosine–melphalan (180 mg)
[g] CSP, cyclosporine; MP, methylprednisolone; FK, tacrolimus (FK 506); MTX, methotrexate.

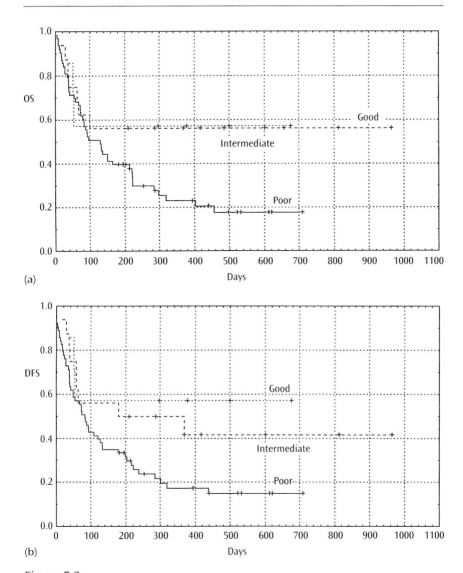

**Figure 5.3**

(a) Overall survival (OS) and (b) disease-free survival (DFS) in patients receiving melphalan/purine analog combinations.

regimen of fludarabine 180 mg/m², busulfan 16 mg/kg, and antithymocyte globulin (ATG) 40 mg/kg.[2] Patients with malignancy had less advanced disease and were younger than the patients who underwent transplantation in Houston. Four patients died of GvHD and 50% of patients had mild to severe veno-occlusive disease (VOD) of the liver. Investigators in Boston used cyclophosphamide 150–200 mg/kg along with ATG and thymic irradiation to treat 15 patients with malignancies. GvHD was seen in 10 patients. Seven patients were alive and free of disease progression 27–475 days after transplantation. Briefly, we can conclude that the more intense non-myeloablative regimens (fludarabine/busulfan and fludarabine/melphalan), although less intense than conventional myeloablative regimens, can still be associated with toxicities in older and heavily pretreated debilitated patients. However, many patients in these categories have benefitted from a treatment strategy that until recently they were considered ineligible for. Therefore physicians should now be tailoring the preparative regimen to the disease and patient rather than trying to treat all patients with the same preparative regimen. The results achieved support the general concept that future regimens may rely less on intensive cytotoxic therapy and more on allogeneic effects to eradicate malignant cells.

## PRETRANSPLANTATION HOST IMMUNOSUPPRESSION COMBINED WITH POST-TRANSPLANTATION IMMUNOSUPPRESSION DIRECTED AT BOTH HOST AND DONOR IMMUNE CELLS

In the last few years, the Seattle group has pioneered studies to determine whether postgrafting immunosuppression (to prevent GvHD) can be used to suppress host immunity, thereby promoting allogeneic engraftment.[11,17] This hypothesis has been tested by Storb et al on healthy dogs who were given marrow grafts and post-grafting immunosuppressive therapy with mofetil mycophenolate (MMF) and cyclosporine (CSP) after conditioning with 4.5 Gy. Marrow and lymph node samples obtained from unirradiated areas showed stable mixed chimerism as early as four weeks after transplantation and lasting for the entire observation period.[19] This finding supports the hypothesis that grafts can create marrow space, most likely through subclinical GvH reactions, and suggests that pretransplantation irradiation can be replaced by more specific and less toxic means of host T-cell suppression.

Based on the efficacy and lack of toxicity of the canine transplants, Storb et al designed an outpatient allografting protocol for human patients older than 50 years with hematologic malignancies.[17] The goal was to establish mixed chimerism that could serve as a platform for subsequent DLI. Immunosuppression consisted of 2 Gy total-body irradiation delivered as a single fraction. Of eight patients treated, five had follow-up of 3–12 months and three were within one month of transplantation. Diagnoses were CLL ($n = 2$), MDS evolving into AML ($n = 1$), AML in CR ($n = 2$), multiple myeloma ($n = 2$) and MDS/refractory anemia with excess blasts (RAEB) ($n = 1$), and ages ranged from 53 to 66 years, except for a 42-year-old male with MDS/RAEB who had advanced liver cirrhosis. Four patients had therapy administered entirely in an outpatient setting. Only one patient's granulocyte count declined to less than 5000/μl for two days, and his platelet nadir was 60 000/μl. Donor T-cell engraftment at days 28 and 56 after transplantation occurred in all patients. Four patients were eligible for initial DLI. Patient 1 developed grade II acute GvHD. After tapering prednisone and CSP, there was a GvL reaction resulting in complete molecular (polymerase chain reaction) remission in marrow and blood by seven months after transplantation. Patient 3 (MDS/AML-CR) developed skin GvHD after DLI, and was treated with corticosteroids. At four months after DLI, his T cells were 69% of donor origin, and he has remained without evidence of AML. Patient 2 has progressive RAEB with loss of donor chimerism, and patients 4 and 5 (both myeloma) had stable disease but rejected their grafts shortly after DLI.

## HIGH-INTENSITY AUTOTRANSPLANTATION FOLLOWED BY AN IMMUNOSUPPRESSIVE NON-MYELOABLATIVE REGIMEN

Having demonstrated that fludarabine-based conditioning regimens can allow engraftment of allogeneic donor HSC, our team has tried to verify whether it is possible to combine high-dose therapy/autografting with protocols appropriate for the underlying disease followed by allografting conditioned by only an immunosuppressive regimen in order to achieve reduction of tumor burden after autografting and control of residual disease with immunologically mediated effects after allografting.[13] Immunosuppression consisted of fludarabine 30 mg/m$^2$ with cyclophosphamide 300 mg/m$^2$, both delivered daily for three days. Cyclosporine 1 mg/kg intravenously from day $-1$ to day 10 (and subsequently orally) and methothrexate 10 mg/m$^2$ intravenously on days 1, 3, and 5 were given. Granulocyte colony-stimulating factor (G-CSF)-mobilized HSC from serologically and molecularly histocompatible sibling donors were reinfused on day 0. Chimerism studies were performed every 10 days for the first month and every 15 days for the subsequent months. The 23 patients treated had a follow-up for 330 days (range 66–780 days) 10 months (range 2–24 months). Diagnoses were metastatic breast cancer ($n = 4$), advanced resistant Hodgkin's disease ($n = 10$) or non-Hodgkin's lymphoma ($n = 5$), refractory anemia with excess blasts in transformation (RAEB-t) ($n = 2$), and accelerated/blastic-phase CML ($n = 2$). The median age was 36 (range 19–60 years) (Table 5.5). In only two patients, did the granulocyte count decline to less than 1000/µl and the platelet nadir was 20 000/µl. Acute GvHD occurred in 10 patients, but was generally mild except for three patients (who experienced gastrointestinal and liver grade III). Fourteen patients achieved complete donor HSC engraftment at a median time of 115 days (range 53–180 days). Seven patients obtained mixed chimerism, and two patients (RAEB and blast-crisis CML) re-engrafted with their autologous stem cells (Table 5.6). Thirteen patients were eligible for DLI at a median dose of $1 \times 10^7$ CD3$^+$ cells/kg. At the present time, the outcome is as follows.

Two of the four breast cancer patients are alive, both in good partial remission (GPR) at 420 and 630 days; both of these patients achieved and maintain

**Table 5.5  Clinical and treatment characteristics of Genoa patients receiving the fludarabine/cyclophosphamide protocol**

| | |
|---|---|
| Number of patients | 23 |
| Age | 36 years (range 19–60 years) |
| Sex: | |
|    Male | 9 |
|    Female: | 14 |
| Diagnosis: | |
|    Hodgkin's disease | 10 |
|    Non-Hodgkin's lymphoma | 5 |
|    Breast cancer | 4 |
|    CML (accelerated/blastic phase) | 2 |
|    RAEB-t | 2 |
| Prior treatment courses | 3 (range 1–5) |
| Autografted (ASCT) | 21 |
| Interval ASCT/mini-Allo | 40 days (range 30–1149 days) |
| Stage at BMT:[a] | |
|    Progressive disease | 4 |
|    Untreated relapse | 2 |
|    1st relapse | 2 |
|    Refractory or ≥2nd relapse | 11 |
|    ≥CR2 | 2 |
|    CP2 CML | 2 |
| Donor age | 38 years (range 19–69 years) |
| Donor gender: | |
|    Male | 13 |
|    Female | 10 |
| Time to transplantation | 20 months (range 6–120 months) |
| GvHD prophylaxis[c] | CSP/MTX |

[a] CR, complete remission; CP, chronic phase.
[b] CMV, cytomegalovirus.
[c] CSP/MTX, cyclosporine/methotrexate.

**Table 5.6  Engraftment after the fludarabine/cyclophosphamide protocol**

| | |
|---|---|
| Number of patients | 23 |
| WBC < 1000/µl | 2/23 |
| Platelets < 20 000/µl | 2/23 |
| Complete chimerism (100% donor) | 14/23 (61%) |
| Mixed chimerism (29–90% donor) | 7/23 (30%) |
| Autologous recovery | 2/23 (9%) |

complete chimerism, they developed gastrointestinal/liver grade III acute GvHD after DLI, and in both cases remarkable reduction of bone metastases was demonstrated.

Seven of the ten Hodgkin's disease patients are alive (Table 5.7). Six patients achieved CR (two for the first time, two for the second time, and two for the

## Table 5.7  Clinical results in Hodgkin's disease (HD) and non-Hodgkin's lymphoma (NHL) receiving the fludarabine/cyclophosphamide protocol

| Patient no. | Diagnosis | Status | | | Outcome (days) |
|---|---|---|---|---|---|
| | | Pre-auto | Post-auto | Post-mini-allo | |
| 1 | HD | PRD | PR | PD | Died in PD/chronic GvHD (liver) (460) |
| 2 | HD | REL2 | PR | CR3 | Alive REL4 (>780) |
| 3 | HD | PRD | PR | PD | Died in PD (66) |
| 4 | HD | REL2 | PR | CR3 | Died in CR3 (brain *Aspergillus*) (120) |
| 5 | HD | REL4 | CR5 | PR | Alive in PR (>600) |
| 6 | HD | PR | CR1 | CR2 | Alive in CR2 (>430) |
| 7 | HD | REL1 | CR2 | CR2 | Alive in CR2 (>330) |
| 8 | HD | PRD | PR | CR1 | Alive in CR1 (>330) |
| 9 | HD | REL4 | PR | PR | Alive in PR (>270) |
| 10 | HD | PRD | PR | CR1 | Alive in CR1 (>210) |
| 11 | NHL | PRD | PR | CR1 | REL2 after 360 days, DLI → alive PD (>630) |
| 12 | NHL | PRD | PR | PD | Died in PD (172) |
| 13 | NHL | REL4 | PR | CR5 | Died in CR5 of extensive chronic GvHD (303) |
| 14 | NHL | REL1 | PR | CR2 | Alive in CR2 (>240) |
| 15 | NHL | REL3 | PR | CR4 | Alive in CR4 (>270) |

*Abbreviations*: auto, autologous transplantation; allo, allogeneic transplantation; PRD, primarily refractory disease; CR, complete remission; PR, partial remission; REL, relapse; PD, progressive disease; GPR, good partial remission; DLI, donor lymphocyte infusion.

## Table 5.8  Outcome for patients receiving the fludarabine/cyclophosphamide regimen

| | |
|---|---|
| Number of patients | 23 |
| Alive | 16 (70%) |
| Follow-up | 330 days (range 66–780 days) |
| Died | 6 |
| Day 100 or earlier | 3 (1 Hodgkin's disease; 2 breast) |
| After day 100 | 4 (2 Hodgkin's disease + chronic GvHD; 2 non-Hodgkin's lymphoma) |

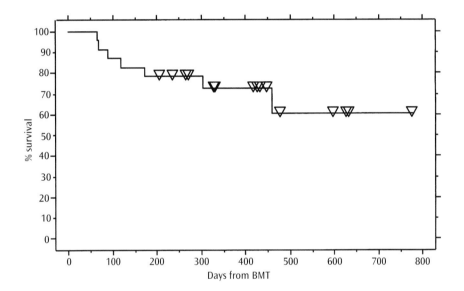

Figure 5.4

Kaplan–Meier survival plot in 23 patients receiving the fludarabine/cyclophosphamide regimen.

third time). The median survival from allografting is 330 days (range 60–780 days).

Three of the five non-Hodgkin's lymphoma patients are alive after 240, 270 and 630 days (Table 5.7). One patient, resistant to first/second-line therapies, achieved his first CR, and has maintained this at 12 months following transplant. Three of the patients achieved a new CR and two of them have maintained it at 240 and 270 days. One patient with large cell lymphoma progressed with his disease and died of lymphoma despite DLI infusion.

Both of the RAEB-t patients are alive at 330 and 450 days. The patient with p190 AP CML developed grade II acute GvHD that was associated with the development of full donor HSC engraftment. After tapering of the CSP, there was granulocytopenia and thrombocytopenia followed by normalization of blood values and complete molecular (polymerase chain reaction) remission in marrow and blood by 780 days after the mini-allografting. Now the patient is off CSP and steroids and has returned tot work[18] (Table 5.8). The Kaplan–Meier survival plot is shown in Figure 5.4.

In conclusion, mini-allografts alone or after tumor debulking with autografting, when employed in older and younger patients resistant to first- or second-line therapies, with the main goal of exploiting GvL effects, is feasible using non-toxic immunosuppressive conditioning regimens. It is extremely important to note that the side-effects of these therapies are uncommon, mixed/complete chimerism has been established in most patients after allografting, and GvL occurred in the same patients. None of our patients has died of acute GvHD. If these results can be confirmed in larger trials, immunosuppressive regimens alone should ultimately be successful in establishing stable engraftment, especially if these regimens are to be preceded by autografting

# REFERENCES

1. Giralt S, Estey E, Albitar M et al, Engraftment of allogeneic hematopoietic progenitor cells with purine analog-containing chemotherapy: harnessing graft-versus-leukemia without myeloablative therapy. Blood 1997; 89: 4531–6.

2. Slavin S, Nagler A, Naparstek E et al, Nonmyeloablative stem cell transplantation and cell therapy as an alternative to conventional bone marrow transplantation with lethal cytoreduction for the treatment of malignant and nonmalignant hematologic diseases. Blood 1998; 91: 756–63.

3. Kolb HJ, Mittermüller J, Clemm C et al, Donor leukocyte transfusions for treatment of recurrent chronic myelogenous leukemia in marrow transplant patients. Blood 1990; 76: 2462–5.

4. Porter DL, Roth MS, McGarigle C et al, Induction of graft-versus-host disease as immunotherapy for relapsed chronic myeloid leukemia. N Engl J Med 1994; 330: 100–6.

5. Kolb HJ, Schattenberg A, Goldman JM et al, Graft-versus-leukemia effect of donor lymphocyte transfusions in marrow grafted patients: European Group for Blood and Marrow Transplantation Working Party Chronic Leukemia. Blood 1995; 86: 2041–50.

6. Slavin S, Ackerstein A, Naparstek E et al, Hypothesis: the graft-versus leukemia (GVL) phenomenon – Is GVL separable from GVHD? Bone Marrow Transplant 1990; 6: 155–61.

7. Mackinnon S, Papadopoulos EB, Carabasi MH et al, Adoptive immunotherapy evaluating escalating doses of donor leukocytes for relapse of chronic myeloid leukemia after bone marrow transplantation: separation of graft-versus-leukemia responses from graft-versus-host disease. Blood 1995; 86: 1261–8.

8. Giralt S, Hester J, Huh Y et al, CD8-depleted donor lymphocyte infusions as treatment for relapsed chronic myelogenous leukemia after allogeneic bone marrow transplantation. Blood 1995; 86: 4337–43.

9. Collins RH Jr, Shpilberg O, Drobyski

WR et al, Donor lymphocyte infusions in 140 patients with relapsed malignancy after allogeneic bone marrow transplantation. *J Clin Oncol* 1997; **15**: 433–44.

10. Van Rhee F, Lin F, Cullis JO et al, Relapse of chronic myeloid leukemia after allogeneic bone marrow transplant: the case for giving donor leukocyte transfusions before the onset of hematologic relapse. *Blood* 1994; **83**: 3377–83.

11. Storb R, Yu C, Wagner JL et al, Stable mixed hematopoietic chimerism in DLA-identical littermate dogs given sublethal total body irradiation before and pharmacological immunosuppression after marrow transplantation. *Blood* 1997; **89**: 3049–54.

12. Sullivan KM, Weiden PL, Storb R et al, Influence of acute and chronic graft-versus-host disease on relapse and survival after bone marrow transplantation from HLA-identical siblings as treatment of acute and chronic leukemia. *Blood* 1989; **73**: 1720–8.

13. Carella AM, Lerma E, Dejana A et al, Engraftment of HLA-matched sibling hematopoietic stem cells after immunosuppressive conditioning regimen in patients with hematologic neoplasias. *Haematologica* 1998; **83**: 904–9.

14. Khouri I, Keating MJ, Przepiorka D et al, Engraftment and induction of GVL with fludarabine (FAMP)-based nonablative preparative regimen in patients with chronic lymphocytic leukemia (CLL) and lymphoma. *Blood* 1996; **88**: 301a (Abst 1194).

15. Khouri IF, Keating M, Körbling M et al, Transplant-lite: induction of graft-versus-malignancy using fludarabine-based nonablative chemotherapy and allogeneic blood progenitor-cell transplantation as treatment for lymphoid malignancies. *J Clin Oncol* 1998; **16**: 2817–24.

16. Giralt S, Estey E, van Besien K et al, Engraftment of allogeneic hematopoietic progenitor cells with purine analog containing nonmyeloablative regimens: harnessing graft-versus-leukemia without myeloablative therapy. *Blood* 1997; **89**: 4531–6.

17. Storb R, Nonmyeloablative preparative regimens: experimental data and clinical practice. In: *Educational Book, 55th Annual Meeting, Am Soc Clin Oncol, May 15–18, 1999, Atlanta, GA* (Perry MC, ed): 241–9.

18. Carella AM, Lerma E, Corsetti MT et al, Evidence of cytogenetic and molecular remission by allogeneic cells after immunosuppressive therapy alone. *Br J Haematol* 1998; **103**: 565–7.

# 6
# Hematopoietic stem cell transplantation in older adults

Arthur J Molina, Rainer F Storb

## INTRODUCTION

Hematopoietic stem cell (HSC) transplantation (HSCT) has emerged as an important and increasingly used treatment modality for patients with malignant and non-malignant diseases. The availability of allogeneic and autologous marrow has allowed clinicians to intensify antitumor therapy well beyond the marrow-toxic range, to a point where dose-limiting non-hematopoietic toxicities have been encountered. Toxicities have restricted the application of transplantation to younger patients, and very few transplants have been reported in patients older than 50–55 years. This is unfortunate given that more than half of patients diagnosed with hematologic malignancies are over 50 years of age. With the advent of improved supportive care strategies developed over the last decade, selected older patients have been able to tolerate autologous HSCT. However, the combined effects of graft-versus-host disease (GvHD) and regimen-related toxicities (RRT) have significantly compromised allogeneic HSCT in older patients. New approaches that eliminate toxic conditioning regimens and rely on graft-versus-leukemia (GvL) effects for tumor eradication afford optimism for applying allogeneic HSCT to older patients.

## DEMOGRAPHIC CONSIDERATIONS IN HSCT

Except for acute lymphoblastic leukemia (ALL) and Hodgkin's disease (HD), there are considerable disparities between median ages of patients undergoing HSCT for hematologic malignancies and median ages at the time of diagnoses (Table 6.1). These disparities are further illustrated in Figure 6.1 (autologous HSCT) and Figure 6.2 (allogeneic HSCT). The data show that a disproportionately high percentage of younger patients and a disproportionately low percentage of older patients have undergone HSCT compared with the patient population at large. The minority of 'older' patients referred for HSCT are likely the result of a rigorous selection, and may not be representative of the patient population as a whole. The issue of patient selection needs to be kept

Table 6.1 The national median ages (in years) at diagnosis for patients with various hematologic malignancies as compared with median ages at the time of allogeneic and autologous HSCT at the Fred Hutchinson Cancer Research Center

| Disease[a] | Median age of related allogeneic HSCT[b] | Median age of unrelated allogeneic HSCT[b] | Median age of autologous HSCT[b] | Median age at diagnosis[c] |
|---|---|---|---|---|
| CML | 36 | 36 | 47 | 67 |
| NHL | 33 | 35 | 44 | 65 |
| MM | 45 | 45 | 55 | 70 |
| CLL | 51 | 46 | 59 | 71 |
| AML | 28 | 33 | 35 | 68 |
| ALL | 16 | 15 | 19 | 12 |
| MDS | 40 | 41 | 45 | 68 |
| HD | 29 | 28 | 32 | 34 |

[a]CML, chronic myelogenous leukemia; NHL, non-Hodgkin's lymphoma; MM, multiple myeloma; CLL, chronic lymphocytic leukemia; AML, acute myelogenous leukemia; ALL, acute lymphoblastic leukemia; MDS, myelodysplastic syndrome; HD, Hodgkin's disease.
[b]Fred Hutchinson Cancer Research Center (1980–1999).
[c]SEER, Cancer Statistics, US National Cancer Institute, 1996.

in mind when analyzing the results of HSCT in older patients that are described in the remainder of this chapter.

Given the age restrictions for conventional HSCT at virtually all transplantation centers, most patients with hematologic malignances cannot be effectively treated. The reluctance with which older patients are referred by physicians for conventional autologous and allogeneic HSCT may be justified given the current toxicity of conventional HSCT. However, this practice may require reconsideration as innovations are developed to reduce the toxicities of HSCT. New and unconventional strategies will likely become important foci of future research. As one of the most effective methods of treating and curing patients with hematologic malignances, developments in HSCT will play a central role in how successfully we treat patients in the future.

## MYELOABLATIVE HSCT

### Autologous HSCT

Four recent studies have dealt with the influence of age on outcomes of autologous HSCT. All but one study showed statistically significant worsening in terms of overall survival, disease-free survival or regimen-related toxicity with increased patient age (Table 6.2). Sweetenham et al[1] were the only authors to

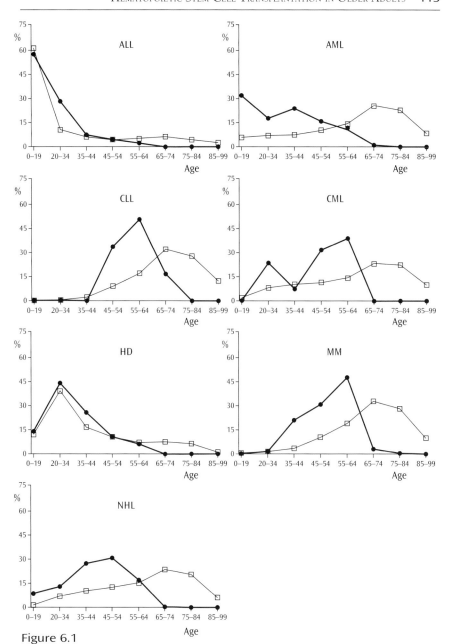

Figure 6.1

Age distribution curves of patients with various hematologic diseases undergoing autologous HSCT at the Fred Hutchinson Cancer Research Center (thick lines/black circles). These are compared with age distribution curves from the US NCI SEER database (thin line/white squares) at the times of diagnoses nationally. Except for patients with ALL and HD, the curves show dramatic differences between the age groups diagnosed and those of patients undergoing conventional HSCT. (ALL, acute lymphoblastic leukemia; AML, acute myelogenous leukemia; CLL, chronic lymphocytic leukemia; CML, chronic myelogenous leukemia; HD, Hodgkin's disease; MM, multiple myeloma; NHL, non-Hodgkin's lymphoma.)

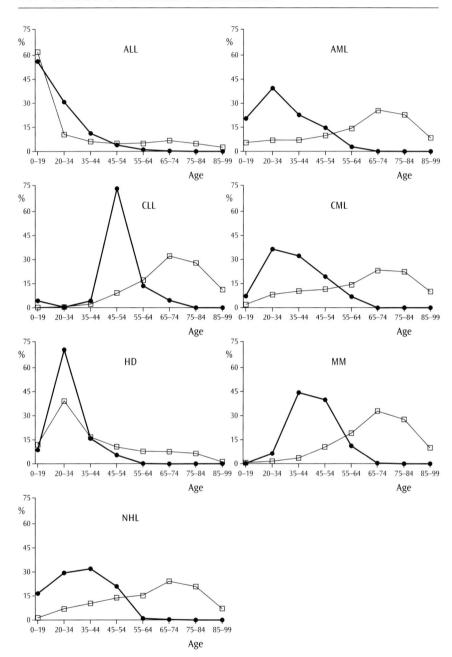

Figure 6.2

Age distribution curves of patients with various hematologic diseases undergoing allogeneic HSCT at the Fred Hutchinson Cancer Research Center (thick lines/black circles). These are compared with age distribution curves from the US NCI SEER database (thin lines/white squares) at the times of diagnoses nationally. There is a large discrepancy between ages at diagnoses and ages at the times of conventional allogeneic HSCT, with the exception of HD and ALL. (For abbreviations, see Figure 6.1.)

**Table 6.2 Summary of studies analyzing the influence of age on autologous HSCT**

| Team | Diseases treated[a] | Study period | No. of patients | | Patients' age range (years)[c] | | OS/DFS (%) | | Regimen related toxicity (%) | |
|---|---|---|---|---|---|---|---|---|---|---|
| | | | Y[b] | O[b] | Y | O | Y | O | Y | O |
| Sweetenham et al[1] | NHL | 1980–93 | 82 | 82 | 16–54 (37) | 55–65 (55) | 39/33 | 38/37 | 11 | 13 |
| Cahn et al[2] | AML (CR1) | 1980–91 | 786 | 111 | 16–49 (35) | 50–63 (53) | 48[d]/43 | 35/34[d] | 14 | 28[d] |
| Miller et al[3] | AML, ALL, NHL, HD, MM, BRCA | 1987–94 | 405 | 101 | 18–48 | 50–65 | —/28 | —/25 | 12 | 28[d] |
| Kusnierz-Glaz et al[4] | NHL, HD, MM, AML | 1988–95 | 387 | 113 | <20–50 | 50–65 | —/46[d] | —/34 | 7 | 13 |

[a]NHL, non-Hodgkin's lymphoma; AML, acute myelogenous leukemia (CR1, 1st complete remission); ALL, acute lymphoblastic leukemia; HD, Hodgkin's disease; MM, multiple myeloma; BRCA, breast cancer.
[b]Y, younger age group; O, older age group.
[c]Median age in parentheses.
[d]Statistically significant difference.

demonstrate equivalent progression-free and overall survivals of older and younger patients who were matched for known prognostic factors at the time of autologous HSCT. Despite this favorable result, there seemed to be a higher regimen-related mortality in older patients. There was a significantly higher toxic death rate observed in the older patients compared with patients less than 55 years of age (38% versus 12%; $p = 0.03$). Kaplan–Meier estimates showed a toxic death rate of 60% for patients aged 55 years or more treated with total-body irradiation (TBI), compared with 11% in the younger age group ($p = 0.02$). Performance status assessments were not available. Selection bias could not be ruled out as a factor in the outcomes noted. A subsequent study by Cahn et al[2] retrospectively analyzed data from the European Bone Marrow Transplant (EBMT) registry for 111 acute myelogenous leukemia (AML) patients over 50 years of age in first complete remission (CR). This group was compared with a younger group of 786 patients with the same diagnosis. Transplant-related mortality was significantly higher in the older age group ($p < 0.0001$), and was mainly due to infection. In a multivariate analysis, age less than 50 years was found to be a favorable prognostic factor for leukemia-free survival (LFS). Four years after transplantation, older patients (>50 years) did worse than younger patients in terms of LFS (34% versus 43%; $p = 0.004$) and overall survival (35% versus 48%; $p = 0.004$). Both groups showed similar relapse rates.

In a study from Johns Hopkins,[3] 101 older patients with multiple hematologic malignancies and solid tumors were found to have a 2.24-fold increased risk of treatment-related mortality (TRM) ($p < 0.001$) compared with 407 younger patients. However, relapse rates were no different. The increased TRM contributed to a slight decrease in overall event-free survival (EFS) in the older patients ($p = 0.15$). Preparative regimen toxicities such as veno-occlusive disease (VOD) of the liver and interstitial pneumonia were the major causes of death in all age groups. Death related to aplasia was relatively uncommon in both age groups. In a similar study of 500 autologous HSCT patients at Stanford Medical Center,[4] disease status at the time of transplant was the strongest predictive factor for EFS and relapse rates. Age less than 50 years had an impact on EFS as well as regimen-related mortality (RRM). EFS at five years for patients less than 50 years of age was significantly higher than for patients older than 50 years ($p = 0.03$; Figure 6.3). The decrease in EFS for the older age group was caused by a 60–70% higher rate of RRM (although the older age group had a higher proportion of patients with AML). The probability of infectious complications was four- to five-fold higher in patients between 50 and 65 years compared with patients 50 years of age or less ($p = 0.01$). The source of progenitor cells, use of low-dose heparin for VOD prophylaxis, and the type of mobilization of the graft did not have significant effects on transplant outcome. There was a trend to a lower RRM in the later years of the study (1992–1995) compared with the period 1988–1991. However, despite the improvement in RRM in the most recent years, a roughly 60% higher RRM in patients 50–65 years of age compared with younger patients was still detectable in the later years of the study.

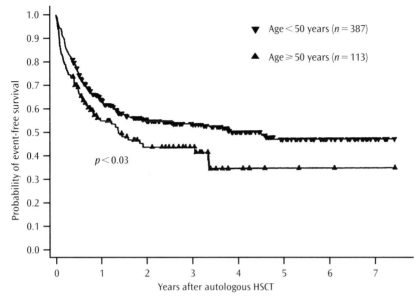

Figure 6.3

Probability of EFS after autologous transplantation in 500 patients <50 and ⩾50 years of age (p <0.03). Adapted from Kusnierz-Glaz et al.[4]

In light of the curative potential of autologous HSCT and decreasing RRM in recent years, age as a sole factor should not be used to exclude patients from this potentially curative therapy. However, most autologous HSCT studies show that older age groups suffer from decreased long-term EFS and higher RRT rates when compared with younger patients.

## Allogeneic HSCT

### Early studies focusing on comparisons between HSCT in adults and children

Initially allogeneic HSCT largely focused on the treatment of children and young adults. As more adults underwent HSCT, worse survival outcomes and an increased incidence of GvHD were observed. Four early reports on allogeneic HSCT described the influence of patient age on outcomes in HSCT (Table 6.3). Thomas[5] initially reported on 75 patients with AML in first remission who were followed at least 2.5 years after allogeneic HSCT. Approximately 75% of patients under the age of 20 years were cured. However, among patients between 30 and 50 years of age, only about 25% were long-term survivors.

**Table 6.3  Early allogeneic bone marrow transplant studies describing outcomes of adults when compared with children. There were increased rates of GvHD, interstitial pneumonia (IP) and lower survival in adults compared with children**

| Team | Diseases treated[a] | Years | No. of patients | Patients' age range (years)[b] | Major findings related to patient age |
|---|---|---|---|---|---|
| Thomas[5] | AML | – | 75 | <10–40+ | • 75% of patients <20 years versus only 25% of patients over the age of 30 were long-term survivors. |
| Storb et al[6] | AA | 1970–81 | 111 | <10–40+ | • Risk of developing chronic GvHD rose by a factor of 2.49 with each decade of patient age.<br>• Chronic GvHD was associated with a mortality of 27%. |
| Barrett et al[7] | ALL | 1978–86 | 690 | 1–49 (20) | • Adults (>16 years) transplanted in 1st and 2nd remissions had a significantly lower leukemia-free survival than children did.<br>• Mortality in adults was principally due to GvHD and IP. |
| Goldman et al[8] | CML | 1978–85 | 405 | 3–53 (31) | • The probability of survival was significantly lower for patients aged ≥20 years. |

[a]AML, acute myelogenous leukemia; AA, aplastic anemia; ALL, acute lymphoblastic leukemia; CML, chronic myelogenous leukemia.
[b]Median age in parenthesis.

The older age group had poorer survival because of a higher incidence of transplant complications, particularly GvHD and interstitial pneumonia. In a study of 110 consecutive aplastic anemia patients, Storb et al[6] found increased patient age, incidence and grade of acute GvHD, and the infusion of donor buffy coat cells in addition to marrow to be associated with an increased risk of chronic GvHD. The odds of developing chronic GvHD were estimated to increase by a factor of 2.49 with each decade of life. Importantly, the mortality rate was 27% for patients with chronic GvHD, while all patients without chronic GvHD survived.

Similarly, in an International Bone Marrow Transplant Registry (IBMTR) study, children aged between 16 years with ALL in first CR had a five-year LFS rate of 56%, whereas adults (16 years of age or older) had a lower probability (39%) of survival ($p < 0.02$).[7] Mortality in adults was principally due to GvHD and interstitial pneumonia. In an IBMTR study of 405 chronic myelogenous leukemia (CML) patients, univariate analysis revealed that patient age was a significant risk factor both when analyzed as a continuous variable (by decade 10–40 years) or as a dichotomous variable.[8] The four-year probability of survival for 65 patients less than 20 years of age was 75%, compared with 52% for 340 older patients ($p < 0.0002$). The relative risk of treatment failure associated with patients 20 years of age or older represented the effect of age over and above its association with acute GvHD. Case fatality rates from interstitial pneumonia and acute GvHD were significantly increased in the older patients.

### Later studies focusing on the influence of age in HSCT between older adults

The previous studies largely considered only patients less than 40 years of age, and made statistical comparisons of disease outcomes between children and young adults. Subsequent studies looked at subgroups of adult HSCT patients (Table 6.4). In general, patients over the age of 50 years performed poorly after allogeneic HSCT. However, patients 40–50 years of age appeared to have outcomes similar to younger adults.

In an early study, Klingemann et al[9] found that CML and AML patients aged over 50 years had high rates of pulmonary complications (8 of 13 patients or 62%) after undergoing allogeneic HSCT. The actuarial incidence of acute GvHD for patients 45–50 years of age was similar to that observed in younger patients. However, in patients over 50 years old, the incidence of acute GvHD was 79.5% (grade II–IV). Only one of 13 patients over the age of 50 years had survived at the time of publication. Blume et al[10] found remission status at the time of transplant to be the major factor affecting outcomes for a group of older HSCT patients. Of note, all four patients between ages 46 and 54 years died.

Conclusions on the influence of age in HSCT are difficult to draw from studies with small numbers of patients, the results of which may be influenced by selection bias. As larger numbers of patients were enrolled in HSCT protocols both in the USA and Europe, it became possible to more accurately assess outcome patterns. Ringden et al[11] performed a retrospective analysis of 2180 HLA-identical sibling bone marrow transplants in adults (>30 years) with leukemia. Patients from the EBMT registry were divided into cohorts based on age: 30–39 years ($n = 1282$), 40–44 years ($n = 527$), 45–49 years ($n = 291$), and 50 years and older ($n = 80$). Patients aged 45 years or over with advanced leukemia had a significantly higher risk of TRM, and the 45–49-year-old cohort had a significantly higher risk of interstitial pneumonia (although overall survival was unaffected). Du et al[12] found the one-month transplant mortality to be significantly higher in patients over 50 years of age when compared

## Table 6.4 Studies comparing outcomes of older adults undergoing allogeneic HSCT

| Team | Diseases[a] | Years | Ages (years) of study group | No. ≥50 years | Outcome for patients ≥50 years[b] |
|---|---|---|---|---|---|
| Klingemann et al[9] | AML, CML, MDS, NHL, AA, MM, other | 1978–84 | 45–62 (n = 63) | 13 | • 62% pulmonary complications.<br>• <10% (1/13) survival.<br>• 80% incidence of acute GvHD (grade II–IV). |
| Blume et al[10] | AML, CML, ALL, other | 1976–85 | 30–54 (n = 86) | ~4 | • All four patients between ages 46 and 54 years died. |
| Ringdén et al[11] | ALL, CML, CLL | 1985–90 | 30–59 (n = 2180) | 80 | • RR of 2.35 for TRM and 1.77 RR for LFS for patients with advanced disease compared with younger patients.<br>• 2-year probability of IP was significantly higher in patients >45 years. |
| Du et al[12] | CML, AML, MDS, ALL, HD, other | 1987–96 | 50–59 (n = 59) | 59 | • The RR of death after adjusting for prognostic factors was 1.654 (p = 0.038) for patients aged over 50 compared with those <40 years.<br>• Transplant mortality was significantly higher in patients >50 years when compared with patients 40 years of age. |
| Clift et al[18] | CML in chronic phase | 1983–94 | 10–60 (n = 328) | 57 | • Age ≥50 was found to be an adverse risk factor (RR = 2.66) relative to age <30 years. |
| Hansen et al[13] | CML in chronic phase (unrelated) | 1985–94 | 6–55 (n = 196) | 13 | • Patients who were over 50 years had a significantly higher risk of death than patients who were 21–50 years of age (RR = 3.4, p = 0.002). |

[a]AML, acute myelogenous leukemia; CML, chronic myelogenous leukemia; MDS, myelodysplastic syndrome; NHL, non-Hodgkin's lymphoma; AA, aplastic anemia; MM, multiple myeloma; ALL, acute lymphoblastic leukemia; CLL, chronic lymphocytic leukemia; HD, Hodgkin's disease.
[b]RR, relative risk; TRM, treatment-related mortality; LFS, leukemia-free survival; IP, interstitial pneumonia.

with patients less than 40 years of age (15% versus 5%; $p < 0.05$). There was also a significantly higher relative risk of death in the oldest patient population when compared with patients aged less than 40 years.

In general, these studies did not show significant differences between patients 40–49 years of age and younger adults (usually compared with groups 20–39 years of age). In the large study reported by Ringden et al,[11] the overall survivals, LFS, risks of GvHD and relapse rates were comparable among the four age cohorts (between 30 and 50 years of age), except for an increased TRM for patients over the age of 45. Blume et al[10] noted that survival was over 40% for the 82 patients aged 30–45 years (independent of disease stage), similar to reported rates in young adults. Hansen et al[13] showed no survival difference in CML patients aged 31–36 who underwent unrelated allogeneic HSCT compared with patients 40–49 years of age. In a pair-matched analysis of 151 AML patients, Cahn et al[14] found no statistical difference in the probability of LFS, TRM, and survival between patients over 40 (median 44) years of age and a group of patients 16–40 (median 29) years old. In other small series (17–20 patients), no differences were found in overall survivals in patients 40–49 years of age when compared with younger adults less than 40 years old.[15–17]

### The influence of age in allogeneic HSCT for CML, MM, CLL, and NHL

The median age of patients diagnosed with CML is 67 years, and there is a steady increase in disease incidence between the third and ninth decades. Median survival is approximately four to five years after diagnosis, and, for almost all patients, allografting is the only curative treatment. More than 1600 allogeneic transplants have been performed for the treatment of CML at the Fred Hutchinson Cancer Research Center (FHCRC), including more than 900 from HLA-identical siblings. Assessment of factors contributing to transplant outcome was facilitated in this relatively homogenous group of patients by a common disease pathogenesis and fairly uniform transplant therapy.

As reported by Clift et al,[18,19] disease phase at the time of transplant was a major factor in outcome. Beyond that, increasing age played an important role in CML in chronic phase. Results from univariate analysis (Figure 6.4) and multivariate analysis (Table 6.5) for chronic-phase patients demonstrated the significant roles of patient age and length of time from diagnosis for non-relapse mortality and survival. Even though our transplant protocols are open to include patients up to age 65 years, we have transplanted few patients aged 50–62 years ($n = 68$). To date, only three CML patients over 62 years old have undergone allogeneic HSCT. As pointed out before, however, these few older patients may be highly selected and not representative of the CML patient population as a whole. Hansen et al[13] found that patients over 50 years of age, undergoing unrelated HLA-matched HSCT, had a significantly higher risk of death than patients who were 21–50 years of age (relative risk 3.4; Figure 6.5). Overall, the ages of recipients appeared to be a significant variable only for patients over 50 years of age, although the number of patients in this age group was small ($n = 13$). These considerations strongly support efforts to develop safe and effective allografting protocols that can be applied to older patients.

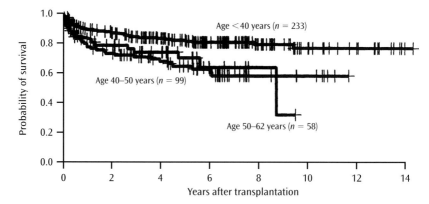

**Figure 6.4**

Kaplan–Meier estimates of survival for patients who received allogeneic HSCT from HLA-identical related donors during the chronic phase of CML within the first two years of diagnosis, categorized by patient age. Adapted from Thomas and Clift.[19]

**Table 6.5 Chronic myelogenous leukemia in chronic phase: multivariable analysis – significant associations with mortality not due to relapse**

| Variable[a] | Relative risk | p-value | 95% confidence interval |
|---|---|---|---|
| Age in years (Ref age <30, n = 78): | | | |
| 30–40 (n = 139) | 1.47 | 0.335 | 0.67–3.18 |
| 40–50 (n = 101) | 2.66 | 0.011 | 1.25–5.65 |
| 50–62 (n = 68) | 2.41 | 0.036 | 1.06–5.46 |
| Diagnosis to transplant (Ref <1 year, n = 294): | | | |
| 1–2 years (n = 50) | 1.41 | 0.286 | 0.75–2.66 |
| >2 years (n = 42) | 2.47 | 0.0023 | 1.38–4.41 |
| Gender of donor and patient (Ref F into F, n = 79): | | | |
| Donor Patient | | | |
| M F (n = 63) | 1.75 | 0.241 | 0.69–4.42 |
| F M (n = 106) | 2.93 | 0.008 | 1.33–6.42 |
| M M (n = 138) | 2.29 | 0.039 | 1.05–5.03 |

[a]Ref, reference group; F, female, M, male.
Not significant: regimen, year of transplant, pretransplant therapy, and CMV serology.

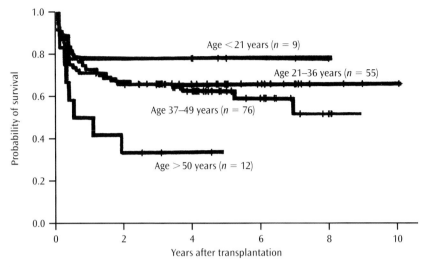

**Figure 6.5**

Probability of survival in 152 patients with CML in chronic phase who received a transplant matched for HLA-A, -B and -DRB1 from an unrelated donor, categorized according to age. Adapted from Hansen et al.[13]

Long-term survivals after allografting for patients with non-Hodgkin's lymphoma (NHL), multiple myeloma (MM), and chronic lymphocytic leukemia (CLL) have been much lower than for patients with CML in chronic phase. This was due in part to significantly higher transplant-related mortalities experienced by patients with NHL, MM, and CLL. A variety of factors contributed to this, including adverse effects of prior chemotherapy, radiation, infections, and the effects of the diseases on organ function, such as renal dysfunction in MM. Early non-relapse mortality was substantial for patients with these three disease categories (Table 6.6). In particular, patients over 50 years old with NHL, MM, or CLL tolerated HSCT poorly. Early transplant-related mortality exceeded 40%, and this was further increased in patients over the age of 50 years.

## Conclusions

In summary, it is clear that both autologous and conventional allogeneic HSCT have been carried out only in small minorities of older patients (>50 years) with malignant hematologic diseases. Those who were transplanted were probably highly selected for good performance status, and thus might not be representative of that age group as a whole. Even so, most published series agree

Table 6.6  Day-100 mortality in patients with non-Hodgkin's lymphoma (NHL), multiple myeloma (MM), and chronic lymphocytic leukemia (CLL) who received allografts at the Fred Hutchinson Cancer Research Center

| Disease | Age (years) | No. of patients | Day-100 mortality after allografting (%) |
|---------|-------------|-----------------|------------------------------------------|
| NHL[a]  |             |                 |                                          |
|         | <30         | 92              | 40                                       |
|         | 30–39       | 68              | 41                                       |
|         | 40–49       | 64              | 45.3                                     |
|         | ≥50         | 6               | 33 (83 by day 140)                       |
| MM      |             |                 |                                          |
|         | <50         | 63              | 41                                       |
|         | ≥50         | 18              | 55                                       |
| CLL[a]  |             |                 |                                          |
|         | <50         | 11              | 27                                       |
|         | ≥50         | 5               | 80 (100 by day 139)                      |

[a]HLA-matched related donors only.

that older patients who underwent conventional HSCT had worse overall survivals compared with their younger counterparts. Clearly, age is the single most serious impediment to efforts at broadening the therapeutic usefulness of conventional high-dose HSCT. While the age ceiling will remain for autologous HSCT given that its success depends on disease eradication by high-dose cytotoxic therapy, stronger reliance on the allogeneic graft-versus-tumor (GvT) effect may allow breaking of the age barrier for allogeneic HSCT.

## NON-MYELOABLATIVE ALLOGENEIC HSCT

The toxicities associated with conventional allogeneic HSCT and a better understanding of how to manipulate both host and donor immune functions have led to a radical rethinking of how HSCT might be done in the future. Specifically, the emphasis has shifted away from trying to eradicate malignant cells through high-dose therapy towards using the donor's immune cells to invoke allogeneic GvT effects.

Several groups of investigators have developed less toxic allotransplantation regimens that rely on graft-versus-host (GvH) effects for complete eradication of malignant cells. Two important facts related to HSC allografts led investigators to develop these less toxic strategies. First, some hematologic malignancies cannot be cured even with the most intensive conditioning regimens. Second, HSC allografts play a role beyond the rescue from severe hematopoietic toxicity of the conditioning regimen.[20,21] Specifically, a graft-versus-leukemia (GvL) effect is responsible for many of the observed cures. This GvL effect was predicted from the murine studies of Barnes et al[20] in 1956, and Mathe et al[21] coined the term 'adoptive immunotherapy' for it in 1965. The first landmark papers describing GvL/GvH effects in human allograft recipients were published by Weiden et al[22,23] in 1979 and 1981. Their observations were confirmed by others,[24–28] and led to the testing of donor buffy coat infusions to augment the GvL effect of marrow allografts[29] and the use of donor lymphocyte infusions (DLI) as therapy for patients whose leukemia had relapsed after transplantation.[29–36]

These two facts have guided the development of less toxic allotransplantation regimens. These non-myeloablative approaches can be roughly divided into two categories:

- reduced-intensity conventional cytotoxic regimens;
- pre- and post-transplantation immunosuppression directed at both host and donor immune cells to establish a state of mixed or full donor hematopoietic chimerism.

In both settings, the allografts serve as platforms for subsequent adoptive immunotherapy of the underlying malignancies using DLI.

## Conventional conditioning regimens of moderate intensity

Several groups have taken a more conventional approach to reducing regimen related-toxicity.[37–42] The intensities of the conditioning regimens in their studies have been decreased, but not sufficiently to carry out the HSC transplantation in the ambulatory care setting. Cyclosporine (CSP) alone, CSP combined with prednisone, methotrexate (MTX)/CSP, or MTX/tacrolimus (FK-506) were used for GvHD prophylaxis. The investigators speculated that the decreased intensity of the conditioning might result in mixed chimerism.

Investigators in Houston used fludarabine- or cladribine-containing regimens. Fludarabine/idarubicin/intermediate-dose adenosine arabinoside was used in 15 high-risk patients aged 27–71 years (median 56 years) with myeloid malignancies or fludarabine/dexamethasone/high-dose cytarabine/platinum or fludarabine/cyclophosphamide (CY) in five patients aged 52–60 years (median 56 years) with lymphoid malignancies.[37,39] Some patients received fludarabine combined with melphalan 140 mg/m². Twelve of 15 patients with myeloid malignancies were assessable, and eight had donor-cell engraftment within 30 days of transplantation. Survivals of recipients were poor, and only one patient achieved a sustained complete response. Similar results were reported in patients with advanced lymphoid malignancies,[39] whereas five of 15 patients aged 45–71 years (median 55 years) with less advanced lymphoid malignancies achieved complete remissions with a median follow-up of six months.[40]

A regimen comparable to the one reported from Houston and consisting of CY/fludarabine was used by investigators in Bethesda to treat patients (ages unspecified) with various malignant diseases,[41] and some complete remissions were observed.

Investigators in Jerusalem reported on 26 patients with ages ranging from 1 to 61 years (median 31 years) who underwent peripheral blood stem cell (PBSC) allografts after a preparative regimen of fludarabine (180 mg/m²), busulfan (8 mg/kg), and antithymocyte globulin (ATG) (40 mg/kg).[38] The study included patients with malignancies and three patients with beta-thalassemia, Blackfan–Diamond anemia, and Gaucher's disease. Patients with malignancy had less advanced disease and, as noted above, were younger than the patients who underwent transplantation in the Houston studies. Overall survival in the study was good (with an event-free survival rate of 77.5% at nine months), although four patients died of GvHD, and 13 patients had mild to severe VOD of the liver. The conditioning regimen was described as non-myeloablative, but no evidence to support this contention was presented.

Investigators in Boston used CY, 150–200 mg/kg, along with ATG and thymic irradiation to treat 15 patients with various malignancies and a median age of 34 years (range 20–51 years). GvHD was seen in 10 patients. Seven patients were alive and free of disease progression 27–475 days after transplantation.[42]

Investigators in Genova treated nine patients with lymphoid malignancies, refractory anemia with excess blasts (RAEB), and CML, first by autologous stem cell transplantation.[43] Then, 30–90 days later, patients were given fludarabine and CY followed by allogeneic transplantation. Three of the nine patients were in remission between two and six months later. Three patients experienced GvHD, including two with remissions. Patients were hospitalized for 16–28 days for the allografts.

In these studies, the investigators concentrated on the concept of moderately intense pretransplantation conditioning regimens combined with the use of PBSC to enhance engraftment. A major goal of the studies was to induce a GvL effect and, accordingly, GvHD was seen in a number of patients. The regimens used were accompanied by significant toxicities, including VOD. The regimens used by the investigators were still sufficiently toxic to require inpatient management, and would probably be unsuitable for outpatient care. All the investigators saw complete remissions in some patients, although follow-up is limited. These results support the general concept that future regimens may rely less on intensive cytotoxic therapy and more on allo-immune effects to eradicate malignant cells.

## Pre- and post-transplantation immunosuppression to establish allogeneic HSCT

GvH and host-versus-graft (HvG) reactions are both mediated by T cells in the setting of major histocompatibility complex (MHC)-identical HSCT. This has engendered studies to explore whether postgrafting immunosuppression that is designed to prevent GvHD can simultaneously be used to suppress host immunity, thereby facilitating allogeneic engraftment. Pregrafting host immunosuppression followed by effective postgrafting immunosuppression would allow for creation of marrow space by allogeneic HSCT through GvH reactions. The net effect would be the establishment of mutual graft–host tolerance, as manifested by stable mixed donor–host hematopoietic chimerism. This state of mixed hematopoietic chimerism could serve as a platform for subsequent adoptive immunotherapy by donor lymphocytes.

### Preclinical studies in dogs

A non-myeloablative transplantation model was developed in preclinical canine studies. This model substitutes post-transplant immunosuppression for the intensive cytotoxic pretransplant conditioning therapy in a stepwise fashion.[44,45]

A random-bred dog model has been used to develop many of the clinical HSCT protocols used in Seattle for more than 35 years.[46–48] TBI has been an integral part of many of the conditioning regimens used. Given this and the simplicity with which TBI can be administered, it has played an important role in the development of non-myeloablative transplantation approaches.

Experiments were initiated to evaluate two drugs commonly used for GvHD prevention, CSP and prednisone, following the barely myeloablative dose of 4.5 Gy of TBI.[44] In this and all subsequent canine studies, postgrafting immunosuppression was discontinued no later than 35 days after transplantation. All seven dogs given CSP were stably engrafted without GvHD – a result that was significantly better than that achieved in 17 controls not given CSP ($p = 0.01$). This was consistent with the hypothesis that post-transplant immunosuppression could be used to control both HvG and GvH reactions. A comparable rate of engraftment in dogs not given CSP was seen only after conditioning with 9.2 Gy of TBI. Surprisingly, high-dose prednisone proved completely ineffective in this setting, in that none of the dogs that underwent transplantation had sustained allogeneic engraftment.

The marrow toxicity of various doses of TBI in dogs given intensive supportive care but no rescue by stem cell grafts is shown in Table 6.7. TBI at 200 cGy was shown to be sublethal, and 18 of 19 dogs survived with spontaneous hematopoietic recovery. When the TBI dose was lowered to this sublethal

| Table 6.7  Marrow toxicity of single-dose TBI in dogs not rescued by marrow infusion | |
|---|---|
| TBI (cGy) (7 cGy/min) | No. of dogs surviving/no. of dogs studied |
| 400 (myeloablative and lethal) | 1/28 |
| 300 | 7/21 |
| 200 (sublethal) | 18/19 |
| 100 | 12/12 |

range of 200 cGy, the addition of CSP alone as post-transplant immunosuppression failed to promote allogeneic engraftment (Table 6.8), and dogs rejected their allografts by four weeks but survived with autologous hematopoietic recovery.[45] Next, CSP was combined with the antimetabolite MTX, given that this drug combination is synergistic in preventing GvHD in both dogs and human patients. Two of the six dogs became stable mixed chimeras, three rejected their grafts, and one mixed chimera was unevaluable because of death at eight weeks. Recent studies showed another antimetabolite, mycophenolate mofetil (MMF), combined with CSP to be superior to MTX combined with CSP for GvHD prevention.[49] Accordingly, MMF/CSP was studied for graft enhancement (Table 6.8).[45] Only 1 of 11 dogs studied rejected the allograft after 12 weeks, whereas 10 dogs became stable mixed chimeras for up to 130 weeks after transplantation, without evidence of GvHD.

Figure 6.6 illustrates the peripheral blood cell changes and the microsatellite marker studies in one of these dogs, and shows persistence of both donor- and host-specific bands among marrow, peripheral blood, and lymph node cells after transplantation.[45,50,51] Mixed chimerism was stable in all dogs, and phosphorimaging analysis estimates of donor-cell contributions ranged from 45% to 85%. The least contributions of donor cells were among the $CD4^+$ and $CD8^+$ T cells, and the highest contribution was among granulocytes. Lymph nodes and lymphocytes also showed a lower percentage of donor cells than granulocytes.

Six dogs conditioned with a TBI dose of only 100 cGy followed by MMF/CSP all rejected their marrow grafts within 3–12 weeks after transplantation.[45] This indicated that 100 cGy was below the threshold of pretransplantation immunosuppression needed for sustained engraftment. However, a recent study involving additional treatment by the T-cell costimulation blocker CTLA4-Ig showed that sustained engraftment was possible after only 100 cGy TBI conditioning.[52]

### Table 6.8 Engraftment of dog leukocyte antigen-identical littermate marrow using a sublethal dose of 200 cGy of TBI before transplantation

| Postgrafting immunosuppression[a] | No. of dogs with stable grafts/no. of dogs studied | Mixed chimerism (weeks) |
|---|---|---|
| CSP | 0/4 | 4, 4, 4, 4 |
| MTX/CSP | 3/6 | 2, 7, 11, >8, >134, >134 |
| MMF/CSP | 10/11 | 12, >49, >55, >56, >57, >62, >63, >73, >104, >130, >130 |

[a]Doses were as follows: cyclosporine (CSP) 15 mg/kg twice daily orally on days −1 to 35; methotrexate (MTX) 0.4 mg/kg intravenously on days 1, 3, 6, and 11; mycophendate mofetil (MMF) 10 mg/kg twice daily subcutaneously on days 0 to 27.

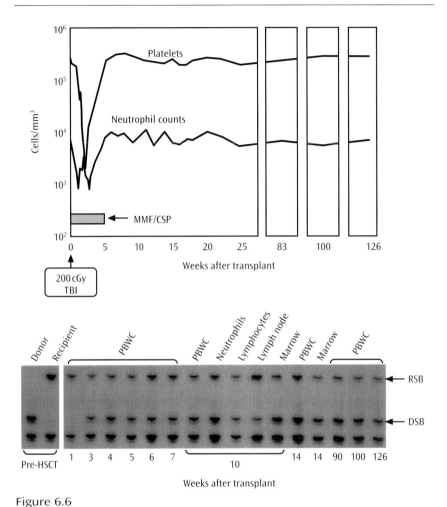

Figure 6.6

Example of stable mixed chimerism: neutrophil count and platelet count changes in dog E219 given 200 cGy of TBI, a marrow graft from a dog leukocyte antigen-identical littermate (E220) on day 0, and postgrafting immunosuppression with mycophenolate mofetil/cyclosporine (MMF/CSP) for more than 35 days. The bottom panel shows the results of testing for microsatellite markers of donor and recipient cells before transplantation (Pre-HSCT) and recipient cells after marrow transplantation (lanes 3–18). (PBWC, peripheral blood white cells; RSB, recipient band; DSB, donor band.) Adapted from Storb et al.[51]

## Allogeneic cell therapy in human patients

Based on the efficacy and lack of toxicity of the non-myeloablative canine transplants, we designed an outpatient allografting protocol for human patients with hematologic malignancies who were more than 50 years of age or who were not conventional HSCT candidates based on medical co-morbidities.[53–55] The goal was to establish mixed chimerism that could serve as a platform for subsequent conversion to complete donor chimerism by DLI (Figure 6.7). DLI was also expected to possess a potential therapeutic utility, given its documented effectiveness in eradicating recurrent malignancy after conventional transplantation, especially in CML, CLL, and MM.[30–36]

In this treatment strategy, pretransplant immunosuppression consisted of TBI 200 cGy delivered as a single fraction at 8 cGy/min, and post-transplant immunosuppression of CSP 6.25 mg/kg twice daily orally from day −1 to day 35, and MMF 15 mg/kg twice daily orally from day 0 to day 27. Granulocyte colony-stimulating factor (G-CSF)-mobilized PBSC from HLA-identical sibling donors were infused on day 0. Chimerism studies (peripheral blood CD3+ T cells, total nucleated bone marrow cells, and peripheral blood granulocytes) were performed on days 28 and 56, and DLI was scheduled for day 65 in those patients with mixed T-cell chimerism.

Of 29 patients transplanted at the FHCRC ($n = 25$) and the Seattle Veterans Administration Hospital ($n = 4$), 27 have been followed for 3–15 months and 2 were within one month of transplant. Diagnoses and patient backgrounds are shown in Table 6.9. Six patients under the age of 50 years were considered ineligible for standard conventional allogeneic HSCT based on medical co-morbidities.

## Engraftment
All patients followed for more than 28 days ($n = 27$) showed mixed donor–host or full donor hematopoietic chimerism by day 28. Ten patients had more than 85% CD3+ T cells of donor origin by day 28, and 18 patients

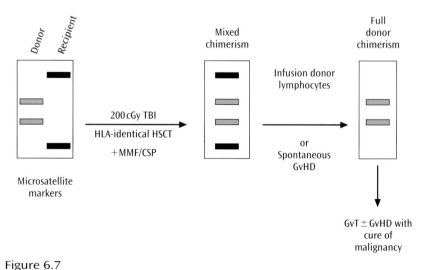

## Figure 6.7
Treatment scheme for patients with malignant hematologic disease by the establishment of mixed chimerism. (MMF/CSP, mycophenolate mofetil/cyclosporine.) Adapted from Storb et al.[51]

## Table 6.9  Background data of patients undergoing non-myeloablative HSCT at the Fred Hutchinson Cancer Research Center

| | No. of patients |
|---|---|
| Age range (years): 31–70 | |
| Decade (years): | |
| 30–39 | 2 |
| 40–49 | 4 |
| 50–59 | 14 |
| 60–69 | 5 |
| 70–79 | 1 |
| Females | 8 |
| Males | 18 |
| Sex-mismatched | 14 |
| Diseases treated:[a] | |
| AML[b] | 4 |
| HD | 3 |
| CLL | 6 |
| CML | 3 |
| MM | 6 |
| WALD | 2 |
| NHL | 1 |
| MDS | 1 |

[a]AML, acute myelogenous leukemia; HD, Hodgkin's disease; CLL, chronic lymphocytic leukemia; CML, chronic myelogenous leukemia; MM, multiple myeloma, WALD, Waldenström's macroglobulinemia; NHL, non-Hodgkin's lymphoma; MDS, myelodysplastic syndrome.
[b]AML patients include treatment-induced aplasia ($n = 1$), 1st complete remission (CR) ($n = 1$), 3rd CR ($n = 1$), MDS/refractory anemia with excess blasts in transformation (RAEB-t) ($n = 1$).

had more than 50% CD3$^+$ donor T-cell engraftment by the same date. Higher degrees of donor engraftment were seen in patients with prior autologous transplants and a history of chemotherapy. The addition of fludarabine (30 mg/m$^2$/day × 3 days) in patients with CML in chronic phase was associated with the first patient attaining full donor chimerism by day 28.

## Rejections

Five patients developed graft rejection (myelodysplastic syndrome (MDS)/refractory anemia with excess blasts in transformation (RAEB-t), $n = 1$; CML, $n = 2$; MM, $n = 2$). All five patients who rejected their grafts had CD3$^+$ T cells less than 50% of donor origin on day 28. Rejection was followed by return to baseline hematologic status in all cases. Graft rejection was associated with a history of little or no prior chemotherapy and multiple transfusions in one case. Because rejections occurred in the initial CML and MM patients, separate modified protocols were written to address this issue. The CML protocol was modified by adding fludarabine to the conditioning regimen, which resulted in full donor chimerism by day 28 in the first patient. Subsequent patients with MM ($n = 4$) underwent autologous transplantation with high-dose melphalan (200 mg/m$^2$), followed 40–120 days later by non-myeloablative allografting. This resulted in more than 90% T-cell engraftment by day 28 post-transplant.

## GvHD

Ten of 27 evaluable patients have developed acute GvHD associated with primary engraftment (before receiving DLI). In all but one, GvHD occurred after discontinuing MMF on day 27. All cases of acute GvHD were grades II–III and were well controlled with corticosteroids. All patients with acute GvHD had CD3$^+$ T cells of greater than 50% donor origin, whereas no patient with less than 50% donor CD3$^+$ T cells developed acute GvHD. GvHD occurred between 30 and 50 days after transplant, except for one patient who developed GvHD at day 125. This patient had CSP maintained through day 110 to allow clearing of a pulmonary fungal infection acquired before transplant.

## Response to treatment

To date, seven patients attained or maintained complete remission during the course of their follow-up: AML ($n = 4$), CLL ($n = 1$), MM ($n = 1$), HD ($n = 1$), and CML ($n = 1$). In other patients, follow-up is too short to allow conclusions regarding remission status. The patient with CLL, a 53-year-old male, had a white blood B-cell count of 70 000/$\mu$L at transplantation, and developed grade II acute GvHD that was associated with the development of full donor T-cell chimerism (Figure 6.8). After tapering of prednisone and CSP, there was a GvL reaction resulting in complete molecular remission in marrow and blood by seven months after transplantation. During the course of his transplant, the patient had no platelet or red blood cell transfusions, and had the procedure performed entirely in an outpatient setting. The case illustrates the potency of the GvL effect and the relative lack of toxicity experienced with allogeneic cell therapy.

## Regimen-related toxicities

None of the patients experienced regimen-induced alopecia or mucositis. The only significant regimen-related toxicity included significant hyperbilirubinemia in two patients. Despite major and minor ABO incompatibilities in several patients, there has been no evidence of overt hemolysis in any patient, although one patient with major ABO incompatibility experienced delayed red blood cell engraftment. Fourteen patients required no platelet transfusions, and nine patients required no red blood cell transfusions during the first 50 days after transplant. Nine patients never became neutropenic during the course of the transplant and 14 of 27 patients had the entire procedure performed in the outpatient setting, with only 3 patients requiring hospitalization for more than one week.

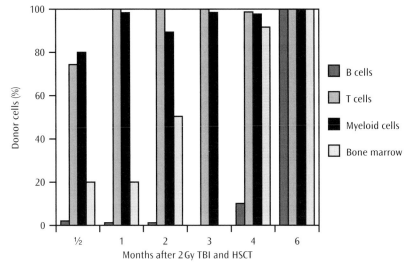

Figure 6.8
Marker studies in a 53-year-old patient with CLL. Results were based on fluorescence in situ hybridization (FISH) analysis for Y- and X-specific microsatellite markers. T and B cells were isolated for analysis by cell sorting. Adapted from Storb.[54]

## Mortality

Despite the older age of this group of patients, only two patients (aged 55 and 53 years) died before day 100 after allografting. The first patient had MM and died of disease progression. The second patient died of a central nervous system hemorrhage. Both patients had acute GvHD. Three other patients, aged 43, 53 and 63 years, died on days 168, 361, and 183, respectively. Causes of death included Gram-positive infection ($n = 1$, CLL), and disease progression ($n = 2$, MDS/RAEB-t, MM).

## Donor lymphocyte infusions

Eight patients have undergone DLI. Two patients evolved to higher degrees of donor chimerism after DLI, although DLI was unable to improve the degree of donor chimerism when patients rejected the donor graft.

## Conclusions

In a patient population with a median age of 56 years, we have demonstrated that allogeneic engraftment is possible without intensive pretransplant conditioning and relying largely on post-transplant immunosuppression to establish the allograft. Furthermore, early responses point to the potency of an allogeneic GvL effect independent of cytoreductive chemoradiotherapy. The establishment of an allograft in a relatively non-toxic and outpatient setting may prove to yield the highest prospect for older patients with hematologic malignancies to achieve permanent cures.

# REFERENCES

1. Sweetenham JW, Pearce R, Philip T et al, High-dose therapy and autologous bone marrow transplantation for intermediate and high grade non-Hodgkin's lymphoma in patients aged 55 years and over: results from the European Group for Bone Marrow Transplantation. *Bone Marrow Transplant* 1994; **14**: 981–7.

2. Cahn JY, Labopin M, Mandelli F et al, Autologous bone marrow transplantation for first remission acute myeloblastic leukemia in patients older than 50 years: a retrospective analysis of the European Bone Marrow Transplant Group. *Blood* 1995; **85**: 575–9.

3. Miller CB, Piantadosi S, Vogelsang GB et al, Impact of age on outcome of patients with cancer undergoing autologous bone marrow transplant. *J Clin Oncol* 1996; **14**: 1327–32.

4. Kusnierz-Glaz CR, Schlegel PG, Wong RM et al, Influence of age on the outcome of 500 autologous bone marrow transplant procedures for hematologic malignancies. *J Clin Oncol* 1997; **15**: 18–25.

5. Thomas ED, Marrow transplantation for malignant diseases (Karnofsky Memorial Lecture). *J Clin Oncol* 1983; **1**: 517–31.

6. Storb R, Prentice RL, Sullivan KM et al, Predictive factors in chronic graft-versus-host disease in patients with aplastic anemia treated by marrow transplantation from HLA-identical siblings. *Ann Intern Med* 1983; **98**: 461–6.

7. Barrett AJ, Horowitz MM, Gale RP et al, Marrow transplantation for acute lymphoblastic leukemia: factors affecting relapse and survival. *Blood* 1989; **74**: 862–71.

8. Goldman JM, Gale RP, Horowitz MM et al, Bone marrow transplantation for chronic myelogenous leukemia in chronic phase: increased risk of relapse associated with T-cell depletion. *Ann Intern Med* 1988; **108**: 806–14.

9. Klingemann H-G, Storb R, Fefer A et al, Bone marrow transplantation in patients aged 45 years and older. *Blood* 1986; **67**: 770–6.

10. Blume KG, Forman SJ, Nademanee AP et al, Bone marrow transplantation for hematologic malignancies in patients aged 30 years or older. *J Clin Oncol* 1986; **4**: 1489–92.

11. Ringdén O, Horowitz MM, Gale RP et al, Outcome after allogeneic bone marrow transplant for leukemia in older adults. *JAMA* 1993; **270**: 57–60.

12. Du W, Dansey R, Abella EM et al, Successful allogeneic bone marrow transplantation in selected patients over 50 years of age – a single institution's experience. *Bone Marrow Transplant* 1998; **21**: 1043–7.

13. Hansen JA, Gooley TA, Martin PJ et al, Bone marrow transplants from unrelated donors for patients with chronic myeloid leukemia. *N Engl J Med* 1998; **338**: 962–8.

14. Cahn J-Y, Labopin M, Schattenberg A et al, Allogeneic bone marrow transplantation for acute leukemia in patients over the age of 40 years. *Leukemia* 1997; **11**: 416–19.

15. Copelan EA, Kapoor N, Berliner M, Tutschka PJ, Bone marrow transplantation without total-body irradiation in patients aged 40 and older. *Transplantation* 1989; **48**: 65–8.

16. Bär BMAM, De Witte T, Schattenberg A et al, Favourable outcome of patients older than 40 years of age after transplantation with marrow grafts depleted of lymphocytes by counterflow centrifugation. *Br J Haematol* 1990; **74**: 53–60.

17. Rapoport AP, DiPersio JF, Martin BA et al, Patients ≥age 40 years undergoing autologous or allogeneic BMT have regimen-related mortality rates and event-free survivals comparable to patients <age 40 years. *Bone Marrow Transplant* 1995; **15**: 523–30.

18. Clift RA, Buckner CD, Storb R et al, The influence of patient age on the outcome of transplantation during chronic

phase (CP) of chronic myeloid leukemia (CML). *Blood* 1995; **86**: 617a.

19. Thomas ED, Clift RA, Allogeneic transplantation for chronic myeloid leukemia. In: *Hematopoietic Cell Transplantation*, 2nd edn (Thomas ED, Blume KG, Forman SJ, eds). Blackwell Science: Boston, 1999: 806–16.

20. Barnes DWH, Corp MJ, Loutit JF, Neal FE, Treatment of murine leukaemia with x-rays and homologous bone marrow. Preliminary communication. *BMJ* 1956; **2**: 626–7.

21. Mathe G, Amiel JL, Schwarzenberg L et al, Adoptive immunotherapy of acute leukemia: experimental and clinical results. *Cancer Res* 1965; **25**: 1525–31.

22. Weiden PL, Flournoy N, Thomas ED et al, Antileukemic effect of graft-versus-host disease in human recipients of allogeneic-marrow grafts. *N Engl J Med* 1979; **300**: 1068–73.

23. Weiden PL, Sullivan KM, Flournoy N et al, Antileukemic effect of chronic graft-versus-host disease. Contribution to improved survival after allogeneic marrow transplantation. *N Engl J Med* 1981; **304**: 1529–33.

24. Horowitz MM, Gale RP, Sondel PM et al, Graft-versus-leukemia reactions after bone marrow transplantation. *Blood* 1990; **75**: 555–62.

25. Butturini A, Bortin MM, Gale RP, Graft-versus-leukemia following bone marrow transplantation. *Bone Marrow Transplant* 1987; **2**: 233–42.

26. Kersey JH, Weisdorf D, Nesbit ME et al, Comparison of autologous and allogeneic bone marrow transplantation for treatment of high-risk refractory acute lymphoblastic leukemia. *N Engl J Med* 1987; **317**: 461–7.

27. Weisdorf DJ, Nesbit ME, Ramsay NKC et al, Allogeneic bone marrow transplantation for acute lymphoblastic leukemia in remission: prolonged survival associated with acute graft-versus-host disease. *J Clin Oncol* 1987; **5**: 1348–55.

28. Sullivan KM, Weiden PL, Storb R et al, Influence of acute and chronic graft-versus-host disease on relapse and survival after bone marrow transplantation from HLA-identical siblings as treatment of acute and chronic leukemia. *Blood* 1989; **73**: 1720–8.

29. Sullivan KM, Storb R, Buckner CD et al, Graft-versus-host disease as adoptive immunotherapy in patients with advanced hematologic neoplasms. *N Engl J Med* 1989; **320**: 828–34.

30. Kolb HJ, Mittermüller J, Clemm Ch et al, Donor leukocyte transfusions for treatment of recurrent chronic myelogenous leukemia in marrow transplant patients. *Blood* 1990; **76**: 2462–5.

31. Porter DL, Roth MS, McGarigle C et al, Induction of graft-versus-host disease as immunotherapy for relapsed chronic myeloid leukemia. *N Engl J Med* 1994; **330**: 100–6.

32. Kolb HJ, Schattenberg A, Goldman JM et al, Graft-versus-leukemia effect of donor lymphocyte transfusions in marrow grafted patients. European Group for Blood and Marrow Transplantation Working Party on Chronic Leukemia. *Blood* 1995; **86**: 2041–50.

33. Slavin S, Ackerstein A, Naparstek E et al, Hypothesis. The graft-versus-leukemia (GVL) phenomenon: Is GVL separable from GVHD? *Bone Marrow Transplant* 1990; **6**: 155–61.

34. Mackinnon S, Papadopoulos EB, Carabasi MH et al, Adoptive immunotherapy evaluating escalating doses of donor leukocytes for relapse of chronic myeloid leukemia after bone marrow transplantation: separation of graft-versus-leukemia responses from graft-versus-host disease. *Blood* 1995; **86**: 1261–8.

35. Giralt S, Hester J, Huh Y et al, CD8-depleted donor lymphocyte infusion as treatment for relapsed chronic myelogenous leukemia after allogeneic bone marrow transplantation. *Blood* 1995; **86**: 4337–43.

36. Collins RH Jr, Shpilberg O, Drobyski WR et al, Donor leukocyte infusions in 140 patients with relapsed malignancy after allogeneic bone marrow transplantation. *J Clin Oncol* 1997; **15**: 433–44.

37. Giralt S, Estey E, Albitar M et al, Engraftment of allogeneic hematopoietic progenitor cells with purine analog-containing chemotherapy: harnessing graft-versus-leukemia without myeloablative therapy. *Blood* 1997; **89:** 4531–6.

38. Slavin S, Nagler A, Naparstek E et al, Nonmyeloablative stem cell transplantation and cell therapy as an alternative to conventional bone marrow transplantation with lethal cytoreduction for the treatment of malignant and nonmalignant hematologic diseases. *Blood* 1998; **91:** 756–63.

39. Khouri I, Keating MJ, Przepiorka D et al, Engraftment and induction of GVL with fludarabine (FAMP)-based nonablative preparative regimen in patients with chronic lymphocytic leukemia (CLL) and lymphoma. *Blood* 1996; **88:** 301a.

40. Khouri IF, Keating M, Körbling M et al, Transplant-lite: induction of graft-versus-malignancy using fludarabine-based nonablative chemotherapy and allogeneic blood progenitor-cell transplantation as treatment for lymphoid malignancies. *J Clin Oncol* 1998; **16:** 2817–24.

41. Childs R, Clave E, Bahceci E et al, Kinetics of engraftment in non-myeloablative allogeneic peripheral blood stem cell transplants: an analysis of hematopoietic-lineage chimerism. *Blood* 1998; **92**(Suppl 1): 520a.

42. Spitzer TR, McAfee SL, Sackstein R et al, Induction of mixed chimerism and potent anti-tumor responses following non-myeloablative conditioning therapy and HLA-matched and mismatched donor bone marrow transplantation (BMT) for refractory hematologic malignancies (HM). *Blood* 1998; **92**(Suppl 1): 519a.

43. Carella AM, Lerma E, Dejana A et al, Engraftment of HLA-matched sibling hematopoietic stem cells after immunosuppressive conditioning regimen in patients with hematologic neoplasias. *Haematologica* 1998; **83:** 904–9.

44. Yu C, Storb R, Mathey B et al, DLA-identical bone marrow grafts after low-dose total body irradiation: effects of high-dose corticosteroids and cyclosporine on engraftment. *Blood* 1995; **86:** 4376–81.

45. Storb R, Yu C, Wagner JL et al, Stable mixed hematopoietic chimerism in DLA-identical littermate dogs given sublethal total body irradiation before and pharmacological immunosuppression after marrow transplantation. *Blood* 1997; **89:** 3048–54.

46. Deeg HJ, Storb R, Canine marrow transplantation models. *Curr Top Vet Res* 1994; **1:** 103–14.

47. Georges GE, Sandmaier BM, Storb R, Animal models. In: *Blood Stem Cell Transplantation* (Reiffers J, Goldman J, Armitage J, eds). Martin Dunitz: London, 1998: 1–17.

48. Wagner JL, Storb R, Preclinical large animal models for hematopoietic stem cell transplantation. *Curr Opin Hematol* 1996; **3:** 410–15.

49. Yu C, Seidel K, Nash RA et al, Synergism between mycophenolate mofetil and cyclosporine in preventing graft-versus-host disease among lethally irradiated dogs given DLA-nonidentical unrelated marrow grafts. *Blood* 1998; **91:** 2581–7.

50. Yu C, Ostrander E, Bryant E et al, Use of $(CA)_n$ polymorphisms to determine the origin of blood cells after allogeneic canine marrow grafting. *Transplantation* 1994; **58:** 701–6.

51. Storb R, Yu C, McSweeney P et al, New strategies for hematopoietic stem cell transplantation. In: *Transplantation in Hematology and Oncology* (Bücher Th et al, eds). Springer-Verlag: Berlin, 2000: 97–111.

52. Storb R, Yu C, Zaucha JM et al, Stable mixed hematopoietic chimerism in dogs given donor antigen, CTLA4Ig, and 100 cGy TBI before and pharmacological immunosuppression after marrow transplant. *Blood* 1999; **94:** 2523–9.

53. McSweeney PA, Wagner JL, Maloney DG et al, Outpatient PBSC allografts using immunosuppression with low-dose TBI before, and cyclosporine (CSP) and mycophenolate mofetil (MMF) after transplant. *Blood* 1998; **92**(Suppl 1): 519a.

54. Storb R, Nonmyeloablative preparative regimens: experimental data and clinical practice. In: *Educational Book, 55th Annual Meeting, Am Soc Clin Oncol, May 15–18, 1999, Atlanta, GA* (Perry MC, ed). 241–9.

55. Storb R, Yu C, McSweeney P, Mixed chimerism after transplantation of allogeneic hematopoietic cells. In: *Hematopoietic Cell Transplantation*, 2nd edn (Thomas ED, Blume KG, Forman SJ, eds). Blackwell Science: Boston, 1999: 287–95.

# 7
# The role of the bone marrow microenvironment in hematopoietic stem cell transplantation

Rodolfo Quarto, Maria Galotto, Andrea Banfi,
Ranieri Cancedda, Giovanni Berisso,
Annamaria Raiola, Andrea Bacigalupo

## INTRODUCTION

In the bone marrow cavity, hematopoiesis occurs in association with a variety of functionally and phenotypically different cell types, which form the bone marrow stromal network.[1,2] Endothelial cells, adipocytes, smooth muscle cells, reticular cells and osteoblasts are included in this system.[3-6] One specific cellular population, namely the stromal fibroblasts, is the cellular component of the microenvironmental network directly involved in the regulation and support of hematopoiesis.[3,7] These cells often are referred to as CFU-f (colony-forming units fibroblast) because of their growth properties in vitro, or mesenchymal stem cells, since they cells have the capability of differentiating into other mesenchymal tissues such as bone, cartilage, and fat.[8-12]

In the 'red' marrow, hematopoietic stem cells, progenitors and precursors are both sustained by cytokines elaborated by stromal cells as well as being supported mechanically by direct contact with surfaces provided by the stromal cells.[13,14] The latter property is a peculiar feature of bone marrow, in which the support is of a cellular nature rather than by an extracellular matrix, such as the collageneous scaffolding present in other organs. Thus the bone marrow stroma is a complex interactive network of cells and cell-derived signals influencing the commitment, differentiation and proliferation of hematopoietic cells.

High-dose chemotherapy with or without total-body irradiation followed by hematopoietic stem cell transplantation is increasingly used for the treatment of both hematologic and solid neoplasms. One of the major points of controversy in transplantation is the effect of the cytotoxic regimens on bone marrow fibroblasts and the marrow microenvironment in the engraftment of donor hematopoietic stem cells. Knowledge of early and late consequences of cytotoxic therapy on the marrow microenvironment is still lacking. Marrow stroma, which constitutes the optimal environment for hematopoietic regeneration, is damaged by high-dose cytotoxic therapy and by radiation exposure.[15–19] Little information is available on the extent of this damage and on the repairability of the stroma.[20] An important question is whether such damage may affect the engraftment of hematopoietic stem cells and the consequent recovery of hematopoietic functions.

## BONE MARROW STROMAL CELLS AND HEMATOPOIETIC RECOVERY

Marrow stromal fibroblasts, owing to their very low turnover rate in vivo, are less radiosensitive than hematopoietic stem cells, and thus would be expected to be relatively more resistant to myeloablative treatments.[21] Many authors have studied the fate of the stromal compartment in hematopoietic stem cell transplantation, and have demonstrated that after high-dose cytotoxic therapy and/or radiation exposure the marrow microenvironment can be seriously damaged.[15–20] One of the variables to be considered in these studies is the pretransplant status of the stromal compartment. No studies have addressed the influence of the underlying hematologic malignancy on CFU-f frequency. Most patients undergo transplantation after the microenvironmental status has already been compromised by previous therapy or by neoplastic marrow invasion.[20,22–24] Further stromal microenvironmental damage has been demonstrated to occur soon after the pretransplant conditioning.[20]

The injury to marrow stroma appears to be significant and irreversible: in fact, several years after transplantation, residual CFU-f barely reach a frequency equal to 10% of the normal age-matched controls.[20] Only in very young patients (less than 4 years of age) can such damage apparently be repaired, since recovery to normal levels can be observed.[20] The marrow microenvironment is also qualitatively damaged, resulting in a decreased capacity to support early hematopoiesis and to secrete cytokines.[25] These effects are reflected by a decrease in long-term culture-initiating cell (LTC-IC) frequency, concomitant with a significant reduction in CFU-f frequency.[20,26]

Marrow fibroblasts do not proliferate in vivo under steady-state conditions, making these cells relatively radioresistant. Osteomedullar biopsies of grafted patients, after an initial period of marrow aplasia, however, do not display significant histologic alterations of the marrow architecture. On the other hand, marrow stroma after hematopoietic stem cell transplantation is both quantitatively and qualitatively defective. In vitro studies show decreased normal hematopoietic cell proliferation when cultured on expanded stromal layers obtained from patients, and marrow fibroblasts may be damaged in their ability to proliferate and elaborate CFU-f. As a result, hematopoietic function (peripheral blood counts) may be abnormal in many patients after transplant. In a recent study, Lamparelli and co-workers[27] have shown that platelet counts remain very low in patients grafted from unrelated donors, especially in those patients with acute graft-versus-host disease (GvHD) or with cytomegalovirus (CMV) infections.[27] Therefore hematopoietic function is subnormal after transplant, but is worsened dramatically in the setting of adverse events.

## POSSIBLE CONSEQUENCES OF HEMATOPOIETIC STEM CELL TRANSPLANTATION ON OTHER TISSUES: BONE

Besides sustaining hematopoiesis,[3,7] CFU-fs also represent a progenitor compartment for endosteal osteoblasts.[8–12] One can expect that damage to this cellular compartment might also have consequences for endosteal bone tissue turnover. There is a relationship between a decrease in CFU-f frequency, advancing age, and osteoporosis outcome.[20,28–30] In transplant patients, osteoporosis has generally been attributed to secondary hypogonadism[31] or to post-transplant chemotherapy.[32,33] In one study, an early decrease in bone mineral density in eugonadic transplant patients has been reported.[34] Furthermore, Galotto and co-workers[20] reported a 20% reduction in bone mineral density and a concomitant decrease of about 90% of CFU-f values in a group of male eugonadic transplant patients (18–40 years old), who were in apparent remission and for whom at least 18 months had elapsed since completion of treatment with cyclosporine and/or corticosteroids.

## IN VITRO PROLIFERATION POTENTIAL OF BONE MARROW STROMAL CELLS

A number of studies have shown that the stromal component of the bone marrow, and in particular the stromal fibroblasts, can be isolated from small marrow samples (5–10 ml).[9,35,36] Upon isolation in culture, these cells generate colonies of fibroblast-like cells (hence their designation as colony-forming units fibroblast, CFU-f). They can be extensively expanded in vitro, yet retain the characteristic features of the original population.[9,35–37] Their phenotype, proliferation, and differentiation potential can be modulated by the action of growth factors, cytokines, and hormones supplemented in the culture medium.[36,38–42] After ex vivo expansion, these cells can be assayed for their differentiation potential either in vitro, using appropriate sets of phenotypic markers or in vivo by means of defined transplantation assays.[28,36,43] The importance of this unique cell population can be determined further using these assays.

## TRANSPLANTATION OF BONE MARROW STROMAL CELLS IN ANIMAL MODELS

The discovery of the enormous potential of stromal cells has prompted increasing attention over the past few years as important potential tools for the development of novel therapeutic approaches in a variety of disorders, including somatic cell therapy and gene therapy.[44–49] Using stromal cells into which a reporter gene has been introduced, it has been possible to investigate the fate of these cells following intravenous infusion. The cells apparently migrate, since after infusion they have been detected in several tissues and organs such as bone marrow, bone, cartilage, lung, spleen, etc.[50,51]

Donor marrow stromal cells have been shown physiologically to contribute to hematopoietic stem cell reconstitution after marrow transplantation. Using a stable clonal stromal cell line (GB1/6) expressing the 'a' isoenzyme of glucose-6-phosphate isomerase (Glu6PI-a), Anklesaria and co-workers[52] have demonstrated that 'conditioned' mice transplanted with culture-expanded GB1/6 cells had detectable Glu6PI-a stromal cells in marrow sinuses. These authors also demonstrated a significantly enhanced hematopoietic recovery in GB1/6-transplanted mice compared with non-stroma-transplanted 'control' mice.[52] Furthermore, marrow cultures derived from stroma-transplanted mice demonstrated Glu6PI-a$^+$ CFU-f and higher production of multipotential stem cells of recipient origin compared with cultures established from irradiated, non-transplanted control mice.[52]

Nolta and co-workers[53] used a cotransplantation system in which human CD34$^+$ progenitor cells, transduced with a reporter gene, were transplanted into immunodeficient mice together with primary human bone marrow stromal cells engineered to express human interleukin-3 (IL-3). In this experimental model, these authors have shown the persistence of circulating levels of human IL-3 for at least four months in the transplanted mice. Furthermore, IL-3-secreting stroma, but not control stroma, were shown to support human hematopoiesis from the cotransplanted human CD34$^+$ progenitors for up to nine months.[53]

These data from animal models demonstrate that stromal cells can be transplanted successfully, and that upon intravenous infusion they are detected in their natural site (bone marrow, bone, cartilage, spleen, etc.). They also suggest a possible therapeutic use of the marrow stromal cells to support reconstitution of hematopoiesis after hematopoietic stem cell transplantation. Finally, the use of gene transfer techniques to 'custom-engineer' bone marrow stromal cells can further improve and extend their potential application.

## TRANSPLANTATION OF BONE MARROW STROMAL CELLS IN HUMANS

In the course of a clinical bone marrow transplant, the intravenous infusion of marrow nucleated cells provides patients with hematopoietic stem cells required for the functional recovery of hematopoiesis. At the same time, a small number of marrow stromal cells are infused as well. The number of stromal cells infused appears to be too small to allow significant colonization of the recipient marrow and the consequent recovery of microenvironmental function. It is even questionable whether the stromal cells administered to the patient during a bone marrow transplant could be detected in the recipient marrow. In fact, the origin of CFU-f after transplantation has been the subject of several controversial studies.[20,54–58] Although our own data indicate that after marrow transplantation residual CFU-f originate from the recipient,[20] the possibility of a small percentage of donor CFU-f engrafting in the host marrow cannot be completely ruled out. Recently, Horwitz and co-workers[49] demonstrated donor osteoblast engraftment after bone marrow transplant in two out of three children with osteogenesis imperfecta. Their experimental evidence implies that, although undetectable, donor CFU-f engraftment does occur, and donor progenitors can give rise to detectable osteoblast progeny. Finally other authors have demonstrated that these cells are indeed transplantable when infused in appropriate numbers.[48,50,51]

Stromal transplants in humans have already been conducted 'de facto'. Patients with chronic myeloid leukemia[59] or acute myeloid leukemia[60] receiving autografts of marrow cells cultured long term ex vivo may receive as many as $3 \times 10^8$ stromal cells. In a true phase I study of stromal cell expansion and infusion, Lazarus and associates[48] reported on 13 'unconditioned' patients receiving escalating doses up to $5 \times 10^7$ stromal cells without side-effects due to the infusion. With the feasibility and safety of stromal cell transplantation, having demonstrated a number of clinical trials have now been initiated.

## CONCLUSIONS

In conclusion, the stromal microenvironment, and in particular the fibroblast component, is severely and irreversibly damaged in adult recipients of hematopoietic stem cell transplants. The marrow microenvironment does not display the ability to repair the injury suffered. Only in very young patients is the marrow stroma capable of self-regeneration potential. In conventional bone marrow transplantation, the dose of donor CFU-f infused together with collected bone marrow is limited, and the percentage of stromal cells homing to the marrow cavity appears to be insufficient to provide detectable colonization of the host marrow space. Residual post-bone marrow transplant stroma appears to be altered in its intrinsic ability to support hematopoiesis. A qualitatively and quantitatively altered microenvironment may not be able to support optimally the full colonization of the marrow space by hematopoietic early progenitors. Finally, medium- and long-term consequences such as osteopenia may be observed in other tissues such as bone.

On the other hand, marrow stromal cells can be easily obtained and extensively expanded in vitro. It has been shown that when culture-expanded stromal cells are intravenously infused, they are well tolerated and do not provoke any toxicity to the recipient organism. Since ex vivo expanded CFU-f are transplantable, it is tempting to entertain the possibility of a clinical use of stromal cells to better support hematopoietic reconstitution after bone marrow transplantation, and for correction or prevention of bone or other stromal disorders.

# REFERENCES

1. Weiss L, The hematopoietic microenvironment of the bone marrow: an ultrastructural study of the stroma in rats. *Anat Rec* 1976; **186**: 161–84.

2. Lichtman MA, The ultrastructure of the hemopoietic environment of the marrow: a review. *Exp Hematol* 1981; **9**: 391–410.

3. Dexter TM, Allen TD, Lajtha LG, Conditions controlling the proliferation of haemopoietic stem cells in vitro. *J Cell Physiol* 1977; **91**: 335–44.

4. Allen TD, Dexter TM, Simmons PJ, Marrow biology and stem cells. *Immunol Ser* 1990; **49**: 1–38.

5. Charbord P, Gown AM, Keating A, Singer JW, CGA-7 and HHF, two monoclonal antibodies that recognize muscle actin and react with adherent cells in human long-term bone marrow cultures. *Blood* 1985; **66**: 1138–42.

6. Strobel ES, Gay RE, Greenberg PL, Characterization of the in vitro stromal microenvironment of human bone marrow. *Int J Cell Cloning* 1986; **4**: 341–56.

7. Dexter TM, Spooncer E, Simmons P, Allen TD, Long-term marrow culture: an overview of techniques and experience. *Kroc Found Ser* 1984; **18**: 57–96.

8. Beresford J, Osteogenic stem cells and the stromal system of bone and marrow. *Clin Orthop Rel Res* 1989; **240**: 270–80.

9. Friedenstein AJ, Osteogenic stem cells in the bone marrow. *Bone Miner Res* 1990; **7**: 243–72.

10. Bennett JH, Joyner CJ, Triffitt JT, Owen ME, Adipocytic cells cultured from marrow have osteogenic potential. *J Cell Sci* 1991; **99**: 131–9.

11. Kuznetsov SA, Krebsbach PH, Satomura K et al, Single-colony derived strains of human marrow stromal fibroblasts form bone after transplantation in vivo. *J Bone Miner Res* 1997; **12**: 1335–47.

12. Pittenger MF, Mackay AM, Beck SC et al, Multilineage potential of adult human mesenchymal stem cells. *Science* 1999; **284**: 143–7.

13. Haynesworth SE, Baber MA, Caplan AI, Cytokine expression by human marrow-derived mesenchymal progenitor cells in vitro: effects of dexamethasone and IL-1. *J Cell Physiol* 1996; **166**: 585–92.

14. Bhatia R, Direct contact with stroma or fibronectin leads to enhanced maintenance and reduced apoptosis of primitive hematopoietic progenitors. *Blood* 1998; **92**(Suppl 2): 168b (Abst 3706).

15. Fried W, Kedo A, Barone J, Effects of cyclophosphamide and of busulfan on spleen colony-forming units and on hematopoietic stroma. *Cancer Res* 1977; **37**: 1205–9.

16. Fried W, Barone J, Residual marrow damage following therapy with cyclophosphamide. *Exp Hematol* 1980; **8**: 610–14.

17. Piersma AH, Ploemacher RE, Brockbank KG. Radiation damage to femoral hemopoietic stroma measured by implant regeneration and quantitation of fibroblastic progenitors. *Exp Hematol* 1983; **11**: 884–90.

18. Tavassoli M, Friedenstein A, Hemopoietic stromal microenvironment. *Am J Hematol* 1983; **15**: 195–203.

19. del Cañizo C, Lopez N, Caballero D et al, Haematopoietic damage persists 1 year after autologous peripheral blood stem cell transplantation. *Bone Marrow Transplant* 1999; **23**: 901–5.

20. Galotto M, Berisso G, Delfino L et al, Stromal damage as consequence of high dose chemo/radio therapy in bone marrow transplant recipients. *Exp Hematol* 1999; **27**: 1460–6.

21. Patt HM, Maloney MA, Bone marrow regeneration after local injury: a review. *Exp Hematol* 1975; **3**: 135–48.

22. Radford JA, Testa NG, Crowther D, The long-term effects of MVPP chemotherapy for Hodgkin's disease on bone marrow function. *Br J Cancer* 1990; **62**: 127–32.

23. Soligo DA, Lambertenghi Deliliers G,

Servida F et al, Haematopoietic abnormalities after autologous stem cell transplantation in lymphoma patients. *Bone Marrow Transplant* 1998; **21**: 15–22.

24. Del Canizo M, Lopez N, Vazquez L et al, Hematopoietic damage prior to PBSCT and its influence on hematopoietic recovery. *Haematologica* 1999; **84**: 511–16.

25. Domenech J, Roingeard F, Herault O et al, Changes in the functional capacity of marrow stromal cells after autologous bone marrow transplantation. *Leuk Lymphoma* 1998; **29**: 533–46.

26. Podesta' M, Piaggio G, Frassoni F et al, Deficient reconstitution of early progenitors after allogeneic bone marrow transplantation. *Bone Marrow Transplant* 1997; **19**: 1011–17.

27. Lamparelli T, Van Lint MT, Gualandi F et al, Bone marrow transplantation for chronic myeloid leukemia (CML) from unrelated and sibling donors: single center experience. *Bone Marrow Transplant* 1997; **20**: 1057–62.

28. Haynesworth SE, Goshima J, Goldberg VM, Caplan AI, Characterization of cells with osteogenic potential from human marrow. *Bone* 1992; **13**: 81–8.

29. Egrise D, Martin D, Vienne A et al, The number of fibroblastic colonies formed from bone marrow is decreased and the in vitro proliferation rate of trabecular bone cells increased in aged rats. *Bone* 1992; **13**: 355–61.

30. Quarto R, Thomas D, Liang CT, Bone progenitor cell deficits and the age-associated decline in bone repair capacity. *Calcif Tissue Int* 1995; **56**: 123–9.

31. Castaneda S, Carmona L, Carvajal I et al, Reduction of bone mass in women after bone marrow transplantation. *Calcif Tissue Int* 1997; **60**: 343–7.

32. Withold W, Wolf HH, Kollbach S et al, Monitoring of bone metabolism after bone marrow transplantation by measuring two different markers of bone turnover. *Eur J Clin Chem Clin Biochem* 1996; **34**: 193–7.

33. Stern JM, Chesnut CH 3rd, Bruemmer B et al, Bone density loss during treatment of chronic GVHD. *Bone Marrow Transplant* 1996; **17**: 395–400.

34. Kelly PJ, Atkinson K, Ward RL et al, Reduced bone mineral density in men and women with allogeneic bone marrow transplantation. *Transplantation* 1990; **50**: 881–3.

35. Goshima J, Golberg VM, Caplan AI, The osteogenic potential of cultured-expanded rat marrow mesenchymal cells assayed in vivo in calcium phosphate ceramic blocks. *Clin Orthop* 1991; **262**: 298–311.

36. Martin I, Muraglia A, Campanile G et al, Fibroblast growth factor-2 supports ex vivo expansion and maintenance of osteogenic precursors from human bone marrow. *Endocrinology* 1997; **138**: 4456–62.

37. Bruder SP, Jaiswal N, Haynesworth SE, Growth kinetics, self-renewal, and the osteogenic potential of purified human mesenchymal stem cells during extensive subcultivation and following cryopreservation. *J Cell Biochem* 1997; **64**: 278–94.

38. Rodan SB, Wesolowski G, Thomas KA et al, Effects of acidic and basic fibroblast growth factors on osteoblastic cells. *Connect Tissue Res* 1989; **20**: 283–8.

39. Gronthos S, Simmons PJ. The growth factor requirements of STRO-1-positive human bone marrow stromal precursors under serum-deprived conditions in vitro. *Blood* 1995; **85**: 929–40.

40. Lennon DP, Haynesworth SE, Young RG et al, A chemically defined medium supports in vitro proliferation and maintains the osteochondral potential of rat marrow-derived mesenchymal stem cells. *Exp Cell Res* 1995; **219**: 211–22.

41. Robinson D, Bab I, Nevo Z, Osteogenic growth peptide regulates proliferation and osteogenic maturation of human and rabbit bone marrow stromal cells. *J Bone Miner Res* 1995; **10**: 690–6.

42. Locklin RM, Williamson MC, Beresford JN et al, In vitro effects of growth factors and dexamethasone on rat marrow stromal cells. *Clin Orthop* 1995; **313**: 27–35.

43. Krebsbach PH, Kuznetsov SA, Satomura K et al, Bone formation in vivo: comparison of osteogenesis by transplanted mouse and human marrow stromal fibroblasts. Transplantation 1997; 63: 1059–69.

44. Krebsbach PH, Mankani MH, Satomura K et al, Repair of craniotomy defects using bone marrow stromal cells. Transplantation 1998; 66: 1272–8.

45. Kadiyala S, Kraus KH, Bruder SP, Canine mesenchymal stem cell-based therapy for the regeneration of bone. Trans Tissue Eng Soc 1996; 1: 20.

46. Kadiyala S, Jaiswal N, Bruder SP, Culture-expanded, bone marrow-derived mesenchymal stem cells can regenerate a critical-sized segmental bone defect. Tissue Eng 1997; 3: 173–85.

47. Bruder SP, Kraus KH, Goldberg VM, Kadiyala S, The effect of implants loaded with autologous mesenchymal stem cells on the healing of canine segmental bone defects. J Bone Joint Surg 1998; 80: 985–96.

48. Lazarus HM, Haynesworth SE, Gerson SL et al, Ex vivo expansion and subsequent infusion of human bone marrow-derived stromal progenitor cells (mesenchymal progenitor cells): implications for therapeutic use. Bone Marrow Transplant 1995; 16: 557–64.

49. Horwitz EM, Prockop DJ, Fitzpatrick LA et al, Transplantability and therapeutic effects of bone marrow-derived mesenchymal cells in children with osteogenesis imperfecta. Nature Med 1999; 5: 309–13.

50. Piersma AH, Ploemacher RE, Brockbank KG, Transplantation of bone marrow fibroblastoid stromal cells in mice via the intravenous route. Br J Haematol 1983; 54: 285–90.

51. Pereira RF, Halford KW, O'Hara MD et al, Cultured adherent cells from marrow can serve as long-lasting precursor cells for bone, cartilage, and lung in irradiated mice. Proc Natl Acad Sci USA 1995; 92: 4857–61.

52. Anklesaria P, Kase K, Glowacki J et al, Engraftment of a clonal bone marrow stromal cell line in vivo stimulates hematopoietic recovery from total body irradiation. Proc Natl Acad Sci USA 1987; 84: 7681–5.

53. Nolta JA, Hanley MB, Kohn DB, Sustained human hematopoiesis in immunodeficient mice by cotransplantation of marrow stroma expressing human interleukin-3: analysis of gene transduction of long-lived progenitors. Blood 1994; 83: 3041–51.

54. Golde DW, Hocking WG, Quan SG et al, Origin of human bone marrow fibroblasts. Br J Haematol 1980; 44: 183–7.

55. Keating A, Singer JW, Killen PD et al, Donor origin of the in vitro haematopoietic microenvironment after marrow transplantation in man. Nature 1982; 298: 280–3.

56. Simmons PJ, Przepiorka D, Thomas ED, Torok-Storb B, Host origin of marrow stromal cells following allogeneic bone marrow transplantation. Nature 1987; 328: 429–32.

57. Agematsu K, Nakahori Y, Recipient origin of bone marrow-derived fibroblastic stromal cells during all periods following bone marrow transplantation in humans. Br J Haematol 1991; 79: 359–65.

58. Santucci MA, Trabetti E, Martinelli G et al, Host origin of bone marrow fibroblasts following allogeneic bone marrow transplantation for chronic myeloid leukemia. Bone Marrow Transplant 1992; 10: 255–9.

59. Barnett MJ, Eaves CJ, Phillips GL et al, Successful autografting in chronic myeloid leukaemia after maintenance of marrow in culture. Bone Marrow Transplant 1989; 4: 345–51.

60. Chang J, Coutinho L, Morgenstern G et al, Reconstitution of haemopoietic system with autologous marrow taken during relapse of acute myeloblastic leukaemia and grown in long-term culture. Lancet 1986; i: 294–5.

# 8

# The status of gene transfer in clinical hematopoietic stem cell transplantation

Christof von Kalle and Roland Mertelsmann

## INTRODUCTION

Since the arrival of the concept of somatic gene therapy, the hematopoietic system has been the most extensively studied target organ for transferring genetic information in attempts to treat and cure human disease at the molecular level (for reviews, see references 1–3). Of the motivations for focusing on hematopoiesis in this respect, three are the most prominent.

First, the hematopoietic system supplies every cell type of the blood-forming and immune systems. It is therefore vitally important for the function of every organ, and defines the biological 'self' of an individual. In addition, as discovered more recently, cells from the bone marrow contribute to different body tissues beyond their previously conceived limits of activity, supplying regenerating stem cells to the vasculature,[4] liver,[5] muscle,[6] and brain (for a review, see reference 7).

Second, the hematopoietic system is the most readily accessible organ of the body. Differentiated peripheral blood cells as well as bone-marrow-derived progenitor cells can be harvested from an organism with very little trauma. Even the direct quantitative harvest of bone marrow sufficient for replacing an entire human's hematopoietic system has few side-effects and is considered a minor surgical procedure.

Third, according to our current understanding, the marrow of an adult human contains a finite number of stem cells with both functional and proliferate plasticity capable of generating vast numbers of progeny cells of many different lineages (for reviews, see references 8 and 9). This supposedly pluripotent hierarchic derivation and their limited number makes stem cells an ideal target for the stable transfer of therapeutic genes. Successful gene transfer in stem cells can achieve the presence of the transgene in a vast number of differentiated progeny leukocytes[10] and, potentially, differentiated regenerating cells in other organ systems.

This concept of stable stem cell gene transfer has been very successful in preclinical mouse models using murine leukemia retrovirus (MLV)-derived ectotropic vector systems. It could be demonstrated that the murine blood-forming system could be repopulated with a very limited number of stem cells.[11] By preselecting the transplant for transgene expression, gene transfer by murine retrovirus vectors could be obtained into close to 100% of leukocytes by pre-enrichment of repopulating stem cells, species-specific (ecotropic) vector exposure, rigorous ex vivo and/or in vivo selection, and transplantation after otherwise-lethal myeloablative conditioning.[11] In that setting, expression of a corrective transgene has been a curative approach for in vitro and murine models of human genetic diseases, including adenosine deaminase (ADA) deficiency (ADA-deficient severe combined immunodeficiency (SCID)), X-linked SCID, arylsulfatase A (ASA) and B (ASB) deficiency, hemophilia A and B, Gaucher's disease, chronic granulomatous disease, Fanconi's anemia, and HIV-1 infection (for reviews, see reference 12).

These results have only been partially reproducible in preclinical large-animal and preclinical human cell xenotransplantation models and in the pioneering clinical studies. Successful transduction and engraftment of hematopoietic stem cells is more difficult in large compared with small mammals for a number of, mostly obvious, reasons. Because of the lack of syngeneic stem cell donors in randomly bred large animals and the susceptibility of the autologous donors to harsh stem cell mobilization treatment, the numbers of stem cells per body weight available for ex vivo treatment is usually much lower compared with the murine model. In mice, syngeneic 'total donor' cells of littermates can be harvested and pooled after 5-fluorouracil (5-FU) conditioning. An ecotropic producer cell line that is known to be capable of substituting as a bone marrow stroma feeder line, such as the ecotropic MLV vector 3T3-based producer cell line, is not yet available in any of the large-animal models or for human clinical applications.[13] The highly efficient co-cultivation of the stem cell preparation on these producer cell lines is considered an uncalculable biological hazard in the clinical setting. Transduction cultures for preclinical and clinical use are therefore usually restricted to repeated exposure to vector-containing media in suspension or nonproductive stromal culture.[14-16] Reinfusion in these murine models is performed after lethal conditioning that completely eliminates endogenous competing stem cells. Mostly, a low number of stem cells close to a limiting dilution of proven engraftment potential are used after harshly selecting for transgene expression. Taken together, the stringent conditions used in the murine retroviral gene transfer model provide a reproducible high transduction efficiency in repopulating stem cells and at the same time are associated with procedure-related toxicity and mortality that is prohibitive outside of the murine model.

Despite the limitations of the available vector systems, significant insights have been gained into the process of ex vivo gene transfer and engraftment of transduced stem cells in patients. Approaches to gene transfer can be grouped into four major categories: gene marking, the transfer of drug resistance, the transfer of prodrug susceptibility, and the transfer of therapeutic genes. This chapter gives an overview of these approaches, together with a discussion of the integrating vector systems that have been employed.

## GENE MARKING: HANDLING AND TRACKING THE HEMATOPOIETIC STEM CELL

Whether a gene of potential therapeutic benefit was transferred or not, all initial clinical gene transfer trials in hematopoietic stem cells were marking trials in that their primary purpose was to quantify the fate of transduced cells following their reinfusion. All but one were performed also to study by molecular marking whether the autologous transplantation of stem cells contributed significant amounts of contaminating tumor cells to a potential relapse in participating patients. These pioneering gene marking studies were performed in the context of acute and chronic myeloid leukemias (AML and CML), neuroblastoma, and breast cancer.

Taken together, the first gene marking trials have universally provided evidence for the integration of retroviral vectors at low efficiency into repopulating hematopoietic stem cells. Gene marking of tumor cells has also been observed in all the entities studied.

To explore the possibility of engrafting transduced cells without prior conditioning, Cynthia Dunbar at the NIH in collaboration with investigators from the National Institute of Neurological Disorders and Stroke and Donald Kohn at the Children's Hospital of Los Angeles investigated in a clinical protocol the safety and feasibility of retroviral transduction of peripheral blood (PB) or bone marrow (BM) CD34$^+$ cells with a vector that expresses human glucocerebrosidase cDNA. Three adult Gaucher patients were followed for up to 15 months. Granulocyte colony-stimulating factor (G-CSF)-mobilized CD34-enriched PB cells were transduced on autologous stroma without (patient 1) or with interleukin (IL)-3, IL-6, and stem cell factor (SCF) (patient 2) or using BM cells in the latter approach (patient 3). After culture, the cells were reinfused immediately. Transduction efficiency was 1%, 10%, and 1%, respectively. Vector-positive cells were detectable at one month (patients 2 and 3) and at two and three months post infusion (patient 2 only) at low levels (<0.02%). There was no measurable difference in glucocerebrosidase activity.[17] This trial suggests cautious optimism that transduced stem cells may be engraftable in the absence of myelosuppressive conditioning, although the efficiency of the process at that time was still too low. Several explanations for the low but reproducible level of marking in the first set of clinical studies have been discussed.

### The influence of cell cycling on retroviral transduction

Genomic integration by oncoretroviruses such as MLV depends on cycling activity. The long terminal repeat (LTR) circle junction as a marker for nuclear entry can only be observed in infected cells after mitosis.[18] In cells arrested prior to mitosis, the cytoplasmic variant of the retroviral preintegration complex has a half-life of approximately 6 hours.[19]

Although in itself hard to prove for a target cell population that cannot be identified by phenotype, it seems obvious that short-term (i.e. <24-hour) exposure of cells to retrovirus vector, which was standard practice in the early marking trials, should fail to achieve vector nuclear entry in the majority of repopulating cells during the permissive 12- to 24-hour time window prior to cell cycling.[2] Unstimulated progenitor cells are supposed to cycle rarely. Jo Anna Reems et al[20] have shown that close to 98% of unstimulated adult CD34$^+$CD38$^-$ marrow cells are in the $G_0$ phase of the cell cycle. Reems et al[20] and Bruemmendorf et al[135] have estimated the cell cycle transit time of CD34$^+$CD38$^-$ cells at over 30 hours. As predicted by these observations of stem cell quiescence, progenitor cell preparations from cord blood and fetal liver with high proliferative potential can be transduced more efficiently with retroviral vectors than preparations from adult mobilized peripheral blood cells and bone marrow, which have been demonstrated to reside predominantly in $G_0$.[21] We and others have demonstrated that extending the vector exposure beyond 72 hours is beneficial for the retroviral transduction of immature progenitor cells – most likely because the chances of a vector preintegration complex being ready for nuclear entry once cycling occurs is greatly increased by multiple or continuous vector exposures of a non-synchronized population.[22–26]

## Timing

Veena et al[27] have used a two-step transduction to study retroviral transduction efficiency in different fractions of cultured CD34$^+$ cells sorted according to the number of cell divisions after five days of culture. Marrow CD34$^+$ cells stained with the membrane dye PKH2 were pre-stimulated for 24 hours with SCF, IL-3, and IL-6. On day 1, a fibronectin-supported transduction with the retroviral vector LNL6 was performed. On day 5, half of the cultured cells were transduced with the retroviral vector G1Na. These cells were then sorted on day 6 into cytokine-responsive (CR) cells (loss of PKH2 fluorescence relative to day 0 sample) and cytokine-none-responsive (CNR) cells that had not divided since day 0. The other half of the cultured cells were sorted on into day 5 CR and day 5 CNR cells before transduction with G1Na. All cells were cultured in secondary long-term cultures and assessed weekly for transduced progenitor cells. After two weeks, transduction efficiency was similar between CR and CNR cells. After three and four weeks, both day 5 and day 6 CNR cells equally produced significantly more G418-resistant colonies compared with CR cells. Polymerase chain reaction (PCR) analysis demonstrated that CR cells had predominantly acquired day 1 vector (LNL6) sequences, while the CNR fractions were transduced on day 5 with G1Na.[27] While not verified in in vivo repopulating cells, these data demonstrate that an extended exposure to stimulating cytokines is necessary for the transduction of primitive progenitor cells. No significant gene transfer into primitive cells occurred on day 1.

To the best of our current knowledge, the uptake of retroviral vector indicates that a cell has cycled in ex vivo culture. It would be tempting to assume inversely that repopulating stem cells resistant to transduction with cycling-dependent vectors even in the presence of mitogenically activating cytokines cycle rarely or not at all. Verfaillie et al and we have demonstrated that long-term culture-initiating cell (LTC-IC) activity is enriched in cells that are functionally resistant to cytokine stimulation and maintain an immature phenotype in ex vivo culture. Cycling in this subpopulation was increasing significantly during culture, and retroviral transduction in LTC-IC was quite efficient. Extending earlier observations by Dexter et al[28] and Verfaillie et al,[29] more recent data by Glimm and Eaves[30] show that the original hypothesis of nearly complete stem cell quiescence as the major obstacle to successful retroviral transduction may need re-evaluation. 5- and 6-carboxyfluorescein diacetate succinimidyl ester (CFSE)-dyed human CD34$^+$ cord blood and fetal liver progenitor cells were sorted according to the number of cell divisions after five days of serum-free ex vivo culture and $(0.7–7.8) \times 10^3$ cells per animal were retransfused in a limiting dilution competitive in vivo engraftment experiment. In this experiment, over 88% of LTC-IC activity was concentrated in those cells that had divided at least once. In vivo repopulation activity was highest in cells that had undergone between three and six divisions during the five-day culture period that preceded transplantation. Almost two-thirds (63%) of the xenotransplant competitive repopulating units (CRU) had cycled three or more times in the five-day interval.[30]

## INTEGRATING VECTOR SYSTEMS IN HEMATOPOIETIC GENE TRANSFER

### Retroviral vectors

About 15 years after successful retroviral gene transfer was first achieved in the mouse, this achievement has still only partially been reproduced in large animals and humans. Within the last two years, however, there has been enormous progress towards that goal.

#### *Vector construction*

MLV-derived vectors are very versatile, stably integrating gene ferries, because the genetic structure of their parent virus is simple and well studied. It has been demonstrated that the complete coding sequence of the viral *gag*, *pol*, and *env* genes can be removed. The resulting vector backbone that has to be transferred consists only of the viral LTRs, the packaging signal *psi*, and the 3' sequence for the initiation of second strand synthesis. Packaging of MLV vectors is achieved by the use of packaging cell lines that carry the viral structural genes in separate coding sequences, supplying the gene products required for viral assembly in *trans*. In early-generation vectors, the *gag/pol/env* genes were used as a single entity and, for reasons of efficiency and convenience, were usually driven by a truncated viral LTR promoter. Further splitting of the proviral cDNA coding regions into *gag/pol* polymerase/integrase and a separate envelope construct has afforded an increase in biosafety and the opportunity to more conveniently pseudotype, i.e. exchange the retroviral vector envelope with a different strain envelope.[31]

Retroviral vectors have been produced in a variety of cell lines from different species for several reasons, mostly because particles budding from the membrane of a cell from an identical species are likely to introduce less foreign protein and nucleic acid than a xenogenic line. Further improvements in vector construction include the elimination of homologous vector sequences from the packaging plasmids and attempts at simplifying the exchange of the transported gene of interest by means of Cre–*lox* recombination.

Determination of vector titers is complicated by methodological and systematic variation.[32] The standard methodology determines the infectious titer of particles that lead to measurable expression of proviral vector in clones of a target cell line. It can vary depending on the type of target cells used and their expression of the corresponding retroviral receptor. Optimized retroviral producer cell lines with amphotropic or gibbon ape leukemia virus (GALV) pseudotype will typically produce $1 \times 10^5$ to $1 \times 10^6$ infectious particles per milliliter in a period of 8–24 hours. Recently, a method for the transient transfection of 293T cells was described to produce high-titer murine recombinant retroviral vectors. Higher titer and infectivity were obtained than with stable murine producer lines. Titers of $(0.3–1) \times 10^7$ infectious units per milliliter for vectors encoding the green fluorescent protein (GFP) were achieved. Virions with amphotropic or GALV pseudotype resulted in gene transfer of 50% in $CD4^+$ human T lymphocytes. The authors describe a protocol for the production of large-scale supernatants using transient transfection up to titers of $1.9 \times 10^7$ IU/ml.[33] Transient producer cells are more difficult to characterize for clinical use, because a genetically stable master cell clone cannot be pre-established and tested for safety.

### Pseudotyping

Of the multiple envelope pseudotypes used with retroviral vectors for experimental purposes, the GALV envelope and the vesicular stomatitis glycoprotein pseudotype (VSV-G) envelope are the most widely used.

Dusty Miller designed the GALV pseudotyped producer cell clone PG13 with the rationale that a primate pseudotype might support viral entry into human cells more efficiently than a murine amphotropic pseudotype, because of a higher expression level.[34] Both *env* genes bind to different varieties of sodium phosphate symporters: GALV to PIT-1 and amphotropic MLV to PIT-2. Sabatino et al[35] compared the levels of PIT-2 and PIT-1 in human tissue culture cell lines. mRNA levels were highest in K562 cells and lowest in HL60 cells. An increase in the level of PIT-2 and PIT-1 mRNA by 4-phorbol-12-myristate 13-acetate (PMA) or IL-1α treatment in HL60 cells correlated with increased transduction efficiency by both amphotropic and GALV retroviral vectors.[35] The low transduction efficiency in the mouse hematopoietic stem cell line FDC-Pmix is limited to the amphotropic envelope and is due to a post-transcriptional problem of receptor expression at normal PIT-2 mRNA levels which suggests that predicting PIT expression on mRNA levels alone may be imprecise in hematopoietic cells.[36] In normal mouse bone marrow, the subpopulation with the highest level of PIT-2 mRNA is more efficiently transduced by amphotropic retrovirus. Populations enriched for human primitive progenitor cells (CD34$^+$CD38$^-$) express low levels of human PIT-2 mRNA. Higher levels are found in committed progenitor cells (CD34$^+$CD38$^+$).[37]

When comparing mRNA expression levels in different sources of human hematopoietic progenitor cells, peripheral blood hematopoietic stem cells had a fourfold higher level of amphotropic retrovirus receptor mRNA and 2.6-fold more cells in the $G_1$ phase of the cell cycle compared with steady-state bone marrow.[38] A freeze–thaw cycle was also demonstrated to increase PIT-2 expression levels.

Taken together, these data suggest that one of the reasons for inefficient gene transfer to human hematopoietic stem cells may be the putatively low to absent PIT-2 expression on these cells. We could already show in 1994 that the GALV pseudotype more efficiently transduces differentiated and primitive (LTC-IC) human hematopoietic progenitor cells.[22] Hans-Peter Kiem et al[39] have used a baboon competitive repopulation assay to verify these results in in vivo repopulating stem cells. CD34$^+$ marrow cells from each animal were divided into two equal portions, which were co-cultivated with either amphotropic or GALV pseudotyped vectors containing the *neo* gene. The vectors contained small sequence differences to allow a comparative PCR analysis. Peripheral blood and marrow cells after engraftment showed the *neo* gene to be present in all four animals in 0.1–5% of cells, with higher results for the GALV pseudotyped vector. The higher GALV *env* gene transfer efficiency correlated with higher levels of GALV receptor RNA.[39]

The VSV-G pseudotype attaches to target cells by membrane glycolipids present on many cell populations in a variety of vertebrate hosts. No specific receptor protein has to be present. In retroviral systems, it is not clear whether the use of VSV-G can significantly improve transduction efficiency compared with amphotropic or GALV pseudotypes. VSV-G pseudotyping does, however, provide superior stability to the coated virus particles, enabling their density-gradient enrichment by two to three orders of magnitude up to titers of $10^9$ cfu/ml.[40] This feature has been used extensively in the study of retroviral vector systems, where, in the first three generations of packaging systems, spontaneous titers have been too low ($10^3$–$10^4$) to allow the use of unconcentrated preparations of vector-containing supernatant.

### Biosafety concerns regarding the clinical use of retroviral vectors

Vectors derived from this virus type are well suited for clinical use, because there is no known pathogenicity of wild-type MLV infection in humans.

The virus is readily inactivated by CH 100, C1q complement fraction, and anti-α-galactosyl natural antibody-mediated mechanisms of human serum. Amphotropic retrovirus vector infectivity is reduced more than 20-fold after 30 minutes in adult human serum. Interestingly, this immunity appears not to be naive, since amphotropic transduction efficiency is maintained after 30 minutes of incubation in umbilical cord serum, supposedly because of lower levels of maternal anti-α-galactosyl antibodies.[41] After infusion in nonhuman primates, high titers of replication-competent retrovirus are rapidly cleared from the circulation.[41-43] The amphotropic and GALV pseudotyped vectors have half-lives of approximately 12–24 hours in medium at 37°C, 24–36 hours at 4°C, and over six months at −80°C. The wild-type envelope is too unstable for enrichment by gradient ultracentrifugation or membrane filtration, and also is not stable in a dry environment and under ultraviolet light.

In applications to gene therapy in humans, there are three areas of potential biohazard associated with the use of retroviral vectors.

First, the vector system is of animal origin, mostly produced in animal cells of defined source, and applied together with media components of animal and/or synthetic origin. It is therefore likely that immune reactions to foreign proteins will interfere with the direct in vivo application, especially if repeated, of these vectors. Such reactions could be the source of potential side-effects, including an anaphylactic reaction or performance failure of transduced cells secondary to immune elimination at or after engraftment.

Whether long-term immune responses against the transgene proteins of ex vivo transduction will occur is related to how the cells are treated after the vector exposure, how many and how many times treated cells will be reinfused, and, most importantly, which route of administration can be used.

A T-cell response against different transgene products has been shown in the follow-up of two trials that included repeated transfusions of gene-modified T cells. In the Seattle immunotherapy trial, individuals seropositive for human immunodeficiency virus (HIV) received CD8$^+$ HIV-specific cytotoxic T cells modified by retroviral transduction to express the hygromycin resistance/HSV thymidine kinase fusion gene (*HyTK*), which permits ex vivo positive and in vivo negative selection of transduced cells. Five of six patients developed cytotoxic T-lymphocyte responses specific for the transgene protein, and eliminated the transduced cytotoxic T cells at increasing speed in subsequent infusions.[44] Also, T- and B-cell responses against the transgene and associated products have been discovered in the participants of the NIH ADA trial. Here, T-cell responses against the transgene as well as immunoglobulins directed against the bovine lipoprotein fraction of the cell culture media could be observed.

As has been extensively studied in preclinical transplantation models, antigen presentation in the context of bone marrow transplantation can tolerize the immune system to no longer reject the antigen. Transfer of an allogeneic MHC class I molecule by gene modification has been described to induce specific tolerance.[45] In contrast to the aforementioned T-cell modification studies, Morgan and colleagues could demonstrate that in a mouse model of partial factor VIII intolerance, autologous bone marrow transplantation with gene-modified cells expressing factor VIII markedly diminished the anti-factor VIII T- and B-cell response.[136] Dunbar and colleagues have extensively studied the influence of expressing different transgenes in the murine and large-animal rhesus model. No difference was observed between the marking efficiency, persistence, and lineage distribution between cells expressing *neo* alone versus *neo* and β-galactosidase.[46] In naive rhesus monkeys, ex vivo transduced *neo*-expressing T cells disappeared from the circulation after 5–10 weeks, while cells with an otherwise-identical non-expression vector persisted for over 12 months. In four out of five myeloablated animals transplanted with transduced marrow cells, *neo*-expressing leukocytes, including T cells, persisted for over 12 months. Secondarily infused *neo*-expressing T cells persisted in animals that had been tolarized by a prior gene-modified marrow transplant.

Second, the integration of the virus may by chance interrupt the function of a cellular gene and may induce apoptosis, malfunction, or growth transformation in single cells. While the incapacitation of a percentage of the treated cells is of little concern other than for the efficiency of the process, cellular transformation would be a serious side-effect severely restricting the applicability of any vector system. Radiation studies in cell lines have demonstrated, however, that single mutational events are not sufficient to transform eukaryotic cells. As retroviral transduction efficiency is well below 50% and, to the best of our knowledge, strictly monoallelic, the chance of a cell receiving a second or third integration and deriving mutational transformation from this event is considered minute at this point. In support of this evaluation, a transformation by the integration of a replication-incompetent retroviral vector has never been observed in any primary cell culture, cell line, small- or large-animal study, or in any of the more than 500 patients worldwide who have been enrolled in trials involving the use of retroviral vectors.

Third, the most prominent biosafety concern for the clinical use of retroviral vectors is the reactivation or concurrence of replication-competent retrovirus (RCR) in the vector preparation or the transduced patient cells. Based on the available animal data, MLV-associated pathogenicity is minimal for immunocompetent individuals. Infusion of $1 \times 10^8$ replication-competent amphotropic retrovirus particles into five rhesus monkeys, two of which had been immunosuppressed, has not led to detectable sequelae in more than four years of follow-up.[47] The virus was no longer detectable in the serum after 15 minutes, and likely underwent complement inactivation.[48,49] All of these animals did develop a temporary lymphadenopathy. In another experiment, immunosuppressed primates received otherwise-lethal total-body irradiation (TBI) followed by the autologous transplantation of ex vivo transduced, heavily helper virus-contaminated peripheral blood progenitor cells derived from an early-generation packaging cell line that produced $10^3$–$10^4$ cfu/ml of RCR. Lymphoma developed after six months in those three of the eight animals that had not developeda measurable antibody titer against viral antigens. A chronically productive RCR infection had developed. In the lymphoma cells from these animals,10–50 copies of the RCR, but no copy of the replication-incompetent vector, could be found.[50] It has to be assumed that the inadvertent infusion of a high titer, even of a murine RCR, could potentially lead to morbidity and mortality in immunocompromised human hosts, for example after myeloablative conditioning.

Fortunately, extremely sensitive assays exist that can detect minimal concentrations (1–5 cfu/tested volume) of infectious retroviruses with the help of multiply passaged amplification cultures on permissive cell lines (3T3, *mus dunni*, 293) followed by indicator gene mobilization assays or focus formation of indicator cells (PG-4, S$^+$/L$^-$ assay).[51] Clinically applied materials are tested three times on the levels of the master cell bank and of the vector-containing media, and, depending on protocol design, before or at reinfusion of the transduced cells. Patient screening for evidence of antiretroviral antibodies followed by confirmatory RCR testing is performed yearly for purposes of toxicity testing. Interestingly, it has been demonstrated that antilentiviral agents for clinical use also inhibit retroviral replication in cell culture.

## Culture conditions for the maintenance of repopulating capacity

The cell cycle dependence of any retroviral and of efficient lentiviral integration has focused investigators on the goal of propagating and maintaining hematopoietic repopulating cells in ex vivo culture. Clear evidence for successful repopulating stem cell cycling has been established by gene marking experiments in large-animal and human autologous stem cell transplantation. Culture conditions have undergone continuous improvement by competitive repopulation assays in the non-obese diabetic (NOD)–SCID human xenograft model and intraindividual canine and simian competitive engraftment studies. The major elements determining the character of an ex vivo culture are the presence or absence of a stromal or other adherent cell feeder layer, and the mixture of growth factors used.

Owing to the lack of phenotypic definition, primitive progenitor and stem cells can only be studied in retrospective functional assays. To assay primitive progenitor cells in vitro, the five-week LTC-IC assay has been used. The NOD–SCID xenotransplant model in immunodeficient mice is currently considered the assay closest to assessing the potential for early human hematopoietic repopulation in vivo.[52]

### Stroma
It is uncontested that the presence of a stromal feeder layer is at least beneficial for the maintenance of repopulating stem cells in the presence of growth factors, and is indispensable in the absence of growth factors. Many investigations focus on defining the physiology of stromal support. One of the main reasons from the perspective of clinical gene therapy to pursue this goal is the absence of a defined and reproducibly growing stromal cell line or other source of a fully functional feeder cell layer that eliminates the variability and the infectious hazard of using primary stromal cells.

In the murine setting, 3T3 fibroblasts and their vector packaging derivatives can replace the function of primary stroma. Co-cultivation on virus packaging cells has also been used successfully in the canine and monkey large-animal models.[53]

For human stem cells, human umbilical vein endothelial cells (HUVEC) and porcine microvascular endothelial cells (PMVEC) have been suggested as a stroma replacement. Chute et al[55] describe that after seven days of co-culture on PMVECs in the presence of granulocyte–macrophage colony-stimulating factor (GM-CSF), IL-3, IL-6, SCF and Flt-3 ligand (Flt-3L), the total $CD34^+$ population and the $CD34^+CD38^-$ subset had increased 8.4- and 67-fold. Fifty-three percent of the $CD34^+CD38^-$ subset were in $G_1$, and 17% were in $G_2$/S/M. In contrast, in the $CD34^+CD38^-$ subset from stroma-free culture, only 22% and 6% were in $G_1$ and $G_2$/S/M phases, respectively. Despite the high level of proliferation, PMVEC co-culture maintained the surface expression of adhesion molecules CD11a and b, CD15s, CD43, CD44 (HCAM), CD49d (VLA4), CD54 (ICAM), CD58, and CD62L (L-selectin).[54]

Moore et al[56] and Wells et al[57] could demonstrate that the presence of a stromal layer significantly increased the extent of glucocerebrosidase gene transfer into 14-day colony-forming cells (CFC), LTC-IC, and non-adherent cells from long-term bone marrow cultures. The addition of IL-3, IL-6, and SCF to the stroma significantly increased the extent of gene transfer into CFC but not LTC-IC.[56] In addition to SCF, Flt-3L is required to sustain long-term in vivo hematopoietic ability of human $CD34^+$ cells. Dao et al[14] hypothesized that Flt-3L might be capable of replacing part of stroma's role in the maintenance of such cells. $CD34^+$ progenitors from human bone marrow were transduced in the presence of IL-3, IL-6, and SCF, with or without stromal support and with or without 100 U/ml of Flt-3L. No significant increase of gene transfer into CFC was obtained by adding Flt-3L. Human primitive hematopoietic cells were determined by recovering human myeloid cells, T cells, and colony-forming progenitors seven or eight months after xenotransplantation of transduced cells. Vector provirus was detected in the marrow recovered from 9 of 10 mice transplanted with human $CD34^+$ cells from stromal transduction, in 5 of 11 mice that received human cells transduced in suspension culture with Flt-3L, but none of the 10 mice that received human suspension cells cultured without Flt-3L.[14]

Recently, stroma-supported culture systems have been described to generate vast amounts of primitive progenitor cells in the presence of IL-3, IL-6, G-CSF, and Flt-3L.[57] If these results truly reflect repopulating stem cell expansion, and the generated cells can be engrafted in vivo, then these conditions should further enhance retroviral and lentiviral gene transfer.

### Growth factors: mandatory versus detrimental

Stroma produces a number of growth factors and expresses surface markers interacting with the homing and regulation of hematopoiesis. It has long been attempted to model this interaction in suspension culture in the absence of stromal cells.

For systematic analysis, the use of cytokines in ex vivo transduction cultures can be structured into factors mainly affecting the maintenance (SCF, Flt-3L, thrombopoietin (TPO)/megakaryocyte growth and development factor (MGDF)), proliferation, or/and differentiation (e.g. IL-3, IL-6, G-CSF, TPO/MGDF) of immature progenitor and stem cells. Combinations are sought that achieve proliferation in the proportion of cells that are initially unresponsive to cytokine stimulation without driving them into differentiation.

SCF is considered indispensable for the survival of stem cells in suspension culture.[58] Arguing that the SCF signal can be delivered directly by the producer cell line, Povey et al[59] simply constructed a retroviral producer line that expresses the membrane-bound form of human SCF on its cell surface. In five-day co-culture, about 20% of LTC-IC derived from 5-FU-resistant highly quiescent adult human bone marrow cells could be transduced using the SCF-expressing producer line. The parent amphotropic producer line gave reduced or no transduction.

Growth factors also influence the kinetics of cell cycling. We found in 1997 that extending the exposure of human adult $CD34^+CD38^-$ bone marrow cells to five days can give substantial (42%) transduction efficiency in immature hematopoietic progenitor cells (LTC-IC) using SCF, IL-3, and IL-6. Hennemann et al[60] recently counted single-cell dilutions of human $CD34^+CD38^-$ cord blood cells exposed to different Flt-3L-containing cytokine combinations. With either Flt-3L plus hyper-IL-6 plus TPO or Flt-3L plus SCF plus IL-3 plus IL-6 plus G-CSF, over 90% of cells that formed clones within six days undertook their first division on days 2–4. Transduction on fibronectin-coated dishes with a GALV pseudotyped GFP/neo vector for two days following prestimulation of the target cells with either cytokine combination increased their susceptibility, resulting in 47–54% GFP+ CD34+ cells and 67–69% G418-resistant CFC. Transplantation of lin− cord blood cells into NOD–SCID mice after a six-day transduction protocol in which virus was added on the third, fourth, and fifth days yielded 0.2–72% readily detectable human lymphoid and myeloid GFP+ cells in 10 of 11 mice that were engrafted with human cells.[59] It will be of great importance to reproduce these data in cell preparations relevant for adult human clinical use.

### Pre-harvest priming

Growth factors can be applied to ex vivo stem cell gene transfer not only during the ex vivo culture but also at the level of preculture mobilization. Bodine et al[36] could show in earlier observations that G-CSF and SCF treatment in mice immediately increases peripheral blood stem cell content, increases retrovirus receptor expression, and produces a 10-fold increase in bone marrow hematopoietic stem cells after 14 days. They went on to show that rhesus monkey repopulating bone marrow cells collected 14 days after G-CSF and SCF priming were transducible with amphotropic retroviruses at levels of approximately 10% by Southern blot analysis.[36]

## Transforming growth factor beta (TGF-β)

Transforming growth factor beta (TGF-β) has different activities at different levels of hematopoiesis. On the level of primitive progenitor and stem cells, it is thought to inhibit proliferation and may compromise long-term repopulating activity in murine models. Yu et al[60] have demonstrated that the elimination of autocrine or paracrine TGF-β by neutralizing antibodies increases transduction efficiency both in progenitor (CFU-C) and W/Wv repopulating murine stem cells after four days of transduction using IL-3, IL-6, and SCF. This effect may be the result of the influence of TGF-β on the intracellular levels of the cyclin-dependent kinase inhibitor p15$^{INK4B}$. This kinase inhibitor in conjunction with others can hold cells in quiescence by blocking the association of cyclin-dependent kinase (CDK) 4 with cyclin D. A second important inhibitor, which blocks CDK2/cyclin A and CDK2/cyclin E activity (both of which are necessary for cell-cycle progression), is called p27$^{kip-1}$ kinase inhibitor. Dao et al[61] could demonstrate that an additional lowering of p27$^{kip-1}$ kinase inhibitor expression levels by antisense oligonucleotides together with neutralization of TGF-β in serum-free medium was capable of increasing transduction of human repopulating cells as assessed in the murine xenograft model.

## Chimeric envelope design

The retroviral envelope molecule is a highly sophisticated structure. On the surface of the vector particle, it functions as a trimeric molecule responsible for vector attachment as well as initiation of the biophysics of cell entry. Most likely owing to the complex dynamics of that process, our current understanding does not permit the very desirable manipulation or exchange of the site responsible for specific attachment without inactivating the ability of the Env complex to initiate cell entry.[62] Nevertheless, the scarcity of retrovirus receptors on the hematopoietic target cells of interest has led several investigators to construct producer systems with chimeric envelope or surface proteins engineered to obtain hematapoiesis-specific vector attachment and hopefully cell entry.[63]

Yajima et al[65] have engineered an ecotropic envelope protein by inserting a sequence encoding the N-terminal 161 amino acids of murine stem cell factor (mSCF), the ligand for murine c-Kit. The chimeric envelope protein was correctly processed and incorporated into viral particles. The chimeric Env virion pseudotype bound preferentially to 293 cells expressing murine c-Kit without transducing any c-Kit-positive cells under normal conditions, although some transduction could be observed in 293KIT and HEL cells expressing human c-Kit in the presence of chloroquine. This transduction could be inhibited by recombinant mSCF in the medium, suggesting that vector mSCF–c-Kit interaction was involved in the infection process.[64]

In contrast to the theoretical ideal, the specific binding of chimeric envelopes can effectively and selectively abrogate infectivity completely. In this setting, Fielding et al[65] have obtained an interesting if unexpected result. Building on their previous observation that vectors with an epidermal growth factor (EGF) chimeric envelope glycoprotein are sequestered upon binding to EGF receptor (EGFR)-positive target cells without achieving infection, SCF chimeras were constructed in the form of a factor Xa protease-cleavable N-terminal extension of the envelope glycoprotein. Viral incorporation of the chimeric Env molecule and specific attachment to SCF receptors (c-Kit) was observed. Here, similar to the EGF observation, the infectivity of SCF-displaying vectors was selectively inhibited on c-Kit-expressing cells. Turning the vice into a virtue for an inverse targeting strategy, the authors went on to show in cell mixtures that EGFR-positive cancer cells were selectively transduced by the SCF-displaying vector and the SCF receptor (c-Kit)-positive hematopoietic cells were selectively transduced by the EGF-displaying vector.[65]

The observation that chimeric envelopes can be incorporated into vector particles and successfully mediate binding but fail to initiate the uptake and integration process has the logical consequence that cell entry and integration currently require the use of a second, functional Env glycoprotein. Maurice et al[66] have fused human IL-2 to the amino terminus of the amphotropic MLV envelope. Retroviral vectors were pseudotyped with both the IL-2 chimeric and the wild-type amphotropic MLV envelope. IL-2-co-displaying vector could infect proliferating cells through amphotropic receptors irrespective of whether the cells expressed the IL-2 receptor (IL-2R). IL-2-co-displaying vector particles could achieve transient cell cycling and proliferation of IL-2-dependent cell lines, and could efficiently transduce $G_0/G_1$-arrested T cells expressing IL-2R at a 34-fold higher efficiency compared with unmodified vectors. Should this strategy be portable to other hematopoietic cell systems, co-display of a ligand could be used to activate the cell cycle of the target cells at the time of virus entry. This strategy might facilitate transgene integration more specifically into otherwise-quiescent cells expressing the corresponding growth factor receptor.[66]

## Fibronectin, integrins, and surface receptors

Localization of stem cells in the medullary cavity appears to involve the local cytokine and growth factor milieu as well as surface receptors for specific components of the extracellular matrix, including both integrin- and proteoglycan-mediated (e.g. fibronectin) cell–cell and cell–matrix interactions. Specifically, Williams et al[67] have established that the adhesion of primitive hematopoietic stem and progenitor cells to the carboxy-terminal 30/35 kDa fragment of the extracellular matrix molecule fibronectin seems to be of central importance for the adhesion and migration of stem cells.

A fibronectin fragment including the recognition sequence Arg-Gly-Asp (RGD) can foster the transduction of murine HSC, suggesting the presence of integrin very late antigen (VLA)-5 on stem cells. van der Loo et al[68] have therefore studied the binding of murine and human hematopoietic cells to recombinant peptides that contained all or one of three fibronectin cell binding domains, the aforementioned VLA-5-binding RGD sequence in repeat 10 of the fibronectin cell binding domain, the VLA-4-binding site CS1 with the alternatively spliced IIICS region, and the high-affinity heparin-binding domain (type III repeat, 12, 13, 14). Murine and human in vivo repopulating stem cells specifically bound fibronectin via integrin VLA-5 in vitro. Preincubation of marrow cells with a 574-amino-acid 63 kDa peptide displaying all domains diminished their engraftment. Intravenous injection of the same peptide (CH-296) increased the spleen progenitor pool.[68] When this fragment was precoated on the culture dish, however, its presence helped to maintain xenografted repopulating human stem cells, supposedly by integrin–receptor interaction, much better than an otherwise identical suspension culture.[69]

The discovery of specific retrovirus particle binding to the high-affinity heparin-binding site of this fragment has been a major achievement for retroviral gene transfer. One of the different recombinant fibronectin fragments tested (CH-296, RetroNectin) has been found ideal for this purpose. Moritz et al could demonstrate in 1996 that transduction of 12-month repopulating murine hematopoietic stem cells on this fragment is similarly effective compared with direct producer co-cultivation. During binding, signs of cellular activation, including proliferation or an increase of protein phosphorylation, were not observed.[70]

Gene transfer into SCF, G-CSF, and MGDF-prestimulated CD34+ bone marrow cells was very stable on CH-296-coated plates against changes in coating and cell concentration. Because the virus vector is immobilized on the culture dish surface, repeated 'preloading' of the dishes with viral vector can be performed, further increasing the local concentration of bound virus prior to the addition of the cells.[71]

## AAV

Adeno-associated virus is a parvovirus, not associated with known pathogenicity in humans, that in its wild-type form depends on adenoviral genes for its replication to occur. The structural simplicity of AAV vectors is comparable to that of retroviruses. The size limit for packaging genes in AAV vectors is somewhat lower than in retroviral vectors at about 5 kbp. The viral inverted repeats (ITR) can mediate genomic integration in the presence of the viral integrase. Intermittently stable high expression levels of the transferred gene have been found to be derived from extrachromosomal viral concatemers, circular multimers of viral DNA present in the nucleosol for weeks after the original transduction. AAV gene transfer can give high levels of transgene expression that for the most part does not seem to be stable long term in vivo.

## Lentiviral vectors

### HIV vectors

Interest in using lentiviruses such as the human immunodeficiency virus (HIV) and its feline (FIV), simian (SIV), and equine (EIAV) counterparts as genetic vectors has been stimulated by the observation that lentiviruses depend less on the cell cycle to become integrated into the host cell genome and may, although at lower efficiency, be independent of it. To study the capacity of HIV-based vectors to deliver genes into nondividing cells, several groups have initially constructed replication-defective HIV type 1 (HIV-1) reporter vectors with inactive *vpr*, *vpu*, and *nef* coding regions that carried various marker genes at the HIV-1 gp160 site. Pseudotyped HIV-1 particles carrying either the amphotropic MLV envelope proteins or the vesicular stomatitis virus (VSV) G protein were found capable of infecting human 293T and monkey COS cells and human skin fibroblasts arrested at the $G_0/G_1$ stage of the cell cycle by density-dependent inhibition of growth.[72] Human CD34[+] cells without prior cytokine stimulation were transduced efficiently using HIV-1 pseudotyped particles. In rats, pseudotyped HIV vectors could mediate in vivo gene transfer into terminally differentiated neurons.[73]

In short succession, HIV vector systems were developed in which the virulence genes *env*, *vif*, *vpr*, *vpu*, and *nef* were deleted.[74] Of the two regulatory genes, *tat* and *rev*, that were considered essential for HIV replication, the *tat* gene could be offset by placing constitutive promoters upstream of the vector construct in the form of a chimeric LTR. Tat-independent vectors transduced postmitotic neurons in vivo at high efficiency. In these third-generation lentivirus vectors, *rev* has to be supplied in *trans*, leaving the HIV *gag*, *pol*, *rev*, Rev-responsive element (RRE), and LTR as the minimal genes required for generating a good-titer HIV vector producer cell line.[75] Cui et al[76] observed more recently that deletion of RRE alone markedly impaired vector function. By contrast, combined deletion of RRE, *gag* (excluding bp 1–40), and *env*, and the SD mutation resulted in increased viral RNA transcription and a vector efficiency up at 50% of the wild-type level. Although the type of producer cell was critical for the function of these mutants, the results showed that lentivirus vector function can be maintained in the absence of most essential and all accessory viral genes.[76]

By replacing the U3 region of the 5' LTR in vector constructs with the cytomegalovirus (CMV) promoter, Tat-independent transcription and expression could also be maintained. A deletion of 133–400 bp in the 3' LTR U3 region removed the promoter function, TATA box, and binding sites for the transcription factors Sp1 and NF-κBA. Because the deletion is transferred to the 5' LTR after reverse transcription and upon integration, a transcriptional self-inactivation (SIN) of the proviral LTR results in infected cells. SIN vectors have titers comparable to those of undeleted vectors. Injection of a SIN GFP vector into the rat brain showed comparable levels of GFP expression as a wild-type vector.[77] The SIN deletion is also supposed to remove LTR sequences previously associated with transcriptional interference.[78]

Lentiviral vector production has always been hampered by the fact that Vpr expression prevents the activation of p34[cdc2] cyclin, arresting (packaging) cells in the $G_2/M$ phase of the cell cycle.[79,80] Besides Vpr, the expression of gp55*** and the frequently used VSV pseudotype are toxic for producer cells, effectively restricting lentivirus vector production to the use of transient transfection systems. Recently, an inducible VSV-G pseudotyped lentivirus packaging cell line was constructed expressing these toxic components of vector assembly under the tight control of the tetracycline-inducible promoter. The producer line could generate $10^6$ cfu/ml of virus particles for three to four days. Because of the stable VSV pseudotype, a further 3 log concentration ($10^9$ cfu/ml) of this vector could be obtained by ultracentrifugation.[81] A stable lentivirus packaging cell line will eventually facilitate research and reliable large-scale production of vector quantities for preclinical in vivo studies.

### Lentiviral transduction of hematopoietic cells: independent of the cell cycle?

The *vpr* gene product of HIV-1 is one of the key elements for nuclear localization of this virus. For the wild-type virus, this protein is essential for effectively replicating in monocytes and macrophages. In the absence of other viral proteins, Vpr localizes to the nucleus. Vpr packaging into viral particles depends on the p6 domain of the Gag precursor polyprotein p55$^{gag}$. Mutational analysis suggests that the N-terminal domain of Vpr is involved in both nuclear localization and virion packaging. Other HIV structures are also involved in nuclear localization, so that this characteristic cannot be transferred to other vector systems by Vpr transfer alone.[79,80]

Efficient HIV-1 virus and vector infection requires target cell activation. Target cell cycling greatly improves the efficiency of integration, but does not seem to be required. Resting T cells are one extensively studied model of lentiviral integration into quiescent cells. In HIV-1 infection of quiescent peripheral CD4$^+$ lymphocytes, reverse transcription is incomplete. Korin et al[82] isolated highly purified quiescent T cells to study the influence of CD3/CD28 activation and cell cycle inhibitors in HIV-1 reverse transcription. CD3 activation led to cycle progression into $G_{1a}$ and incomplete reverse transcription. Co-stimulation of the CD28 receptor for the transition into $G_{1b}$ also led to complete reverse transcription.[82]

Resting T cells as a model of lentivirus-refractory cells could also be transduced with an HIV-1 vector after culture in IL-2, IL-4, IL-6, IL-7, or IL-15, demonstrating that cytokine signals alone permit transduction of a resting cell population with these vectors.[83]

The exact kinetics of lentivirus vector integration still remain to be established. When comparing the transduction of primitive, quiescent human hematopoietic progenitor cells between an HIV-1 lentiviral vector and an MLV retroviral vector, Case et al[84] found that only the lentiviral vector expressed GFP in nondivided CD34$^+$ cells and in $G_0$ CD34$^+$CD38$^-$ cells 48 hours after transduction. Interestingly, short-term GFP expression could also be detected after transduction with a mutation-disabled-integrase lentiviral vector, suggesting transcriptional activity of the preintegration complex. Integrated vector activity could only be detected after extended long-term bone marrow culture.

Both lentiviral and MLV vectors efficiently transduced cytokine-stimulated

CD34$^+$ cells. As expected from the in vitro data and the MLV vector experience, use of SCF, Flt-3L, IL-3, and IL-6 in serum-free media in human umbilical-cord-derived CD34$^+$CD38$^-$ cells for five days improved lentiviral transduction efficiency in CD34$^+$CD38$^-$ cells (59%) as determined by flow cytometry. Erythroid and myeloid colonies derived from transduced CD34$^+$CD38$^-$ cells were EGFR-positive at a high frequency (66% ± 9%).[85] Lentiviral transduction of CD34$^+$CD38$^-$ cells stable over 15 weeks of extended long-term culture (9.2% ± 5.2%, $n = 7$) was less efficient and failed with MLV vectors at lower titers. Without growth factors, only the lentiviral vector was able to transduce CD34$^+$ and CD34$^+$CD38$^-$ cells at all. Gene transfer into these primitive progenitor cells was clearly easier with a lentiviral vector – but much less efficient than in cycling cells.[84] In another lentiviral vector system, HIV-2 vector DNA could be detected in HIV-2 vector-transduced nondividing CD34$^+$CD38$^-$ human hematopoietic progenitor cells, whereas stable integration and expression of the reporter gene could not be detected in these hematopoietic progenitors, leaving open the question of the accessibility of these cells to stable lentivirus transduction.[86]

Several reports indicate that in vivo repopulating cells are also reached with this vector system. Miyoshi et al[87] report that transduction of human CD34$^+$ cord blood cells without cytokine stimulation resulted in transgene expression in multiple lineages for up to 22 weeks after xenotransplantation into NOD–SCID mice. Currently, several groups are attempting to reproduce this data in large-animal models.

### Feline, simian, and equine immunodeficiency virus vectors

Although HIV infection is likely of primate origin, there is a good degree of species adherence in lentiviruses. Its molecular basis is not well understood, but obviously a key issue for the generation of safer lentiviral vectors. Nonprimate lentiviruses are therefore of special interest to vector designers. The highly restricted tropism of feline immunodeficiency virus (FIV) can be overcome by promoter substitution to generate a pseudotyped three-plasmid lentiviral vector system in a human cell line. Pseudotyped FIV vectors could transduce dividing, growth-arrested, and postmitotic human target cells.[88,89]

Another approach to reduce sequence homologies in order to decrease the likelihood of homologous recombination is to combine elements of multiple lentiviruses in a single packaging system. White et al[90] describe encapsidation of an HIV-1-vector backbone by nonvirulent SIVmac1A11 core particles pseudotyped with VSV glycoprotein G. Like a normal HIV vector, this 'HIV/SIVpack/G' could achieve gene transfer into human lymphocytes, human primary macrophages, human bone-marrow-derived CD34$^+$ cells, and primary mouse neurons.[90]

### The biosafety of lentiviral vector systems

As in other retroviral vector systems, the most prominent safety concern for the in vitro and in vivo preclinical use of lentiviral vectors arises mainly from the possibility of recombination between vector and packaging genes of the vector system, which may give rise to replication-competent viruses with pathogenic potential.

A self-inactivating (SIN) deletion in parts of the 3' LTR reduces but does not abolish the possibility of homologous recombination to generate a replication-competent lentivirus with vector elements in the vector producer cells or in a wild-type HIV-infected host.

Nonprimate lentiviral vectors may offer safety advantages, but a simple promoter substitution can overcome their species restriction. Even without genetic modifications, the species restriction can be leaky. The infectivity of two FIV strains, V1CSF and Petaluma, was compared in human cells after cell-free infection. Up to 12% of cells showed immunocytological evidence for infection. FIV genome, reverse-transcriptase activity, and increased cell death were detected in infected human peripheral blood mononuclear cells (PBMC) and macrophages. Antibodies binding the CCR3 chemokine receptor maximally inhibited infection of human PBMC by both FIV strains compared with antibodies to CXCR4, the original receptor, or CCR5. FIV can productively infect primary human cell lines and viral strain specificity should be considered in FIV vectors for gene therapy.[91]

# TRANSFER OF DRUG RESISTANCE: IN VITRO AND IN VIVO SELECTION

Drug-resistance genes are desirable tools for manipulating the hematopoietic system by gene transfer in two major application groups. Transferred as single genes, drug-resistance genes can potentially increase the resistance of the hematopoietic system against specific agents, reducing the hematopoietic toxicity of repeated or long-term chemotherapy. The second group of applications uses co-transferred resistance gene as a means of distinguishing and selecting transduced cells in vitro and in vivo. If successful, ex vivo and in vivo selection of stem cells is hoped to overcome an otherwise insufficient gene transfer by eliminating competing non-transduced stem cells before and after engraftment.

## MDR1: Multidrug resistance

Physiologic multidrug resistance (MDR) is provided by the adenosine triphosphate (ATP)-dependent multidrug membrane transporter P-glycoprotein (P-gp) MDR1. MDR1 expression or overexpression protects cells against natural-product anticancer drugs, including paclitaxel. Overexpression of human MDR1 has been reported to confer an in vivo selectable drug resistance to murine hematopoietic stem cells.[92, 93] To select transduced cells on the basis of MDR1, Aran et al have constructed functional bicistronic expression vectors by linking the MDR1 gene via an internal ribosomal entry site (IRES) to other (reporter) genes of interest, including β-galactosidase and the red-shifted green fluorescent protein (GFP).[94]

The potential problems of *MDR1* gene transfer, however, are manifold. The gene is large (4 kb), using up about half of the overall theoretical capacity of MLV vector systems. In addition, and probably inherent to its size, therapeutic applications of the *MDR1* gene are hampered by cryptic splicing of the mRNA before and after vector packaging and transfer. Spliced inactive variants of *MDR1* vector RNA are being packaged and transferred from the packaging line as well as being spliced from transcripts of successfully transferred full-length cDNA. Conservative mutations of prominent splice donor and acceptor sites have been used to control this problem.[95]

Murine and human hematopoietic progenitor and stem cells are supposed to express high physiologic levels of MDR1 as detectable by their characteristic rhodamine 123-low phenotype. In the murine system where the overexpressed human MDR1 is active on a background of its murine analogue, selection could be achieved. In large-animal and human models, that situation may be different in terms of what additional benefit a constitutive transferred expression of MDR1 may confer to an already high native expression in hematopoietic target cells and a probably inducible expression in the treated tumor cells.

In common marmosets, a non-human primate model, Hibino et al[96] performed ex vivo transduction with an *MDR1*–vector. Proviral DNA was detectable by PCR in granulocytes and lymphocytes for up to 400 days post transplantation. When recipient marmosets were challenged with docetaxel, the <1% level of in vivo gene transfer did not prevent docetaxel-induced neutropenia.[96]

In a first clinical protocol, Cowan et al at the NIH have conducted a clinical gene therapy trial of retroviral-mediated *MDR1* gene transfer. One-third of both peripheral blood apheresis and bone marrow product obtained after mobilization with single-dose cyclophosphamide (4 g/m²), G-CSF (10 µg/kg/day), and CD34 enrichment from patients with metastatic breast cancer was transduced ex vivo for 72 hours with *MDR1* retroviral vector (G1MD), SCF, IL-3, and IL-6. Manipulated and non-manipulated cells were reinfused following ifosfamide, carboplatin, and etoposide conditioning chemotherapy. After hematopoietic recovery, patients received six cycles of paclitaxel (175 mg/m² every 3 weeks). Bone marrow and peripheral blood were tested for presence of the *MDR1* transgene by PCR. The ex vivo transduction efficiency, estimated by the PCR assay, ranged from 0.1% to 0.5%. Three out of the four patients engrafted transduced cells, with a range of marker-positive peripheral mononuclear cells from 0.01% to 9%. Two of these three patients lost all detectable *MDR1* marking.[97,98] Neither in this nor in the other two trials reported in the literature by Hanania et al[93] and Hesdorffer et al[99] was selection of *MDR1*-transduced leukocytes or stem cells observed at any level. The second NIH *MDR1* trial performed a direct side-by-side comparison of a total-transplant transduction with half of the transplant transduced on stroma without cytokines with an *MDR1*–vector and the other half with a *neo*–vector. At transplantation, on average only 0.26% of cells contained the *MDR1* gene from the G1MD vector, whereas *neo* transduction efficiency with G1Na was 30.3%. All six patients had detectable gene marking at some point after recovery.

Interestingly, in those three patients where the marking was not detected initially, granulocytes were selected to a vector-positive percentage of around 1% during the post-transplantation paclitaxel chemotherapy. Also, despite the high pretransplantation levels of *neo* marking, in vivo *neo* signal was only detectable in three out of the six patients, and became undetectable during chemotherapy in two of these three.

A modification of this approach has been proposed to circumvent low expression and selectability of the *MDR1* gene in vivo. Machiels et al[100] have used multidrug-resistance-associated protein (MRP) instead of MDR1. MRP function is not affected by MDR1 reversal agents. After murine ex vivo trans-duction, long-term MRP expression and function was detectable for over five months. In vivo selection of MRP-transduced cells was achieved by doxoru-bicin administration, and chemoprotection was improved after the second chemotherapy cycle.[100]

Currently, a new development in the field of *MDR1* gene transfer is the focus of interest. Bunting et al[101] observed dramatic ex vivo stem cell expansion in the presence of the early-acting hematopoietic cytokines IL-3, IL-6, and SCF. After transducing bone marrow cells with retroviral vectors and subse-quent 'expansion culture' over 12 days, high levels of long-term engraftment occurred, and progressive expansion of *MDR1*-transduced repopulating cells over the expansion period was observed, with a 13-fold overall increase in stem cells after 12 days. Mice transplanted with expanded *MDR1*-transduced stem cells developed a myeloproliferative disorder/leukemia characterized by high peripheral white blood cell counts and splenomegaly.[101] It is currently the subject of intense study whether the overexpression of *MDR1* itself can repro-ducibly induce myeloproliferation when it is transferred by other vectors or into other animal models. It is conceivable that the increase in MDR1 function together with the cytokines used may produce proliferation of early cells; how-ever, the phenomenon may also be related to the vector system used. Interest-ingly, Bunting et al[101] did not observe this phenomenon when transplanting the cells without the 'expansion culture' step or when transferring the dihydro-folate reductase (*DHFR*) gene instead of the *MDR1* gene.

## DHFR: methotrexate resistance

The Tyr22, Arg22, Ser31, Trp31, or Ser34 *DHFR* mutants confer resistance to methotrexate (MTX) by decreasing drug binding, while enzymatic activity remains sufficient for physiologic folate metabolism. It has not been entirely clear whether mutant *DHFR* protection allows a selective advantage at the right cell level. Single-dose MTX up to 250 mg/kg did not reduce CFU-C numbers in mice after one to three days, while non-clonogenic precursor cells declined. Preceding systemic SCF administration also could not recruit progenitor cells into MTX or trimetrexate susceptibility, which is the case for alkylating agents. In theory, folate analogues may therefore be less than ideal for selection of primitive progenitor cells in vivo.[102]

Kwok et al[103] could demonstrate successful retroviral transfer of the *DHFR* gene in a large-animal model as early as 1986. Flasshove et al[104] could show later that transduced human Ser31 *DHFR* rendered CFU-GM resistant against a toxic level of $2 \times 10^{-8}$ mol/L MTX, leading to a twofold selective advantage. In the same year, May et al[105] could confer a survival advantage to mice against lethal doses of MTX by transplanting large doses of bone marrow from transgenic animals expressing either the Arg22 or Trp31 *DHFR* mutants. Allay et al[106] could then define conditions where trimetrexate treatment could select vector-expressing peripheral blood erythrocytes, platelets, granulocytes, and lymphocytes in vivo. Secondary transplants demonstrated that this selection occurred at the level of hematopoietic stem cells.[106]

To model the therapeutic benefit of high dose MTX treatment, Zhao et al[107] used the transplanted breast cancer E0771 tumor. After cyclophosphamide conditioning and transplantation of Ser31 *DHFR*-transduced marrow, tumor-bearing mice were treated with otherwise-lethal doses of methotrexate. Forty-four percent of the mice had no demonstrable tumor on day 52. The control group of mice transplanted but not treated with MTX died of tumor regrowth.[107]

To demonstrate a possible application in a gene-therapeutic setting, the same authors[108] used transfer of a vector that combines a Tyr22 *DHFR* gene with anti-*BCR/ABL* b3a2 *BCR/ABL* antisense sequences, enabling post-transplant chemotherapy to decrease persistent CML disease while rendering inadvertently transduced CML stem and progenitor cells functionally normal. b3a2 *BCR/ABL* containing 32D and MO7e cells were transduced with this vector and selected in MTX for 14 days. *BCR/ABL* mRNA and p210[BCR/ABL] protein levels were reduced by six- to tenfold, cell growth was slowed, and cytokine independence was reverted. Tumorigency of 32D *BCR/ABL* cells in vivo decreased by 3–4 logs.[108]

## $O^6$-MGMT: chloroethylnitrosourea/$O^6$-benzylguanine resistance

Chloroethylnitrosourea (CENU) chemotherapeutic alkylating agents such as 1,3-bis(2-chloroethyl)-1-nitrosourea (BCNU, carmustine) can ablate hematopoietic progenitor and stem cells. CENU cytotoxicity is effected by alkylation at the $O^6$ position of guanine and subsequent interstrand DNA crosslinking. Repair of CENU-induced DNA damage occurs by removal of alkyl groups from the $O^6$ position of $O^6$-alkylguanine by the eukaryotic methyl-guanine DNA methyltransferase (MGMT). Williams and co-workers have previously demonstrated that a retroviral vector expressing MGMT driven by the human phosphoglycerate kinase promoter (PGK–MGMT) protects transplantated murine bone marrow in vivo from acute CENU toxicity. Even the profound carmustine-induced CD4$^+$CD8$^+$ lymphocyte deficiency observed in control mice was prevented in mice transplanted with PGK–MGMT-transduced bone marrow. Molecular studies suggest a selection at the level of transduced lymphoid cells.[109]

MGMT repair of CENU-induced damage can be suppressed and thus CENU cytotoxicity can be potentiated by addition of a specific MGMT inhibitor, $O^6$-benzylguanine ($O^6$-BG). MGMT mutants have been identified that have a greatly reduced affinity for the $O^6$-BG suppressor molecule while retaining their repair activity. Retroviral transfer of $O^6$-BG-insensitive MGMT mutants can be used to enhance the effects of CENU selection. In this strategy, the presence of $O^6$-BG increases the CENU sensitivity of nontransduced cells by suppressing the natural background of MGMT DNA repair without affecting the MGMT function of the mutant transgene. Hickson et al[110] performed retroviral transduction of an $O^6$-BG-inhibitable and an $O^6$-BG-insensitive MGMT mutant into K562 human erythroleukemic cells and human cord-blood-derived CD34$^+$ hematopoietic cells. Significant protection in the presence of 20 μm $O^6$-BG against mitozolomide- ($p < 0.05$) and temozolomide- ($p < 0.001$) induced toxicity was only present in cells harboring the cDNA encoding an $O^6$-BG-insensitive MGMT mutant. Chinnasamy et al found simultaneously that the increased selectivity of this approach extended to transplantable murine hematopoietic progenitors.[110]

By random sequence mutagenesis and subsequent systematic study in the murine hematopoietic transplant model, the P140A and especially the P140K mutants have recently been identified as those $O^6$-BG refractory mutants of mammalian MGMT with the best protective MGMT activity (twice that of wild-type MGMT) in mammalian hematopoietic cells in vivo.[111]

Currently, the use of combinations of a CENU and $O^6$-BG is the subject of intense preclinical and clinical studies, both with respect to their improved antitumor activity (therapeutic index) and, in the field of gene therapy, their suitability for the in vivo selection of human hematopoietic stem cells transduced with $O^6$-BG refractory MGMT mutants. In the murine system, recent data suggest that carmustine/$O^6$-BG in vivo selection can effectively eliminate all nontransduced  hematopoietic stem cells, resulting in 100% stem cell transduction in second- and third-generation transplants in the murine model (S Ragg, personal communication).

## Glutathione-S-transferase: glutathione transfer inhibits alkyl transfer

To protect bone marrow cells from the toxicity of alkylating agents, including cyclophosphamide, and doxorubicin, the glutathione-S-transferase *pi* gene (*GST-pi*) can be transduced. Its gene product is thought to conjugate many alkylating agents with glutathione and to remove a toxic peroxide product of doxorubicin. *GST-pi* gene-transduced CD34$^+$ cells formed 2.5- to 3-fold more CFU-GM than *neo* gene-transduced CD34$^+$ cells in the presence of 2.5 μg/ml of 4-hydroperoxycyclophosphamide (4-HC) and 30 ng/ml of doxorubicin. Colony formation could be observed at up to twice that drug concentration (5.0 µg/ml of 4-HC, 50 ng/ml of doxorubicin) that killed all *neo*-transduced control cells.[112]

## TRANSFER OF PRODRUG SUSCEPTIBILITY: PUTTING THE GENIE BACK INTO THE BOTTLE

One of the new functions that can be added to a cell by gene transfer is the regulation of cell death. Different approaches have been tested to control apoptosis in tumor cells, with mixed results. At less than 100% gene transfer efficiency in vivo, this concept is burdened with a conceptual flaw that still has to be overcome.[113] With relation to gene therapy in stem cell transplantation, however, suicide gene transfer has developed into a very interesting therapeutic application.

### HSV thymidine kinase (HSV-TK): ganciclovir prodrug activation

Observations in clinical transplantation that a moderate degree of graft-versus-host disease (GvHD) was associated with a favorable prognosis after allogeneic marrow transplantation[114] suggested early that allogeneic leukocytes confer immunological control of the tumor cell clone in leukemia.[115] Therapeutic application of this concept began about 10 years ago with the use of donor lymphocyte infusions for the treatment of CML relapse after allogeneic transplantation.[116] Since then, there has been increasing evidence that the therapeutic efficacy of allogeneic stem cell transplantation in myeloid leukemias and other disease entities does not require aggressive conditioning regimens but is mostly the result of allo immune surveillance exerting a graft-versus-leukemia/tumor effect over the residual malignant recipient cells.

By systematic and elegant studies in murine and dog models, it has further been established that myeloablation is not necessary for establishing an allograft, and that the mixed donor/host chimerism resulting from low-intensity conditioning before transplantation can be converted into full donor chimerism by the additional infusion of donor T cells.[117,118] In this setting, the recognition of the importance of donor/host chimerism and the ability to manipulate the degree of tolerance have added adoptive immunotherapy by transfer of donor lymphocytes to the oncological arsenal of relapse treatment. In the first series of 135 patients treated with donor lymphocyte infusions reported by Kolb et al for the European Group for Blood and Marrow Transplantation (EBMT), complete remissions were re-induced by donor lymphocyte transfusions in 54/84 patients (64%) with CML, in 2/2 patients with polycythemia vera and myelodysplastic syndrome (MDS), and in 5/29 patients (17%) with AML.[116,119] As a result of these and other observations, the intensity of conditioning and immunosuppression have been reduced substantially, affording feasibility of allogeneic transplantation to patients with more advanced age or intensive pretreatment.[120,121] With the reduction of acute conditioning treatment toxicity, GvHD – the unwanted immune reaction of the transplant against donor organs, notably gut, liver, and skin – is rapidly becoming the most frequent and dangerous complication of reduced-toxicity allogeneic stem cell transplantation. In the EBMT series reported above, 52/135 patients (39%) developed acute GvHD of grade 2 or more. Fourteen patients died from GvHD and/or myelosuppression.

The herpes simplex virus thymidine kinase (HSV-TK) phosphorylates the low-toxicity prodrug ganciclovir into a highly toxic metabolite, ganciclovir triphosphate. DNA incorporation during the S phase of dividing cells will lead to DNA strand breaks and apoptosis. This toxicity is sufficient to reliably kill over 98% of cells expressing the gene in an environment with a ganciclovir concentration of no acute toxicity that can be obtained by systemic infusion in vivo. The HSV-TK gene can easily be incorporated into a retroviral vector. It can be combined with a gene that allows for the positive selection of transduced cells, for example neomycin or hygromycin phophotransferase for toxin selection or a truncated nerve cell growth factor receptor for immunological selection. The resulting combination vector can be used for initial positive selection of the transduced target cell population and subsequent ablation of that population in vivo should the target cell population be the source of an unwanted side-effect (GvHD) at a later time point.[122]

Bordignon and co-workers have pioneered the use of these vector systems in clinical studies. Successful reversal of acute GvHD could be obtained in 3/3 patients out of the 8-patient study cohort. After evaluating the therapeutic success of the first clinical application of the suicide gene approach, vector design and application can be improved further. As in other studies, a strong immune response against the vector gene product was detectable in two patients. This is interesting for our understanding of transplantation-induced induction of immune tolerance. Also, immunoselection against T cells with the transgene may result in a functional 'leakiness' of the suicide gene function that may result from the survival advantage of nontransduced, i.e. non-ablatable alloreactive, T-cell clones. Further, ganciclovir ablation of T cells did not fully remit the only case of chronic GvHD among the 8 study patients. Verzeletti et al[123] have meanwhile proposed and tested the reduction of transgene immunogenicity by removal of the neomycin phophotransferase resistance gene that was still present in the original vector. Positive selection is now performed by using the truncated low-affinity nerve cell growth factor receptor cDNA to express a cell surface selectable marker of little or no immunogenicity. The lack of long-term efficiency against thus selected and transduced alloreactive GvH T cells is hypothesized to be related to in vivo promoter inactivation that may be overcome by use of different retroviral promoter/enhancer combinations.[123] A similar approach has also been proposed for a more specific use of human HLA-specific T-cell clones by Gallot et al.[124]

## TRANSFER OF THERAPEUTIC GENES

### Preclinical animal models of hematopoietic gene transfer

Spontaneous murine β-glucuronidase deficiency (mucopolysaccharidosis VII) has been one of the most extensively studied early models for therapeutic gene transfer into the hematopoietic system.[125] The feasibility of murine knockouts has vastly expanded the availability of murine monogenetic defect models of human inherited diseases that can be cured by the appropriate gene transfer.

Chronic granulomatous disease (CGD) is a disorder where the phagocytes of affected patients are unable to kill microorganisms owing to a functional defect in the phagocytic nicotinamide adenine dinucleotide phosphatase (NADPH) oxidase (phox) enzyme complex. Bjorgvinsdottir, Dinauer, and Grez, and their colleagues have demonstrated functional reconstitution of burst activity in models of CGD by transfer of a retroviral vector containing the coding sequences of gp91-phox.[126–128]

While there is an ever-expanding list of monogenetic leukocyte disorders that can be treated by retroviral gene transfer in the murine system, thus far no large-animal system has been described where gene transfer has had a major therapeutic impact.

### Long-term expression: approaches to vector design

The murine retroviral LTR is one of the strongest constitutive promoters available. Long-term in vivo expression is not easily achieved using this LTR, however. Grez et al[129] were able to demonstrate that the LTR from the myeloproliferative sarcoma virus (MPSV) can be used for more stable expression in a murine embryonic stem cell vector.

Baum et al[130] and Robbins et al[131] have proposed and tested further modifications of this system. It is mostly consensus that three viral elements may act as repressors of expression by Mo-MuLV: enhancer, the primer binding site, and the negative-control region. Significantly higher quantities (>80 times) of vector-specific transcripts in embryonic stem cells and embryonic carcinoma cells and greater expression of secondary murine CFU-S were detected in those cells transduced with the vector modified in *cis*-acting transcriptional factors.

### Human clinical trials of hematopoietic gene transfer

As already mentioned, several clinical gene transfer trials have been reported in ADA-deficient SCID, X-linked SCID, Gaucher's disease, Fanconi's anemia, CGD and HIV-1 (for a review, see reference 132). The level of gene transfer has overall been as low as in the earlier gene marking trials, usually in or well below the 0.1–0.01% range. However, in many of these trials, evidence for long-term engraftment of transduced cells has been described. Two pediatric trials impress as the most effective to date. Kohn et al[133] described cord blood transplants in three newborns with ADA-deficient SCID. Four years after the initial transplants, the frequency of gene-containing T lymphocytes has risen to 1–10%, whereas the frequency of other marked hematopoietic cells remained at 0.01–0.1%. This led the authors to carefully and temporarily discontinue the enzyme replacement therapy with polyethylene glycol-conjugated adenosine deaminase. A further selective accumulation of gene-containing T lymphocytes was observed. Unfortunately, independence of enzyme replacement therapy could not be maintained despite the relatively high transduction efficiency obtained in this protocol. The authors concluded that further improvements in gene transfer efficiency will be required for a therapeutic benefit.[133]

Recently, Alain Fischer's French trial for a very similar disease (X-linked human SCID, SCID-X1) has reported even more striking results.[134] Two patients were reinfused with 30 and $13 \times 10^6$ CD34$^+$ bone marrow cells per kilogram that had been transduced with an MFG γ-chain vector in three cycles using standard culture conditions (SCF, MGDF, Flt3-L, IL-3, and fibronectin). At retransfusion, 20% of CD34$^+$ cells were vector-positive. In this disease, transfer of the defective IL-2R γ-chain reconstitutes the IL-2, IL-4, IL-7, IL-9, and IL-15 receptor function of blood leukocytes, especially T and natural killer (NK) cells. These cell fractions were hardly detectable in the peripheral blood of the untreated patients (patient 1: lymphocyte count 3000/μl, CD3$^+$ 3%, CD19$^+$ 97%, and CD16$^+$ 1%; patient 2: lymphocyte count 700/μl, CD3$^+$ 0%, CD19$^+$ 95%, and CD16$^+$ 0.1%). In theory, there should be a major growth advantage of transduced blood lymphocytes. Days 75–90 after transplantation, lymphocyte counts started rising. On day 150, the blood of patient 1 contained polyclonal, IL-2, and antigen-proliferating T cells/μl (1800 CD3$^+$ cells/μl, 1250 CD4$^+$ cells/μl and 500 CD8$^+$ cells/μl) that expressed the γ-chain transgene. The second patient had 450 CD3$^+$ cells/μl in the peripheral blood on day +120. Vector-positive NK cells were also detectable. Both patients are currently clinically stable and could be discharged home. It will depend upon long-term observation whether this 'natural selection' will stably maintain T-cell replacement and function over prolonged periods of time.

## CONCLUSIONS

More than 10 years after the beginning of the first clinical application, progress has been made in many areas of hematopoietic gene transfer, including hematopoietic stem cell transduction, selection, and transplantation.

With increasing momentum, the field is moving closer to the possibility of therapeutic hematopoietic gene transfer, with integrating vector systems for a number of diseases. Both as a prerequisite and as a spin-off, our understanding of normal marrow physiology in the adult human will rapidly increase.

# REFERENCES

1. Dunbar CE, Tisdale J, Yu JM et al, Transduction of hematopoietic stem cells in humans and in nonhuman primates. *Stem Cells* 1997; **15**(Suppl 1): 135–9; discussion 139–40.

2. Kohn DB, Gene therapy for haematopoietic and lymphoid disorders. *Clin Exp Immunol* 1997; **107**: 54–7.

3. Nienhuis AW, Bertran J, Hargrove P et al, Gene transfer into hematopoietic cells. *Stem Cells* 1997; **15**(Suppl 1): 123–34.

4. Shi Q, Rafii S, Wu MH et al, Evidence for circulating bone marrow-derived endothelial cells. *Blood* 1998; **92**: 362–7.

5. Petersen BE, Bowen WC, Patrene KD et al, Bone marrow as a potential source of hepatic oval cells. *Science* 1999; **284**: 1168–70.

6. Ferrari G, Cusella-De Angelis G, Coletta M et al, Muscle regeneration by bone marrow-derived myogenic progenitors. *Science* 1998; **279**: 1528–30 [Erratum 1998; **281**: 923].

7. Moore MA, 'Turning brain into blood' – clinical applications of stem-cell research in neurobiology and hematology. *N Engl J Med* 1999; **341**: 605–7.

8. Cross MA, Heyworth CM, Dexter TM, How do stem cells decide what to do? *Ciba Found Symp* 1997; **204**: 3–14; discussion 14–18.

9. Eaves C, Miller C, Conneally E et al, Introduction to stem cell biology in vitro. Threshold to the future. *Ann NY Acad Sci* 1999; **872**: 1–8.

10. Dick JE, Magli MC, Huszar D et al, Introduction of a selectable gene into primitive stem cells capable of long-term reconstitution of the hematopoietic system of W/Wv mice. *Cell* 1985; **42**: 71–9.

11. Lemischka IR, Raulet DH, Mulligan RC, Developmental potential and dynamic behavior of hematopoietic stem cells. *Cell* 1986; **45**: 917–27.

12. Cornetta K, Fan Y, Retroviral gene therapy in hematopoietic diseases. *J Clin Apheresis* 1997; **12**: 187–93.

13. Marandin A, Dubart A, Pflumio F et al, Retrovirus-mediated gene transfer into human CD34+38low primitive cells capable of reconstituting long-term cultures in vitro and nonobese diabetic-severe combined immunodeficiency mice in vivo. *Hum Gene Ther* 1998; **9**: 1497–511.

14. Dao MA, Hannum CH, Kohn DB et al, Flt3 ligand preserves the ability of human cd34(+) progenitors to sustain long-term hematopoiesis in immune-deficient mice after ex vivo retroviral-mediated transduction. *Blood* 1997; **89**: 446–56.

15. Kiem HP, Heyward S, Winkler A et al, Gene transfer into marrow repopulating cells: comparison between amphotropic and gibbon ape leukemia virus pseudotyped retroviral vectors in a competitive repopulation assay in baboons. *Blood* 1997; **90**: 4638–45.

16. Tisdale JF, Hanazono Y, Sellers SE et al, Ex vivo expansion of genetically marked rhesus peripheral blood progenitor cells results in diminished long-term repopulating ability. *Blood* 1998; **92**: 1131–41.

17. Dunbar CE, Kohn DB, Schiffmann R et al, Retroviral transfer of the glucocerebrosidase gene into CD34+ cells from patients with Gaucher disease: in vivo detection of transduced cells without myeloablation. *Hum Gene Ther* 1998; **9**: 2629–40.

18. Lewis PF, Emerman M, Passage through mitosis is required for oncoretroviruses but not for the human immunodeficiency virus. *J Virol* 1994; **68**: 510–16.

19. Miller DG, Adam MA, Miller AD, Gene transfer by retrovirus vectors occurs only in cells that are actively replicating at the time of infection. *Mol Cell Biol* 1990; **10**: 4239–42.

20. Reems JA, Torok-Storb B, Cell cycle and functional differences between $CD34^+CD38^{hi}$ and $CD34^+38^{lo}$ human marrow cells after in vitro cytokine exposure. *Blood* 1995; **85**: 1480–7.

21. Hao QL, Thiemann FT, Petersen D et al, Extended long-term culture reveals a highly quiescent and primitive human hematopoietic progenitor population. *Blood* 1996; **88**: 3306–13.

22. von Kalle C, Kiem HP, Goehle S et al, Increased gene transfer into human hematopoietic progenitor cells by extended in vitro exposure to a pseudotyped retroviral vector. *Blood* 1994; **84**: 2890–7.

23. Glimm H, Kiem HP, Darovsky B et al, Efficient gene transfer in primitive CD34+/CD38lo human bone marrow cells reselected after long-term exposure to GALV-pseudotyped retroviral vector. *Hum Gene Ther* 1997; **8**: 2079–86.

24. Conneally E, Eaves CJ, Humphries RK, Efficient retroviral-mediated gene transfer to human cord blood stem cells with in vivo repopulating potential. *Blood* 1998; **91**: 3487–93.

25. Henneman B, Conneally E, Leboulch P et al, Efficient gene transfer into human CD34+ cord blood cells and progenitors using a GALV pseudotyped recombinant retrovirus containing the neomycin resistance and the green fluorescent protein (GFP) genes. *Proc Am Soc Gene Ther Meeting* 1998; Abst a342.

26. Williams SF, Lee WJ, Bender JG et al, Selection and expansion of peripheral blood CD34+ cells in autologous stem cell transplantation for breast cancer. *Blood* 1996; **87**: 1687–91.

27. Veena P, Traycoff CM, Williams DA et al, Delayed targeting of cytokine-nonresponsive human bone marrow CD34(+) cells with retrovirus-mediated gene transfer enhances transduction efficiency and long-term expression of transduced genes. *Blood* 1998; **91**: 3693–701.

28. Dexter TM, Allen TD, Lajtha LG, Conditions controlling the proliferation of hematopoietic cells in vitro. *J Cell Physiol* 1977; **91**: 335–44.

29. Verfaillie CM, Miller JS, A novel single-cell proliferation assay shows that long-term culture-initiating cell (LTC-IC) maintenance over time results from the extensive proliferation of a small fraction of LTC-IC. *Blood* 1995; **86**: 2137–45.

30. Glimm H, Eaves CJ, Direct evidence for multiple self-renewal divisions of human in vivo repopulating hematopoietic cells in short-term culture. *Blood* 1999; **94**: 2161–8.

31. Miller AD, Rosman GJ, Improved retroviral vectors for gene transfer and expression. *Biotechniques* 1989; **7**: 980–2.

32. Miyao Y, Shimizu K, Tamura M et al, A simplified general method for determination of recombinant retrovirus titers. *Cell Struct Funct* 1995; **20**: 177–83.

33. Yang S, Delgado R, King SR et al, Generation of retroviral vector for clinical studies using transient transfection. *Hum Gene Ther* 1999; **10**: 123–32.

34. Miller AD, Garcia JV, von Suhr N et al, Construction and properties of retrovirus packaging cells based on gibbon ape leukemia virus. *J Virol* 1991; **65**: 2220–4.

35. Sabatino DE, Do B, Pyle LC et al, Amphotropic or gibbon ape leukemia virus (galv) retrovirus binding and transduction correlates with the level of receptor mrna in human hematopoietic cell lines. *Blood Cells Mol Dis* 1997; **23**: 422–33.

36. Bodine DM, Dunbar CE, Girard LJ et al, Improved amphotropic retrovirus-mediated gene transfer into hematopoietic stem cells. *Ann NY Acad Sci* 1998; **850**: 139–50.

37. Orlic D, Girard LJ, Jordan CT et al, The level of mRNA encoding the amphotropic retrovirus receptor in mouse and human hematopoietic stem cells is low and correlates with the efficiency of retrovirus transduction. *Proc Natl Acad Sci USA* 1996; **93**: 11097–102.

38. Horwitz ME, Malech HL, Anderson SM et al, Granulocyte colony-stimulating factor mobilized peripheral blood stem cells enter into G1 of the cell cycle and express higher levels of amphotropic retrovirus receptor mRNA. *Exp Hematol* 1999; **27**: 1160–7.

39. Kiem HP, Heyward S, Winkler A et al, Gene transfer into marrow repopul-

ating cells: comparison between amphotropic and gibbon ape leukemia virus pseudotyped retroviral vectors in a competitive repopulation assay in baboons. *Blood* 1997; **90**: 4638–45.

40. Friedmann T, Yee JK, Pseudotyped retroviral vectors for studies of human gene therapy. *Nature Med* 1995; **1**: 275–7.

41. Agrawal RS, Karhu K, Laukkanen J et al, Complement and anti-alpha-galactosyl natural antibody-mediated inactivation of murine retrovirus occurs in adult serum but not in umbilical cord serum. *Gene Ther* 1999; **6**: 146–8.

42. Shimizu K, Miyao Y, Tamura M et al, Infectious retrovirus is inactivated by serum but not by cerebrospinal fluid or fluid from tumor bed in patients with malignant glioma. *Jpn J Cancer Res* 1995; **86**: 1010–13.

43. Rollins SA, Birks CW, Setter E et al, Retroviral vector producer cell killing in human serum is mediated by natural antibody and complement – strategies for evading the humoral immune response. *Hum Gene Ther* 1996; **7**: 619–26.

44. Riddell SR, Elliott M, Lewinsohn DA et al, T-cell mediated rejection of gene-modified HIV-specific cytotoxic T lymphocytes in HIV-infected patients. *Nature Med* 1996; **2**: 216–23.

45. Sachs DH, Smith CV, Emery DW et al, Induction of specific tolerance to MHC-disparate allografts through genetic engineering. *Exp Nephrol* 1993; **1**: 128–33.

46. Sellers SE, Tisdale JF, Bodine DM et al, No discrepancy between in vivo gene marking efficiency assessed in peripheral blood populations compared with bone marrow progenitors or CD34+ cells. *Hum Gene Ther* 1999; **10**: 633–40.

47. Cornetta K, Morgan RA, Gillio A et al, No retroviremia or pathology in long-term follow-up of monkeys exposed to a murine amphotropic retrovirus. *Hum Gene Ther* 1991; **2**: 215–19.

48. Russell DW, Berger MS, Miller AD, The effects of human serum and cerebrospinal fluid on retroviral vectors and packaging cell lines. *Hum Gene Ther* 1995; **6**: 635–41.

49. Rother RP, Fodor WL, Springhorn JP et al, A novel mechanism of retrovirus inactivation in human serum mediated by anti-alpha-galactosyl natural antibody. *J Exp Med* 1995; **182**: 1345–55.

50. Donahue RE, Kessler SW, Bodine D et al, Helper virus induced T cell lymphoma in nonhuman primates after retroviral mediated gene transfer. *J Exp Med* 1992; **176**: 1125–35.

51. Morgan RA, Anderson WF, PCR and other test systems in human gene therapy. *Dev Biol Stand* 1992; **76**: 171–7.

52. Larochelle A, Vormoor J, Hanenberg H et al, Identification of primitive human hematopoietic cells capable of repopulating NOD/SCID mouse bone marrow: implications for gene therapy. *Nature Med* 1996; **2**: 1329–37.

53. Nolta JA, Smogorzewska EM, Kohn DB, Analysis of optimal conditions for retroviral-mediated transduction of primitive human hematopoietic cells. *Blood* 1995; **86**: 101–10.

54. Chute JP, Saini AA, Kampen RL et al, A comparative study of the cell cycle status and primitive cell adhesion molecule profile of human CD34+ cells cultured in stroma-free versus porcine microvascular endothelial cell cultures. *Exp Hematol* 1999; **27**: 370–9.

55. Moore KA, Deisseroth AB, Reading CL et al, Stromal support enhances cell-free retroviral vector transduction of human bone marrow long-term culture-initiating cells. *Blood* 1992; **79**: 1393–9.

56. Wells S, Malik P, Pensiero M et al, The presence of an autologous marrow stromal cell layer increases glucocerebrosidase gene transduction of long-term culture initiating cells (LTCICs) from the bone marrow of a patient with Gaucher disease. *Gene Ther* 1995; **2**: 512–20.

57. Piacibello W, Sanavio F, Severino A et al, Engraftment in nonobese diabetic severe combined immunodeficient mice of human CD34(+) cord blood cells after ex vivo expansion: evidence for the amplification and self-renewal of repopu-

lating stem cells. *Blood* 1999; **93**: 3736–49.

58. Povey J, Weeratunge N, Marden C et al, Enhanced retroviral transduction of 5-fluorouracil-resistant human bone marrow (stem) cells using a genetically modified packaging cell line. *Blood* 1998; **92**: 4080–9.

59. Hennemann B, Conneally E, Pawliuk R et al, Optimization of retroviral-mediated gene transfer to human NOD/SCID mouse repopulating cord blood cells through a systematic analysis of protocol variables. *Exp Hematol* 1999; **27**: 817–25.

60. Yu J, Soma T, Hanazono Y et al, Abrogaton of TGF-beta activity during retroviral transduction improves murine hematopoietic progenitor and repopulating cell gene transfer efficiency. *Gene Ther* 1998; **5**: 1265–71.

61. Dao MA, Taylor N, Nolta JA, Reduction in levels of the cyclin-dependent kinase inhibitor p27(kip-1) coupled with transforming growth factor beta neutralization induces cell-cycle entry and increases retroviral transduction of primitive human hematopoietic cells. *Proc Natl Acad Sci USA* 1998; **95**: 13006–11.

62. Zhao Y, Zhu L, Lee S et al, Identification of the block in targeted retroviral-mediated gene transfer. *Proc Natl Acad Sci USA* 1999; **96**: 4005–10.

63. Benedict CA, Tun RY, Rubinstein DB et al, Targeting retroviral vectors to CD34-expressing cells: binding to CD34 does not catalyze virus–cell fusion. *Hum Gene Ther* 1999; **10**: 545–57.

64. Yajima T, Kanda T, Yoshiike K et al, Retroviral vector targeting human cells via c-Kit-stem cell factor interaction. *Hum Gene Ther* 1998; **9**: 779–87.

65. Fielding AK, Maurice M, Morling FJ et al, Inverse targeting of retroviral vectors: selective gene transfer in a mixed population of hematopoietic and non-hematopoietic cells. *Blood* 1998; **91**: 1802–9.

66. Maurice M, Mazur S, Bullough FJ et al, Efficient gene delivery to quiescent interleukin-2 (IL-2)-dependent cells by murine leukemia virus-derived vectors harboring IL-2 chimeric envelope glycoproteins. *Blood* 1999; **94**: 401–10.

67. Williams DA, Rios M, Stephens C et al, Fibronectin and VLA-4 in haematopoietic stem cell–microenvironment interactions. *Nature* 1991; **352**: 438–41.

68. van der Loo JC, Xiao X, McMillin D et al, VLA-5 is expressed by mouse and human long-term repopulating hematopoietic cells and mediates adhesion to extracellular matrix protein fibronectin. *J Clin Invest* 1998; **102**: 1051–61.

69. Dao MA, Shah AJ, Crooks GM et al, Engraftment and retroviral marking of CD34+ and CD34+CD38− human hematopoietic progenitors assessed in immune-deficient mice. *Blood* 1998; **91**: 1243–55.

70. Hanenberg H, Xiao XL, Dilloo D et al, Colocalization of retrovirus and target cells on specific fibronectin fragments increases genetic transduction of mammalian cells. *Nature Med* 1996; **2**: 876–82.

71. Hanenberg H, Hashino K, Konishi H et al, Optimization of fibronectin-assisted retroviral gene transfer into human CD34+ hematopoietic cells. *Hum Gene Ther* 1997; **8**: 2193–206.

72. Reiser J, Harmison G, Kluepfel-Stahl S et al, Transduction of nondividing cells using pseudotyped defective high-titer HIV type 1 particles. *Proc Natl Acad Sci USA* 1996; **93**: 15266–71.

73. Naldini L, Blomer U, Gallay P et al, In vivo gene delivery and stable transduction of nondividing cells by a lentiviral vector. *Science* 1996; **272**: 263–7.

74. Blomer U, Naldini L, Kafri T et al, Highly efficient and sustained gene transfer in adult neurons with a lentivirus vector. *J Virol* 1997; **71**: 6641–9.

75. Dull T, Zufferey R, Kelly M et al, A third-generation lentivirus vector with a conditional packaging system. *J Virol* 1998; **72**: 8463–71.

76. Cui Y, Iwakuma T, Chang LJ, Contributions of viral splice sites and cis-

regulatory elements to lentivirus vector function. *J Virol* 1999; **73**: 6171–6.

77. Miyoshi H, Blomer U, Takahashi M et al, Development of a self-inactivating lentivirus vector. *J Virol* 1998; **72**: 8150–7.

78. Zufferey R, Dull T, Mandel RJ et al, Self-inactivating lentivirus vector for safe and efficient in vivo gene delivery. *J Virol* 1998; **72**: 9873–80.

79. Di Marzio P, Choe S, Ebright M et al, Mutational analysis of cell cycle arrest, nuclear localization and virion packaging of human immunodeficiency virus type 1 Vpr. *J Virol* 1995; **69**: 7909–16.

80. Mahalingam S, Ayyavoo V, Patel M et al, Nuclear import, virion incorporation, and cell cycle arrest/differentiation are mediated by distinct functional domains of human immunodeficiency virus type 1 Vpr. *J Virol* 1997; **71**: 6339–47.

81. Kafri T, van Praag H, Ouyang L et al, A packaging cell line for lentivirus vectors. *J Virol* 1999; **73**: 576–84.

82. Korin YD, Zack JA, Progression to the G(1)B phase of the cell cycle is required for completion of human immunodeficiency virus type 1 reverse transcription in T cells. *J Virol* 1998; **72**: 3161–8.

83. Unutmaz D, Kewal Ramani VN, Marmon S et al, Cytokine signals are sufficient for HIV-1 infection of resting human T lymphocytes. *J Exp Med* 1999; **189**: 1735–46.

84. Case SS, Price MA, Jordan CT et al, Stable transduction of quiescent CD34(+)CD38(−) human hematopoietic cells by HIV-1-based lentiviral vectors. *Proc Natl Acad Sci USA* 1999; **96**: 2988–93.

85. Evans JT, Kelly PF, O'Neill E et al, Human cord blood CD34+CD38− cell transduction via lentivirus-based gene transfer vectors. *Hum Gene Ther* 1999; **10**: 1479–89.

86. Poeschla E, Gilbert J, Li X et al, Identification of a human immunodeficiency virus type 2 (HIV-2) encapsidation determinant and transduction of nondividing human cells by HIV-2-based lentivirus vectors. *J Virol* 1998; **72**: 6527–36.

87. Miyoshi H, Smith KA, Mosier DE et al, Transduction of human CD34+ cells that mediate long-term engraftment of NOD/SCID mice by HIV vectors. *Science* 1999; **283**: 682–6.

88. Poeschla EM, Wong-Staal F, Looney DJ, Efficient transduction of nondividing human cells by feline immunodeficiency virus lentiviral vectors. *Nature Med* 1998; **4**: 354–7.

89. Johnston JC, Gasmi M, Lim LE et al, Minimum requirements for efficient transduction of dividing and nondividing cells by feline immunodeficiency virus vectors. *J Virol* 1999; **73**: 4991–5000.

90. White SM, Renda M, Nam NY et al, Lentivirus vectors using human and simian immunodeficiency virus elements. *J Virol* 1999; **73**: 2832–40.

91. Johnston J, Power C, Productive infection of human peripheral blood mononuclear cells by feline immunodeficiency virus: implications for vector development. *J Virol* 1999; **73**: 2491–8.

92. Sorrentino BP, Brandt SJ, Bodine D et al, Selection of drug-resistant bone marrow cells in vivo after retroviral transfer of human MDR1. *Science* 1992; **257**: 99–103.

93. Hanania EG, Giles RE, Kavanagh J et al, Results of MDR-1 vector modification trial indicate that granulocyte/macrophage colony-forming unit cells do not contribute to posttransplant hematopoietic recovery following intensive systemic therapy. *Proc Natl Acad Sci USA* 1996; **93**: 15346–51 [Erratum 1997; **94**: 5495].

94. Licht T, Aran JM, Goldenberg SK et al, Retroviral transfer of human MDR1 gene to hematopoietic cells: effects of drug selection and of transcript splicing on expression of encoded P-glycoprotein. *Hum Gene Ther* 1999; **10**: 2173–85.

95. Eckert HG, Stockschlader M, Just U et al, High-dose multidrug resistance in primary human hematopoietic progenitor cells transduced with optimized retroviral vectors. *Blood* 1996; **88**: 3407–15.

96. Hibino H, Tani K, Ikebuchi K et al, The common marmoset as a target preclinical primate model for cytokine and gene therapy studies. *Blood* 1999; **93**: 2839–48.

97. Cowan KH, Moscow JA, Huang H et al, Paclitaxel chemotherapy after autologous stem-cell transplantation and engraftment of hematopoietic cells transduced with a retrovirus containing the multidrug resistance complementary DNA (MDR1) in metastatic breast cancer patients. *Clin Cancer Res* 1999; **5**: 1619–28.

98. O'Shaughnessy JA, Cowan KH, Nienhuis AW et al, Retroviral mediated transfer of the human multidrug resistance gene (MDR-1) into hematopoietic stem cells during autologous transplantation after intensive chemotherapy for metastatic breast cancer. *Hum Gene Ther* 1994; **5**: 891–911.

99. Hesdorffer C, Ayello J, Ward M et al, Phase I trial of retroviral-mediated transfer of the human MDR1 gene as marrow chemoprotection in patients undergoing high-dose chemotherapy and autologous stem-cell transplantation. *J Clin Oncol* 1998; **16**: 165–72.

100. Machiels JP, Govaerts AS, Guillaume T et al, Retrovirus-mediated gene transfer of the human multidrug resistance-associated protein into hematopoietic cells protects mice from chemotherapy-induced leukopenia. *Hum Gene Ther* 1999; **10**: 801–11.

101. Bunting KD, Galipeau J, Topham D et al, Transduction of murine bone marrow cells with an MDR1 vector enables ex vivo stem cell expansion, but these expanded grafts cause a myeloproliferative syndrome in transplanted mice. *Blood* 1998; **92**: 2269–79.

102. Blau CA, Neff T, Papayannopoulou T, The hematological effects of folate analogs – implications for using the dihydrofolate reductase gene for in vivo selection. *Hum Gene Ther* 1996; **7**: 2069–78.

103. Kwok WW, Schuening F, Stead RB et al, Retroviral transfer of genes into canine hemopoietic progenitor cells in culture: a model for human gene therapy. *Proc Natl Acad Sci USA* 1986; **83**: 4552–5.

104. Flasshove M, Banerjee D, Mineishi S et al, Ex vivo expansion and selection of human CD34+ peripheral blood progenitor cells after introduction of a mutated dihydrofolate reductase cDNA via retroviral gene transfer. *Blood* 1995; **85**: 566–74.

105. May C, Gunther R, McIvor RS, Protection of mice from lethal doses of methotrexate by transplantation with transgenic marrow expressing drug-resistant dihydrofolate reductase activity. *Blood* 1995; **86**: 2439–48.

106. Allay JA, Persons DA, Galipeau J et al, In vivo selection of retrovirally transduced hematopoietic stem cells. *Nature Med* 1998; **4**: 1136–43.

107. Zhao SC, Banerjee D, Mineishi S et al, Post-transplant methotrexate administration leads to improved curability of mice bearing a mammary tumor transplanted with marrow transduced with a mutant human dihydrofolate reductase cdna. *Hum Gene Ther* 1997; **8**: 903–9.

108. Zhao RC, McIvor RS, Griffin JD et al, Gene therapy for chronic myelogenous leukemia (CML): a retroviral vector that renders hematopoietic progenitors methotrexate-resistant and CML progenitors functionally normal and nontumorigenic in vivo. *Blood* 1997; **90**: 4687–98.

109. Maze R, Kapur R, Kelley MR et al, Reversal of 1,3-bis(2-chloroethyl)-1-nitrosourea-induced severe immunodeficiency by transduction of murine long-lived hemopoietic progenitor cells using O6-methylguanine DNA methyltransferase complementary DNA. *J Immunol* 1997; **158**: 1006–13.

110. Chinnasamy N, Rafferty JA, Hickson I et al, Chemoprotective gene transfer II: multilineage in vivo protection of haemopoiesis against the effects of an antitumour agent by expression of a mutant human O6-alkylguanine–DNA alkyltransferase. *Gene Ther* 1998; **5**: 842–7.

111. Maze R, Kurpad C, Pegg AE et al, Retroviral-mediated expression of the P140A, but not P140A/G156A, mutant

form of O6-methylguanine DNA methyl-transferase protects hematopoietic cells against O6-benzylguanine sensitization to chloroethylnitrosourea treatment. *J Pharmacol Exp Ther* 1999; **290**: 1467–74.

112. Kuga T, Sakamaki S, Matsunaga T et al, Fibronectin fragment-facilitated retroviral transfer of the glutathione-S-transferase pi gene into CD34+ cells to protect them against alkylating agents. *Hum Gene Ther* 1997; **8**: 1901–10.

113. Bachier CR, Deisseroth AB, Gene therapy of solid tumors and hematopoietic neoplasms. *Cancer Treat Res* 1997; **77**: 3–26.

114. Fefer A, Sullivan KM, Weiden P et al, Graft versus leukemia effect in man: the relapse rate of acute leukemia is lower after allogeneic than after syngeneic marrow transplantation. *Prog Clin Biol Res* 1987; **244**: 401–8.

115. Butturini A, Gale RP, The role of T-cells in preventing relapse in chronic myelogenous leukemia. *Bone Marrow Transplant* 1987; **2**: 351–4 [Erratum 1988; **3**: 245].

116. Kolb HJ, Mittermuller J, Clemm C et al, Donor leukocyte transfusions for treatment of recurrent chronic myelogenous leukemia in marrow transplant patients. *Blood* 1990; **76**: 2462–5.

117. Slavin S, Gurevitch O, Zhu J et al, Deletion of donor-reactive cells followed by stem cell transplantation in recipients treated with total lymphoid-irradiation as a means for induction of transplantation tolerance to organ allografts and xenografts. *Transplant Proc* 1998; **30**: 4021–2.

118. Storb R, Yu C, Wagner JL et al, Stable mixed hematopoietic chimerism in DLA-identical littermate dogs given sublethal total body irradiation before and pharmacological immunosuppression after marrow transplantation. *Blood* 1997; **89**: 3048–54.

119. Kolb HJ, Schattenberg A, Goldman JM et al, Graft-versus-leukemia effect of donor lymphocyte transfusions in marrow grafted patients. European Group for Blood and Marrow Transplantation

Working Party Chronic Leukemia. *Blood* 1995; **86**: 2041–50.

120. Storb R, Yu C, Barnett T et al, Stable mixed hematopoietic chimerism in dog leukocyte antigen-identical littermate dogs given lymph node irradiation before and pharmacologic immunosuppression after marrow transplantation. *Blood* 1999; **94**: 1131–6.

121. Sykes M, Preffer F, MacAfee S et al, Mixed lymphohaemopoietic chimerism and graft-versus-lymphoma effects after non-myeloablative therapy and HLA-mismatched bone-marrow transplantation. *Lancet* 1999; **353**: 1755–9.

122. Tiberghien P, 'Suicide' gene for the control of graft-versus-host disease. *Curr Opin Hematol* 1998; **5**: 478–82.

123. Verzeletti S, Bonini C, Marktel S et al, Herpes simplex virus thymidine kinase gene transfer for controlled graft-versus-host disease and graft-versus-leukemia: clinical follow-up and improved new vectors. *Hum Gene Ther* 1998; **9**: 2243–51.

124. Gallot G, Hallet MM, Gaschet J et al, Human HLA-specific T-cell clones with stable expression of a suicide gene: a possible tool to drive and control a graft-versus-host–graft-versus-leukemia reaction? *Blood* 1996; **88**: 1098–103.

125. Wolfe JH, Sands MS, Barker JE et al, Reversal of pathology in murine mucopolysaccharidosis type VII by somatic cell gene transfer. *Nature* 1992; **360**: 749–53.

126. Bjorgvinsdottir H, Ding C, Pech N et al, Retroviral-mediated gene transfer of gp91phox into bone marrow cells rescues defect in host defense against *Aspergillus fumigatus* in murine X-linked chronic granulomatous disease. *Blood* 1997; **89**: 41–8.

127. Li LL, Dinauer MC, Reconstitution of NADPH oxidase activity in human X-linked chronic granulomatous disease myeloid cells after stable gene transfer using a recombinant adeno-associated virus 2 vector. *Blood Cells Mol Dis* 1998; **24**: 522–38.

128. Becker S, Wasser S, Hauses M et al,

Correction of respiratory burst activity in X-linked chronic granulomatous cells to therapeutically relevant levels after gene transfer into bone marrow CD34+ cells. *Hum Gene Ther* 1998; 9: 1561–70.

129. Grez M, Akgun E, Hilberg F et al, Embryonic stem cell virus, a recombinant murine retrovirus with expression in embryonic stem cells. *Proc Natl Acad Sci USA* 1990; 87: 9202–6.

130. Baum C, Hegewisch-Becker S, Eckert HG et al, Novel retroviral vectors for efficient expression of the multidrug resistance (mdr-1) gene in early hematopoietic cells. *J Virol* 1995; 69: 7541–7.

131. Robbins PB, Yu XJ, Skelton DM et al, Increased probability of expression from modified retroviral vectors in embryonal stem cells and embryonal carcinoma cells. *J Virol* 1997; 71: 9466–74.

132. Kohn DB, Gene therapy for haematopoietic and lymphoid disorders. *Clin Exp Immuno* 1997; 107(Suppl 1): 54–7.

133. Kohn DB, Hershfield MS, Carbonaro D et al, T lymphocytes with a normal ADA gene accumulate after transplantation of transduced autologous umbilical cord blood CD34+ cells in ADA-deficient SCID neonates. *Nature Med* 1998; 4: 775–80.

134. Cavazzana-Calvo M, Hacien-Bey S, Basile CD et al, Gene therapy of human severe combined immunodeficiency (SCID)-X1 disease. *Science* 2000; 288: 669–72

135. Brummendorf TH, Holyoake TL, Rufer N et al, Prognostic implications of differences in telomere length between normal and malignant cells from patients with chronic myeloid leukemia measured by flow cytometry. *Blood* 2000; 95: 1883–90

136. Evans GL, Morgan RA, Genetic induction of immune tolerance to human clotting factor VIII in a mouse model for hemophilia A. *Proc Natl Acad Sci USA* 1998; 95: 5734–9.

# 9
# Allogeneic transplantation of hematopoietic stem cells: Blood versus bone marrow

Peter Dreger, Norbert Schmitz

## INTRODUCTION

For a long time, bone marrow (BM) was the only source of hematopoietic tissue that could be used for allogeneic stem cell transplantation. During recent years, however, mobilized peripheral blood stem cells (PBSC) have increasingly come to be used instead of BM for allogeneic transplantation.

Attempts to use blood instead of marrow for allogeneic transplantation were made over 30 years ago.[1] Experience from autologous transplantation showed that PBSC obtained during steady state could be used for hematopoietic reconstitution of a myeloablated host; however, such PBSC did not have striking advantages over autologous BM stem cells, because extensive leukapheresis was required in order to collect a sufficient number of progenitor cells.[2,3] Therefore the use of unmobilized PBSC for allogeneic transplantation was not an attractive alternative to BM transplantation (BMT).[4]

With the availability of hematopoietic growth factors, however, the harvesting of large numbers of PBSC with only a few leukapheresis procedures became possible, allowing rapid reconstitution of marrow function after autologous transplantation.[5,6] Given these promising results, trials were initiated in the early 1990s to determine whether the main advantages of mobilized PBSC, namely improving the convenience for the donor while providing larger stem cell numbers and faster hematopoietic recovery, could be transferred to the allogeneic setting. After publication of the first series of patients successfully allografted with mobilized PBSC, allogeneic PBSC transplantation (PBSCT) rapidly gained worldwide acceptance; in Europe already in 1997 PBSCT accounted for 30% of all allogeneic stem cell transplants performed (versus fewer than 1% in 1993).[7] Although major features of allogeneic PBSCT, such as donor safety, rapid and durable engraftment, an incidence of acute graft-versus-host-disease (GvHD) similar to that with allogeneic BMT, and an increased frequency of chronic GvHD now appear to be well recognized, these and a number of additional issues, including the optimum regimen for PBSC mobilization and harvesting, the immunological characteristics of the graft in terms of graft-versus-host (GvH) and graft-versus-leukaemia (GvL) reactivity, and approaches to manipulate the functional components of PBSC grafts ex vivo ('graft engineering') are not completely settled.

In this chapter, we shall describe the current status of allogeneic PBSCT with particular focus on the critical issues mentioned above. The main topics that will be discussed are:

- PBSC harvesting and donor safety;
- reconstitution of hematopoiesis and the immune system;
- GvHD;
- GvL effects of PBSC;
- graft engineering and cell component therapy.

## PBSC HARVESTING AND DONOR SAFETY

The most important points that have to be considered in order to design an optimum strategy for stem cell mobilization and harvesting in healthy donors are:

- selection of suitable mobilizing agents;
- timing of leukapheresis;
- dose and timing of cytokine administration;
- technique of PBSC collection;
- donor safety.

### Selection of suitable cytokines

Although PBSC grafts can be obtained without mobilization (i.e. during 'steady-state' hematopoiesis), the pool of circulating stem cells should be expanded by exogenous stimulation prior to stem cell harvesting to allow for reasonable yields of stem cells with acceptable collection effort. To date, granulocyte colony-stimulating factor (G-CSF) and granulocyte–macrophage-stimulating factor (GM-CSF) are the only growth factors for which relevant experience with priming of healthy individuals is available.

The stem cell-mobilizing effects of G-CSF and GM-CSF were first described in 1988 by Dührsen et al[8] and Socinski et al.[9] Both cytokines can be used for expansion of the peripheral blood progenitor cell pool in patients with cancer as well as in healthy donors.[5,6,10–12] G-CSF is routinely used for this purpose because of its superior mobilization efficacy in comparison to GM-CSF (Table 9.1),[11,12] and, more importantly, because it is the safest among the agents available for PBSC priming. The predominant side-effect of G-CSF is bone pain, which usually responds well to peripheral analgetics like acetaminophen (paracetamol) and quickly disappears after withdrawal of G-CSF. In contrast, GM-CSF has a higher risk of inducing systemic adverse effects. Another disad-

## Table 9.1  Cytokines in clinical use for PBSC mobilization

| Cytokine | CD34+ enrichment | Days to CD34+ peak | Side effects |
|---|---|---|---|
| Granulocyte colony-stimulating factor (G-CSF) | 30–100× | 4–5 | Bone pain, headache |
| Granulocyte–macrophage colony-stimulating factor(GM-CSF) | 3–15× | 7–10 | Fever, erythema, fluid retention, anaphylaxis |
| Interleukin-3 (IL-3) | 2–5× | 7–14 | Fever, erythema |

## Table 9.2  Cytokines of potential value for PBSC mobilization

| Cytokine | CD34+ enrichment | | Side effects |
|---|---|---|---|
| | Alone | In combination with G-CSF | |
| Thrombopoietin (Tpo) | 1–7× | = G-CSF alone | Thrombocytosis |
| Stem cell factor (SCF) | None | 1–4× G-CSF alone | Mast cell activation, urticaria, erythema |
| Flt3 ligand (Flt3L) | 2–5× | 5–20× G-CSF alone | |

vantage of GM-CSF is that it must be administered for a longer period of time until the PBSC peak is reached (Table 9.1).[13]

Other growth factors, including interleukin (IL)-3 (Table 9.1), thrombopoietin (Tpo), and Flt3 ligand (Flt3L) may have some stem-cell-mobilizing capacity when administered alone or in combination with G-CSF (Table 9.2).[14–16] Another interesting agent is IL-8, which appears to play a critical role also in G-CSF-triggered mobilization.[17,18] Because there is as yet no evidence that any of these agents is superior to G-CSF in terms of efficacy and safety, and because the use of all of these cytokines for mobilization is still experimental, however, they may not be utilized outside of controlled clinical trials.

The combined use of G-CSF and GM-CSF does not significantly increase the PBSC yield in comparison to G-CSF alone, while exposing the patient to the toxicities of both cytokines.[12] A more promising combination may be G-CSF plus stem cell factor (SCF);[19,20] however, at the present time this regimen is still not approved for clinical use in healthy donors.

## Timing of leukapheresis

With a G-CSF dose of 10 µg/kg/day, the peripheral blood CD34$^+$ count does not rise before three days after the start of G-CSF administration, whereas the peak of CD34$^+$ cells in the peripheral blood usually occurs on day 5 and lowers afterwards despite continued cytokine administration.[10,21] This means that the PBSC yield will be highest on day 5, followed by day 6, day 4, and day 7. Accordingly, leukapheresis should be commenced not earlier than after three days of mobilization, and should not be continued after six days of mobilization (=day 7 after the start of G-CSF administration).

## Dose and timing of cytokine administration

Although the rise in PBSC numbers in the peripheral blood may occur a little bit earlier and last slightly longer with intensified G-CSF stimulation, the described CD34$^+$ cell kinetics are reproducible with a variety of G-CSF doses between 3 and 24 µg/kg in patients and healthy donors.[10,22–26] G-CSF at a dose of 10 µg/kg gave significantly higher CD34$^+$ cell yields than 3–5 µg/kg,[10,24,27] suggesting that the mobilization efficacy depends on the amount of G-CSF used (Figure 9.1). Employing doses as high as 30 µg/kg may further increase the PBSC yield.[25,26,28] Since the adverse effects of G-CSF also appear to be dose-dependent,[10,21,26,28,29] today 10–16 µg/kg are accepted as the standard dose by the majority of clinicians, and a dose of 10 µg/kg has been recommended by investigators representing the European Bone Marrow Transplant (EBMT) registry and the National Marrow Donor Program (NMDP).[30,31]

There is increasing evidence that splitting the daily G-CSF dose into two aliquots may enhance PBSC mobilization.[26,32,33] The findings concerning the optimum timing of leukapheresis in relation to the administration of G-CSF are contradictory, but, taken together, the available data indicate that leukapheresis should be performed within 12 hours after the preceding G-CSF dose to ensure optimum yield,[34,35] implying that the cytokine should be administered in the evening or immediately before PBSC collection. Another factor that may affect mobilization efficacy is higher donor age.[10,26]

At present, two forms of recombinant human G-CSF are available for clinical use: an *Escherichia coli*-derived non-glycosylated form (filgrastim) and a Chinese hamster ovary cell-derived glycosylated form (lenograstim). Provided that bioequivalent doses are administered, both forms appear to have similar PBSC mobilizing efficacy.[36,37]

In conclusion, mobilization should be performed with G-CSF 10–16 µg/kg split into two aliquots. Leukapheresis should start on day 4 or day 5 of G-CSF administration, and should not be continued after day 7 of G-CSF administration.

(a)

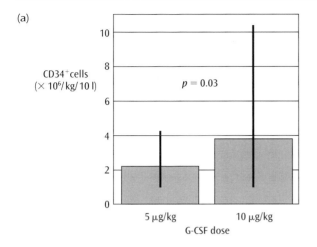

Figure 9.1
The PBSC yield in healthy donors is dependent on the dose of G-CSF (data from 53 healthy individuals harvested at the University of Kiel).
(a) CD34$^+$ cell yield per 10-liter apheresis volume. (b) Percentage of donors achieving more than $4 \times 10^6$/kg CD34$^+$ cells with a single apheresis.

(b)

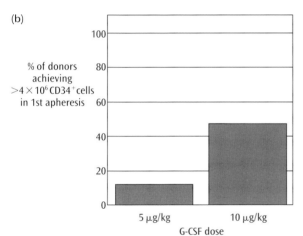

## Technique of PBSC collection

The PBSC collection facilities should meet the requirements listed in the standards adopted by the Joint Accreditation Committee of the International Society of Hematotherapy and Graft Engineering (ISHAGE) and the EBMT (JACIE standards, Sections C2.100 and C2.300).

Apheresis of mononuclear cells is the standard procedure for collecting circulating PBSC. Leukapheresis is performed with continuous-flow cell separators, such as Baxter CS3000, Cobe Spectra, or Fresenius AS104. The donor needs adequate double-lumen venous access to allow a blood flow rate of at least 30 ml/min. In most healthy individuals, this can be achieved by peripheral venous access. Usually, 10 liters of blood are processed daily at a flow rate of 30–80 ml/min, but the collection volume can be reduced or increased to up to 16 liters, according to the patient's needs. Leukapheresis can be repeated on consecutive days, provided that growth factor administration is continued. For anticoagulation during cytapheresis, citrate solutions, commonly ACD-A, are used at a recommended anticoagulant-to-whole blood ratio greater than 1 : 12.[38]

## Donor safety

As mentioned earlier, the use of G-CSF for PBSC mobilization in healthy donors is usually associated with mild to moderate bone pain, which occurs in the vast majority of individuals receiving G-CSF doses of 10 μg/kg/day or more. In addition, 10–40% of healthy donors treated with G-CSF suffer from symptoms such as headache, fatigue, and nausea[21,24,26] (Table 9.3). More severe adverse events have been observed very rarely; however, individual cases of life-threatening complications have been reported, mainly involving thromboembolic incidents, including myocardial infarction,[39] cerebrovascular disorder,[31] splenic rupture,[40] and anaphylactoid reactions.[41] Since acute iritis has occurred in a healthy donor in association with G-CSF administration, it has been speculated that G-CSF might be able to trigger autoimmune phenomena.[42]

The effects of G-CSF on blood counts are essentially restricted to leukocytosis which occurs rapidly and in a dose-dependent fashion (up to $(50–70) \times 10^9/l$ with 10 μg/kg/day). After G-CSF has been stopped, a transient mild neutropenia may occur, which might be due to the inhibitory activity of other cytokines involved in the regulation of granulopoiesis or to suppression of endogenous G-CSF production.[43]

G-CSF has no apparent influence on haemoglobin levels and platelet counts.[10,29,44] However, some investigators have observed a delayed moderate decrease in platelets, which can occur six to nine days after the start of G-CSF administration in individuals with a steady-state hematopoiesis.[21,28,45,46] The mechanisms responsible for the negative effect of G-CSF on thrombocyte numbers in healthy individuals are not clear; it has been suggested that platelet

## Table 9.3  G-CSF-related toxicity in donors of allogeneic PBSC

| Symptom | Frequency (%) |
|---|---|
| Bone pain | 50–100 |
| Headache | 10–40 |
| Flu-like symptoms | 10–25 |
| Severe toxicity (vascular complications, anaphylactoid reactions) | ≤1 |

production might be downregulated by a direct or indirect effect of higher doses of G-CSF. Another possible explanation is that the expanding granulopoiesis stimulated by G-CSF suppresses the thrombopoiesis in healthy donors. There is some evidence that G-CSF interferes with platelet activity and plasmatic hemostasis,[27,47] although a clear-cut procoagulatoric effect of G-CSF has not been demonstrated to date. However, these phenomena may be of some importance in the pathogenesis of the thromboembolic events mentioned earlier.

Whereas the serum levels of sodium, calcium, urea, creatinine, uric acid, and bilirubin remain unchanged during G-CSF administration, reversible moderate increases in alkaline phosphatase and lactate dehydrogenase are observed in some donors. Serum potassium tends to decline to subnormal levels under G-CSF, necessitating occasional oral potassium substitution. These phenomena are probably due to the increased neutrophil turnover induced by G-CSF.[10,48]

Although long-term adverse effects cannot be definitely ruled out at this point of time, G-CSF has been administered safely to large cohorts of patients for the treatment of neutropenia and for PBSC mobilization, and to a considerable number of healthy subjects such as granulocyte and PBSC donors. BM analysis of normal donors who had received G-CSF five years earlier showed no evidence of morphological or cytogenetic abnormalities.[49] Even though G-CSF can stimulate leukemic blasts under certain conditions in vitro, and development of leukemia has been observed in children with congenital neutropenia who had been treated with G-CSF, there is at present no evidence that G-CSF is leukemogenic in vivo.[50,51]

One of our donors, a 54-year old woman, developed breast cancer six years after PBSC collection. Interestingly, her syngeneic recipient who suffered from acute lymphoblastic leukemia, is still alive and well, without evidence of cancer, although she was treated with high-dose radiochemotherapy and received G-CSF for acceleration of neutrophil recovery post transplant. It is clear that neoplastic diseases will occur in PBSC donors as they do in the normal population. However, the available data do not suggest that the incidence of malignancy might be increased in individuals exposed to G-CSF. It is noteworthy that strongly elevated G-CSF levels can also occur owing to endogenous release of G-CSF, for example during severe infections.[52]

Provided that the time interval between the collections is not too short, second PBSC harvests can be performed in healthy individuals without apparent difference from first collections in terms of side-effects and stem cell yield, indicating no long-lasting impact on the progenitor cell pool.[53,54]

Similarly, long-term effects on neutrophil and platelet counts appear to be absent.[53,55] In one study, persistent reductions in blood lymphocyte numbers have been observed in stem cell donors subjected to extensive leukapheresis; these findings were not confirmed by other investigators.[43,49,55]

The risks of leukapheresis are low when carried out in an appropriate setting. Among the 348 patients from the pooled data of 10 studies reviewed earlier, one case of myocardial infarction shortly after leukapheresis for PBSC collection has been reported, and two other donors had angina pectoris-like symptoms during leukapheresis.[56] The most common problems consist in complications associated with placement of central venous catheters (i.e. pneumothorax and arterial puncture) and transient hypocalcemia induced by the ACD-A used for anticoagulation during the separation.[57] The latter problem can be successfully alleviated by infusion of supplemental calcium into the return line. Some donors complain of headache or fatigue occurring during cytapheresis, but these symptoms rarely require therapeutic intervention.

Depending on the cell separation system employed, leukapheresis results in a variable depletion of platelets, which can reduce the platelet count to 50% of the precollection value (average 30% reduction per leukapheresis procedure[21,31] and unpublished observations, P Dreger). As a consequence, the thrombocyte count prior to and after the leukapheresis procedure should be carefully monitored and raised by means of retransfusion of the autologous platelets contained in the collection products if necessary.[58] Apheresis should be avoided if the platelet count is below $70 \times 10^9/l$.[31]

On the other hand, BM harvesting under general anesthesia has been reported to be associated with an up to 0.4% incidence of life-threatening complications, which may be reduced to 0.1–0.2% by excluding donors with risk factors such as cardiovascular disease, obesity, or higher age.[59,60] In addition, BM collection can result in considerable morbidity due to soft tissue and bone trauma; nausea and associated symptoms occur in a large proportion of donors as a consequence of general anesthesia. Taken together, the risks of G-CSF priming and leukapheresis in healthy donors appear to be acceptable compared with those of BM collection.

In conclusion, G-CSF priming and subsequent stem cell harvesting by leukapheresis is not a trivial procedure without any risk, but appropriate selection of donors should allow one to avoid serious complications. The joint ad hoc Workshop of the International Bone Marrow Transplant Registry (IBMTR), the EBMT registry and the NMDP has identified a number of conditions that do not appear to be perfectly compatible with PBSC donation. These include cardiovascular risk factors, a history of thromboembolic events, inflammatory or autoimmune disorders, a history of malignancy, and poor peripheral veins.[31] Furthermore, all efforts should be undertaken to assure long-term monitoring of healthy donors of both PBSC and BM via national and international transplant registries.

## RECONSTITUTION OF HEMATOPOIESIS AND THE IMMUNE SYSTEM

### Reconstitution of hematopoiesis

Numerous studies have demonstrated that all subsets of progenitor cells or stem cell equivalents that can be assayed in vitro or in vivo are present in

G-CSF-mobilized PBSC products, and there is no evidence that components essential for engraftment are lacking or critically reduced in PBSC grafts obtained from healthy donors.[27,61–63] In particular, the numbers of cells expressing the CD34 antigen have been found – similar to observations in the autologous setting[64] – to be more than twofold higher in peripheral blood allografts than in marrow grafts.[10,65–67]

As a consequence of this, and because of the striking advantages of autologous PBSC over marrow grafts in terms of speed of engraftment, one of the main expectations prompting investigators to pursue allogeneic PBSCT was the possibility of accelerating hematopoietic recovery with mobilized blood grafts.

First experience obtained in identical twins indeed confirmed that primary transplantation of G-CSF-primed PBSC consistently resulted in rapid and sustained restoration of hematopoiesis, which was considerably faster than the engraftment of historical controls from the same center receiving syngeneic BM.[68,69] The speed of hematopoietic recovery after allogeneic PBSCT, however, turned out to be much more variable than what is seen after syngeneic or autologous transplantation. The main reason for this seems to be the genetic difference between graft and recipient, which may delay engraftment per se, causes complications such as GvHD and viral infections, and necessitates the use of cytotoxic drugs like methotrexate. Nevertheless, the reconstitution of hematopoiesis after allogeneic PBSCT tended to be more rapid than in historical BM controls.[70–72] These first data were confirmed by randomized trials and matched-pair analyses reported recently. Table 9.4 lists the results of six of these studies. The IBMTR and the EBMT registry compared the engraftment data of 288 patients with leukemia who were allografted with PBSC from an HLA-identical sibling donor with the results of 536 matched recipients of BM. A highly significant difference in favor of the PBSC group was found with regard to neutrophil and platelet engraftment ($p < 0.001$ for both).[73]

An important factor adversely affecting engraftment is the use of methotrexate post transplant,[74] while a striking correlation between the speed of engraftment and the number of CD34$^+$ cells infused could not be shown. Although unaffected engraftment was seen with CD34$^+$ cell numbers less than $2 \times 10^6$/kg, the minimum target dose to ensure engraftment is currently regarded as $(4–5) \times 10^6$/kg.[30,75]

The engraftment of allogeneic PBSC is durable, as shown by molecular analysis of chimerism and blood group typing.[70,71,76] The strong hematopoietic capacity of G-CSF-mobilized PBPC is also underlined by successful PBSC rescue of patients with non-engraftment after BMT.[77–80]

## Reconstitution of the immune system

Compared with values observed in allogeneic marrow grafts, PBSC harvests contain about one log more T cells.[10,67,81] This is not only important with regard to potential GvH and GvL activities of the graft, but also has implica-

**Table 9.4 Hematopoietic recovery after stem cell transfusion: results of controlled studies**

| Investigator (date) | No. per cohort | Days to ANC[a] $> 0.5 \times 10^9/l$ | | Days to platelets $> 20 \times 10^9/l$ | |
| --- | --- | --- | --- | --- | --- |
| | | PBSC | BM | PBSC | BM |
| Bensinger (1996)[88b] | 37/37 | 14 | 16* | 11 | 15* |
| Hägglund (1998)[128c] | 23/23 | 12 | 16.5* | 15 | 19*† |
| Powles (1997)[129d] | 20/20 | 18 | 23* | 15 | 21* |
| Vigorito (1998)[89e] | 18/19 | 16 | 18 | 12 | 17* |
| Schmitz (1998)[65f] | 33/33 | 14 | 15 | 15 | 19 |
| Ringden (1999)[67g] | 45/45 | 16 | 20 | 23 | 29*‡ |

[a]ANC, absolute neutrophil count.
[b]Single center, matched-pair analysis.
[c]Single center, matched-pair analysis.
[d]Single center, double-blind randomized study.
[e]Single center, open-label randomized study.
[f]Multicentre, open-label randomized study.
[g]Multicentre, matched-pair analysis.
*$p < 0.05$.
†Recovery to $30 \times 10^9/l$.
‡Recovery to $50 \times 10^9/l$.

tions for the reconstitution of the immune system post transplant. Recent studies suggest that T-cell regeneration in adult recipients after allogeneic transplantation is mainly determined by the number of mature T cells contained in the allograft.[82,83] Thus allogeneic PBSCT may be associated with acceleration of both hematopoietic and immune engraftment. Two consecutive studies from a single center indicated that the recovery of T-cell numbers and function after allogeneic PBSCT is indeed faster than after BMT, resulting in a normalization of the CD4$^+$ : CD8$^+$ ratio as early as six months after transplant.[76,84] Accelerated lymphocyte recovery after PBSCT in comparison with BMT was also observed by others; however, immunoglobulin recovery does not appear to be faster in recipients of PBSC.[85,86]

Similar to the situation after BMT, the natural killer (NK)-cell compartment is the first lymphocyte subset recovering to normal levels after PBSC graft infusion. In spite of this, NK-cell function may be impaired for prolonged periods of time post transplant. Whether this has to do with the reduced functional capacity of the NK cells present in mobilized PBSC collection products that was observed by different investigators remains to be determined.[86,87]

# GvHD

## Acute GvHD

Since T cells are the effector cells of both acute and chronic GvH reactions (GvHR), it was a major concern that the large numbers of T cells contained in PBSC grafts might give rise to an increased incidence or severity of GvHR. However, the initial impression was that the incidence of acute GvHR was lower rather than higher compared with allogeneic BMT.[70-72] With higher patient numbers, it became evident that, with standard immunosuppression, there is no striking difference between PBSCT and BMT in terms of acute GvHR. In the controlled studies mentioned earlier, grade II–IV disease was observed in 23–54% of PBSC recipients, compared with 19–56% in BM recipients (Table 9.5).[65-67,88,89] The IBMTR/EBMT registry matched-pair analysis also failed to demonstrate an increase in acute GvHD after allogeneic PBSCT.[73]

It is not understood why the large numbers of T cells infused with the PBSC grafts do not correlate with an increase of acute GvHR. However, it has been shown that the absolute number of T cells in an allogeneic graft may not be the crucial factor determinating the severity of GvHR.[81,90] Thus, provided that a critical number of T cells are present in the graft, the quality (i.e. specificity) rather than the quantity of donor T cells seems to be the more important determinant influencing GvHR frequency and severity.

Another explanation may be that the T cells contained in PBSC products are not only quantitatively but also qualitatively different from those in BM grafts: murine studies have demonstrated that the T cells in G-CSF-mobilized PBSC grafts express predominantly a Th2 cytokine pattern (IL-4 production), whereas the majority of peripheral blood T cells of mice not exposed to G-CSF

**Table 9.5 Acute and chronic GvHD: results of controlled studies**

| Investigator (date) | No. per cohort | Grade II–IV/III–IV acute GvHD (%) | | Overall/extensive chronic GvHD (%) | |
| --- | --- | --- | --- | --- | --- |
| | | PBSC | BM | PBSC | BM |
| Bensinger (1996)[88a] | 37/37 | 37/14 | 56/33 | na | |
| Hägglund (1998)[128b] | 23/23 | 23 | 22 | 68 | 61 |
| Vigorito (1998)[89c] | 18/19 | 27/13 | 19/13 | 71/71 | 53/27* |
| Schmitz (1998)[65d] | 33/33 | 54/21 | 48/18 | na | |
| Ringden (1999)[67e] | 45/45 | 29/14 | 20/16 | 53/9 | 68/11 |

[a] Single-center, matched-pair analysis.
[b] Single-center, matched-pair analysis, includes 11/11 unrelated donors.
[c] Single-center, open-label randomized study.
[d] Multicenter, open-label randomized study.
[e] Multicenter, matched-pair analysis.
*$p < 0.05$.
na, not available

shows a Th1 pattern (IL-2/interferon-γ production).[91] Interestingly, Th2 cells can attenuate acute GvHR after allogeneic BMT.[92] Reduced Th1 function and predominance of L-selectin expression patterns associated with decreased alloreactivity were also observed in G-CSF-mobilized blood from humans.[93,94] Moreover, the development of GvHR may be modulated by regulatory T-cell subsets or other bystander cells predominating in PBSC grafts.[95]

## Chronic GvHD

There is increasing evidence that chronic GvHD occurs in a significantly higher proportion of recipients of unmanipulated PBSC compared with marrow recipients.[96] Vigorito et al[89] reported that 71% of patients allografted with PBSC developed extensive chronic GvHR, which was significantly more than the 27% incidence in the marrow recipients. Similarly, the relative risk of developing chronic GvHD was significantly increased after PBSCT also in the IBMTR/EBMT registry series (cumulative probability 66% at 12 months post transplant).[73] In contrast to this, the one-year cumulative incidence of chronic GvHD was not different after PBSCT and BMT, respectively, in a recent series of 90 recipients of allografts from unrelated volunteer donors (65% versus 70%).[67] The currently ongoing randomized studies will help in understanding the cause and extent of excess chronic GvHD occurring after allogeneic PBSCT.

## Alternative donors and GvHD

The experience with transplantation of unmanipulated allogeneic PBSC from donors other than HLA siblings is still limited. The Essen group reported 24 PBSC recipients allografted from zero to two-antigen-mismatched related donors. As expected, the cumulative probability of grade II–IV acute GvHD was significantly higher in the 19 patients receiving mismatched grafts than in 41 control recipients of HLA-matched PBSC (86% versus 25%; $p < 0.003$). Similar differences were observed in terms of chronic GvHD, although exact figures on this issue were not reported. There was no influence of donor match, however, on treatment-related mortality, event-free survival, and overall survival.[76]

Owing to the complex ethical and regulatory implications, G-CSF-mobilized PBSC have been used less frequently in the setting of stem cell transplantation from unrelated donors. In 1997, 12% of all unrelated volunteer donor transplants were performed with mobilized blood. The national German donor registry (DKMS) is currently undertaking a prospective trial on PBSC harvesting from unrelated donors. So far, 40 donations have been reported. In general, the procedures were tolerated well, and the toxicity of PBSC mobilization and collection appeared at least acceptable when compared with the side-effects of 245 marrow harvests organized by the same registry.[97] The first larger series of unrelated PBSC transplants has been described recently by Ringden and co-workers.[67] As already mentioned, the incidence of acute and chronic GvHD, treatment-related mortality, and overall survival were not significantly different between 45 PBSC recipients and a matched cohort of patients grafted with marrow.

## GvL effects

Since the antileukemic activities of allogeneic stem cell grafts are mediated predominantly by T cells and NK cells,[98,99] the large numbers of lymphocytes contained in PBSC allografts may result in increased GvL effects after primary PBSCT. Although it is far too early for definite conclusions, recent data observed in patients with chronic myelogenous leukemia (CML) suggest that complete disease eradication as revealed by *bcr/abl* PCR may indeed occur more often after PBSCT than after BMT.[100] In this series, the 29 patients with PBSCT also had a superior outcome in terms of freedom from cytogenetic or clinical relapse. This is in accordance with our own experience obtained in a mouse model comparing the GvL activity of PBSC and BM allografts respectively: in an MHC-matched setting, transplantation of unmanipulated PBSC into lethally irradiated recipients who had been injected with cells from the B-lymphoblastic leukemia A20 resulted in a reduction of the relapse rate to 29%, which was significantly better than the leukemia incidence observed after identical numbers of unmanipulated marrow cells (60%; $p < 0.05$).[62]

On the other hand, preliminary analysis failed to disclose a decreased incidence of relapse after PBSCT in the IBMTR/EBMT registry series, although leukemia-free survival may be better for PBSC recipients in certain unfavorable subgroups.[73]

Another line of evidence for stronger antitumor activities of PBSC allografts comes from studies aiming at the treatment of leukemia relapse after BMT using allogeneic PBSC boosts. In comparison with the infusion of unmobilized donor leukocytes (DLI), the potential advantages of PBSC are:

- rapid recovery of donor hematopoiesis without prolonged cytopenias;
- the possibility of reducing patients' tumor cell load by myelosuppressive chemotherapy prior to PBSC infusion;
- possible competition of donor-derived progenitor cells with the malignant clone;[101]
- reduction of DLI-associated GvHR due to the immune-modulating effects of G-CSF during mobilization.[91]

Preliminary data obtained by us and others indicate that indeed durable remissions can be achieved after transfusion of donor-derived mobilized PBSC in patients relapsing with CML or AML after allogeneic BMT. Even in patients who received additional chemotherapy, extensive cytopenias as observed after conventional DLI could be largely avoided, whereas devastating GvH reactions did not occur.[102,103]

A more straightforward approach to this concept is to attempt immune-mediated elimination of residual neoplastic cells by transfusing mobilized PBSC products after non-myeloablative conditioning ('minitransplants'). Preliminary data suggest that complete remissions are achieved by this strategy in a large proportion of patients, implying that strong GvL activity can be conferred with the stem cell grafts.[104,105] The GvL activity of mobilized peripheral blood may be further increased by activation effector cells with appropriate cytokines.[106]

In comparison with marrow grafts, PBSC harvests are also characterized by an increased proportion of NK cells, which could be used to induce GvL effects.[107] Since donor-derived NK cells recover very early post transplant, NK-mediated GvL effects may be important for the elimination of residual disease, particularly in the mismatch setting, as shown by the Perugia group in a series of patients with acute myelogenous leukemia receiving heavily T-cell-depleted stem cells from haplo-identical related donors.[108]

Altogether, these observations suggest that mobilized allogeneic PBSC products are a promising tool for immunotherapy approaches in patients with neoplastic diseases.

## GRAFT ENGINEERING AND CELL COMPONENT THERAPY

Successful attempts to manipulate allogeneic stem cell grafts for eliminating GvH-reactive cells were undertaken as long ago as the 1970s.[109] In the clinical situation, however, T-cell depletion (TCD) of marrow grafts has been hampered by two major drawbacks, which are responsible for its overall disappointing results: the reduction of mortality due to GvHR was offset by (1) a dramatic rise in the incidence of engraftment failure and (2) a strongly increased relapse rate[110] due to unspecific stem cell loss and elimination of GvL activity from the graft.

PBSC can be expected to avoid these problems because of the 'unlimited' numbers of stem cells and GvH/GvL effector cells that can be harvested from mobilized blood as opposed to BM. This hypothesis was confirmed by a recent retrospective study that compared hematopoietic recovery after TCD PBSCT and BMT, respectively, showing that TCD PBSC engrafted significantly faster and more completely than TCD BM.[111] Thus, in conjunction with the recent progress in cell separation technology, PBSC appear to be the perfect source for ex vivo graft engineering.

Soon after we had reported for the first time that 3–4 log of T-cells can be depleted from PBSC grafts by CD34$^+$ cell selection,[112] a number of investigators reported clinical results on HLA-identical recipients of PBSC products that were T-cell-depleted by CD34$^+$ cell selection using either the Ceprate immunoadsorption system (Cellpro, Bothell, USA) or the immunomagnetic Isolex system (Nexell Therapeutics, Irvine, USA). Although immunoselection reduced the median T-cell content of the grafts by 2.5–4 log to

$1 \times 10^5 – 1 \times 10^6$/kg, the incidence of grade II–IV acute GvHD was surprisingly high if GvHD prophylaxis consisted of TCD only ($\pm$ cyclosporin A).[58,113,114] With the addition of methotrexate or steroids, however, elimination of both acute and chronic GvHD could be largely achieved in the HLA-identical but not in the mismatched setting if TCD was accomplished with the Ceprate or Isolex systems.[113,115–117] Table 9.6 gives an overview of the CD34[+] selection devices currently in use for clinical TCD.

It was concluded from these results that in the mismatch situation, more vigorous TCD might be necessary for effective GvHD prevention: the Perugia group employed a double TCD combining E-rosetting with Ceprate CD34[+] cell selection and achieved a TCD efficacy of more than 4 log. Fifty-three haplo-identical patients were reinfused with extensively TCD PBSC containing a mean of only $3.5 \times 10^4$/kg CD3[+] T cells in addition to TCD marrow. With the only additional GvHD prophylaxis consisting of pretransplant antithymocyte globulin (ATG), both acute and chronic GvHD were virtually completely eliminated.[108] Although the incidence of primary graft failure was low in this preliminary trial (5%), the overall outcome was affected by frequent life-threatening opportunistic infections, suggesting that immune recovery is critically impaired after heavily TCD stem cell transplantation in adults, where T-cell regeneration after BMT is largely dependent on the number of mature T-cells present in the graft.[82,83]

Another approach to 'Mega' TCD relies on the use of more effective CD34[+] cell selection devices. The Clinimacs system is based on immunomagnetic selection, and allows a highly efficient purification of progenitor cell preparations, which is associated with 4–5 log of TCD.[118] In a pediatric study, 20 children received Clinimacs-selected PBSC grafts (T-cell content 1.4 (range 0.1–13) $\times 10^4$/kg) from haplo-identical parent donors after myeloablative conditioning including ATG. Clinically relevant acute or chronic GvHD was not observed, despite the lack of additional prophylaxis. Failure of primary engraftment occurred in a considerable number of patients at risk, but could be overcome with immunosuppressive reconditioning in almost all instances. Probably owing to functioning lymphocyte maturation pathways, immune reconstitution appeared to be uncomplicated in these pediatric recipients of heavily TCD allografts.[119] In contrast, a high incidence of opportunistic infections was observed in a Japanese study on pediatric mismatch transplants of extensively TCD PBSC grafts, indicating that impairment of immune recovery after Mega-TCD may be a problem also in children.[120]

Taken together, modern cell separation systems allow the preparation of PBSC grafts that are devoid of GvHD effector cells and can be successfully used for allografting of three-loci-mismatched recipients, but the problem of insufficient restoration of the immune system remains to be settled.

Another unsolved issue with TCD allografts consists in the increased incidence of leukemia relapse, which will obviously not be overcome with the use of CD34[+] cell selected PBSC alone. However, the large quantities of lymphocytes that can be segregated from PBSC grafts might be used for adding GvL

**Table 9.6 CD34+ selection systems for clinical TCD**

| System | Capture system | CD34+ purity | CD34+ recovery | log TCD (T cells left) | References |
|---|---|---|---|---|---|
| Ceprate[a] | Immunoadsorption | 50–80% | 30–50% | 2–3 ($5$–$15 \times 10^5$/kg) | 88, 113 |
| Isolex | Immunomagnetic | >90% | 30–70% | 3–4 ($0.5$–$3 \times 10^5$/kg) | 114 |
| Clinimacs[b] | Immunomagnetic | >95% | 50–70% | 4–5 (<$0.5$–$3 \times 10^5$/kg) | 119 |

[a]System no longer commercially available.
[b]System not approved for clinical use in the US.

activity to the hematopoietic potential conferred with the isolated CD34$^+$ cells. Supplementing TCD allografts with delayed T-cell addbacks, cytokine-activated NK cells, or leukemia-specific T-cell clones is currently under investigation.[107,121,122] Similarly, specific immunity against critical infectious agents may be restored by the addition of appropriate T-cell clones.[123-125]

In summary, the availability of PBSC has opened a broad spectrum of possibilities for allograft engineering. Designing an allograft tailored to the individual needs of the recipient by distinct selection of progenitor cells, GvL effector cells, and cells with specific anti-infectious activity appears to be feasible in the near future.

## CONCLUSIONS

Transplantation of allogeneic peripheral blood stem cells has become an attractive alternative to allogeneic bone marrow transplantation. Controlled trials suggest that engraftment is faster than after allogeneic BMT, whereas the incidence and severity of acute GvHR appear to be not significantly different. There is some evidence that chronic GvHD is increased after PBSCT, but this may translate into enhanced GvL activity and – up to now – does not appear to have a detrimental effect on survival. Regardless of the features of unmanipulated PBSC in comparison with marrow grafts, a major advantage of allogeneic PBSC over BM is their excellent suitability for graft engineering, such as T-cell depletion, ex vivo expansion, and generation of GvL effector cells.

If the main biological problems of allogeneic stem cell transplantation – namely GvHR, relapse, engraftment failure, and infection – could be overcome by using ex vivo manipulated PBSC, haplo-identical donors could also be considered for stem cell donation. Accordingly, a suitable stem cell graft would be available for almost every patient who needs it. On the other hand, the possibility of donating PBSC instead of BM and thus avoiding general anesthesia and an operative procedure, should also facilitate the recruitment of unrelated stem cell donors. Furthermore, future improvements in stem cell mobilization procedures, for example by using additional cytokines or monoclonal antibodies against adhesion molecules,[126,127] may allow one to obtain a sufficient progenitor cell number by simple collection of 500 ml peripheral blood and to eliminate the need for leukapheresis.

## REFERENCES

1. Epstein RB, Graham TC, Buckner CD et al, Allogeneic marrow engraftment by cross circulation in lethally irradiated dogs. Blood 1966; 28: 692–707.

2. Kessinger A, Armitage JO, Landmark JD et al, Reconstitution of human hematopoietic function with autologous cryopreserved circulating stem cells. Exp Hematol 1986; 14: 192–6.

3. Juttner CA, Blood stem cell transplants in acute leukemia. In: Blood Stem Cell Transplants (Gale RP, Juttner CA,

Henon P, eds). Cambridge University Press: Cambridge, 1994: 101–16.

4. Kessinger A, Smith DM, Strandjord SE et al, Allogeneic transplantation of blood-derived, T cell-depleted hemopoietic stem cells after myeloablative treatment in a patient with acute lymphoblastic leukemia. *Bone Marrow Transplant* 1989; **4**: 643–6.

5. Sheridan WP, Begley CG, Juttner CA et al, Effect of peripheral-blood progenitor cells mobilized by filgrastim (G-CSF) on platelet recovery after high-dose chemotherapy. *Lancet* 1992; **339**: 640–4.

6. Schmitz N, Linch DC, Dreger P et al, Randomised trial of filgrastim-mobilised peripheral blood progenitor cell transplantation versus autologous bone-marrow transplantation in lymphoma patients. *Lancet* 1996; **347**: 353–7.

7. Gratwohl A, Passweg J, Baldomero H et al, Blood and marrow transplantation activity in Europe 1997. *Bone Marrow Transplant* 1999; **24**: 231–45.

8. Dührsen U, Villeval J-L, Boyd J et al, Effects of recombinant human granulocyte colony-stimulating factor on hematopoietic progenitor cells in cancer patients. *Blood* 1988; **72**: 2074–81.

9. Socinski MA, Elias A, Schnipper L et al, Granulocyte–macrophage colony stimulating factor expands the circulating haemopoietic progenitor cell compartment in man. *Lancet* 1988; **ii**: 1194–8.

10. Dreger P, Haferlach T, Eckstein V et al, G-CSF-mobilized peripheral blood progenitor cells for allogeneic transplantation: safety, kinetics of mobilization, and composition of the graft. *Br J Haematol* 1994; **87**: 609–13.

11. Fritsch G, Fischmeister G, Haas OA et al, Peripheral blood hematopoietic progenitor cells of cytokine-stimulated healthy donors as an alternative for allogeneic transplantation. *Blood* 1994; **83**: 3420–1.

12. Lane TA, Law P, Maruyama M et al, Harvesting and enrichment of hematopoietic progenitor cells mobilized into the peripheral blood of normal donors by granulocyte–macrophage

colony-stimulating factor (GM-CSF) or G-CSF: Potential role in allogeneic marrow transplantation. *Blood* 1995; **85**: 275–82.

13. Haas R, Ho AD, Bredthauer U et al, Successful autologous transplantation of blood stem cells mobilized with recombinant human granulocyte–macrophage colony-stimulating factor. *Exp Hematol* 1990; **18**: 94–8.

14. Rosenfeld CS, Bolwell B, LeFever A et al, Comparison of four cytokine regimens for mobilization of peripheral blood stem cells: IL-3 alone and combined with GM-CSF or G-CSF. *Bone Marrow Transplant* 1996; **17**: 179–83.

15. Rasko JE, Basser RL, Boyd J et al, Multilineage mobilization of peripheral blood progenitor cells in humans following administration of PEG-rHuMGDF. *Br J Haematol* 1997; **97**: 871–80.

16. Brasel K, McKenna HJ, Charrier K et al, Flt3 ligand synergizes with granulocyte–macrophage colony-stimulating factor or granulocyte colony-stimulating factor to mobilize hematopoietic progenitor cells into the peripheral blood of mice. *Blood* 1997; **90**: 3781–8.

17. Laterveer L, Lindley IJD, Heemskerk DPM et al, Rapid mobilization of hematopoietic progenitor cells in rhesus monkeys by a single intravenous injection of interleukin-8. *Blood* 1996; **87**: 781–8.

18. Watanabe T, Kawano Y, Kanamaru S et al, Endogenous interleukin-8 (IL-8) surge in granulocyte colony-stimulating factor-induced peripheral blood stem cell mobilization. *Blood* 1999; **93**: 1157–63.

19. Moskowitz CH, Stiff P, Gordon MS et al, Recombinant methionyl human stem cell factor and filgrastim for peripheral blood progenitor cell mobilization and transplantation in non-Hodgkin's lymphoma patients – results of a phase I/II trial. *Blood* 1997; **89**: 3136–47.

20. Weaver A, Chang J, Wrigley E et al, Randomized comparison of progenitor-cell mobilization using chemotherapy, stem-cell factor, and filgrastim or chemotherapy plus filgrastim alone in

patients with ovarian cancer. *J Clin Oncol* 1998; **16**: 2601–12.

21. Stroncek DF, Clay ME, Petzoldt ML et al, Treatment of normal individuals with granulocyte-colony-stimulating factor: donor experiences and the effects on peripheral blood CD34+ cell counts and on the collection of peripheral blood stem cells. *Transfusion* 1996; **36**: 601–10.

22. DeLuca E, Sheridan WP, Watson D et al, Prior chemotherapy does not prevent effective mobilisation by G-CSF of peripheral blood progenitor cells. *Br J Cancer* 1992; **66**: 893–9.

23. Aversa F, Tabilio A, Terenzi A et al, Successful engraftment of T-cell-depleted haploidentical 'three-loci' incompatible transplants in leukemia patients by addition of recombinant human granulocyte colony-stimulating factor-mobilized peripheral blood progenitor cells to bone marrow inoculum. *Blood* 1994; **84**: 3948–55.

24. Grigg AP, Roberts AW, Raunow H et al, Optimizing dose and scheduling of filgrastim (granulocyte colony-stimulating factor) for mobilization and collection of peripheral blood progenitor cells in normal volunteers. *Blood* 1995; **86**: 4437–45.

25. Zeller W, Gutensohn K, Stockschläder M et al, Increase of mobilized CD34-positive peripheral blood progenitor cells in patients with Hodgkin's disease, non-Hodgkin's lymphoma, and cancer of the testis. *Bone Marrow Transplant* 1996; **17**: 709–13.

26. Engelhardt M, Bertz H, Afting M et al, High- versus standard-dose filgrastim for mobilization of peripheral blood progenitor cells from allogeneic donors and CD34+ immunoselection. *J Clin Oncol* 1999; **17**: 2160–72.

27. Harada M, Nagafuji K, Fujisaki T et al, G-CSF-Induced mobilization of peripheral blood stem cells from healthy adults for allogeneic transplantation. *J Hematother* 1996; **5**: 63–71.

28. Weaver CH, Birch R, Greco FA et al, Mobilization and harvesting of peripheral blood stem cells: randomized evaluations of different doses of filgrastim. *Br J Haematol* 1998; **100**: 338–47.

29. Höglund M, Smedmyr B, Simonsson B et al, Dose-dependent mobilisation of haematopoietic progenitor cells in healthy volunteers receiving glycosylated rHuG-CSF. *Bone Marrow Transplant* 1996; **18**: 19–27.

30. Russell NH, Gratwohl A, Schmitz N, The place of blood stem cells in allogeneic transplantation. *Br J Haematol* 1996; **93**: 747–53.

31. Anderlini P, Korbling M, Dale D et al, Allogeneic blood stem cell transplantation: considerations for donors [editorial]. *Blood* 1997; **90**: 903–8.

32. Somlo G, Sniecinski I, Odom-Maryon T et al, Effect of CD34+ selection and various schedules of stem cell reinfusion and granulocyte colony-stimulating factor priming on hematopoietic recovery after high-dose chemotherapy for breast cancer. *Blood* 1997; **89**: 1521–8.

33. Kröger N, Zeller W, Hassan HT et al, Schedule-dependency of granulocyte colony-stimulating factor in peripheral blood progenitor cell mobilization in breast cancer patients. *Blood* 1998; **91**: 1828–9.

34. Stroncek DF, Clay ME, Herr G et al, The kinetics of G-CSF mobilization of CD34+ cells in healthy people. *Transfus Med* 1997; **7**: 19–24.

35. Watts MJ, Addison I, Ings SJ et al, Optimal timing for collection of PBPC after glycosylated G-CSF administration. *Bone Marrow Transplant* 1998; **21**: 365–8.

36. Höglund M, Smedmyr B, Bengtsson M et al, Mobilization of CD34+ cells by glycosylated and nonglycosylated G-CSF in healthy volunteers – a comparative study. *Eur J Haematol* 1997; **59**: 177–83.

37. de Arriba F, Lozano ML, Ortuno F et al, Prospective randomized study comparing the efficacy of bioequivalent doses of glycosylated and nonglycosylated rG-CSF for mobilizing peripheral blood progenitor cells. *Br J Haematol* 1997; **96**: 418–20.

38. Burger SR, Fautsch SK, Stroncek DF

et al, Concentration of citrate anticoagulant in peripheral blood progenitor cell collections. *Transfusion* 1996; **36**: 798–801.

39. Bensinger WI, Buckner CD, Rowley S et al, Treatment of normal donors with recombinant growth factors for transplantation of allogeneic blood stem cells. *Bone Marrow Transplant* 1996; **17**(Suppl 2): S19–21.

40. Becker PS, Wagle M, Matous S et al, Spontaneous splenic rupture following administration of granulocyte colony-stimulating factor (G-CSF): occurrence in an allogeneic donor of peripheral blood stem cells. *Biol Blood Marrow Transplant* 1997; **3**: 45–9.

41. Adkins DR, Anaphylactoid reaction in a normal donor given granulocyte colony-stimulating factor. *J Clin Oncol* 1998; **16**: 812–13.

42. Parkkali T, Volin L, Siren M-K et al, Acute iritis induced by granulocyte colony-stimulating factor used for mobilization in a volunteer unrelated peripheral blood progenitor cell donor. *Bone Marrow Transplant* 1996; **17**: 433–4.

43. Anderlini P, Przepiorka D, Seong D et al, Transient neutropenia in normal donors after G-CSF mobilization and stem cell apheresis. *Br J Haematol* 1996; **94**: 155–8.

44. Martinez C, Urbano-Ispizua A, Mazzara R et al, Granulocyte colony-stimulating factor administration and peripheral blood progenitor cells collection in normal donors: analysis of leukapheresis-related side effects. *Blood* 1996; **87**: 4916–17.

45. Okamoto S, Ishida A, Wakui M et al, Prolonged thrombocytopenia after administration of granulocyte colony-stimulating factor and leukapheresis in a donor of allogeneic peripheral blood stem cells. *Bone Marrow Transplant* 1996; **18**: 482–3.

46. Anderlini P, Przepiorka D, Champlin R et al, Biologic and clinical effects of granulocyte colony-stimulating factor in normal individuals. *Blood* 1996; **88**: 2819–25.

47. LeBlanc R, Roy J, Demers C et al, A prospective study of G-CSF effects on hemostasis in allogeneic blood stem cell donors. *Bone Marrow Transplant* 1999; **23**: 991–6.

48. Fossa SD, Poulsen JP, Aaserud A, Alkaline phosphatase and lactate dehydrogenase changes during leucocytosis induced by G-CSF in testicular cancer. *Lancet* 1992; **340**: 1544.

49. Sakamaki S, Matsunaga T, Hirayama Y et al, Haematological study of healthy volunteers 5 years after G-CSF. *Lancet* 1995; **346**: 1432–3.

50. Kawase Y, Akashi M, Ohtsu H et al, Effect of human recombinant granulocyte colony-stimulating factor on induction of myeloid leukemias by X-irradiation in mice. *Blood* 1993; **82**: 2163–8.

51. Imashuku S, Hibi S, Nakajima F et al, A review of 125 cases to determine the risk of myelodysplasia and leukemia in pediatric neutropenic patients after treatment with recombinant human granulocyte colony-stimulating factor. *Blood* 1994; **84**: 2380–1.

52. Kawakami M, Tsutsumi H, Kumakawa T et al, Levels of serum granulocyte colony-stimulating factor in patients with infections. *Blood* 1990; **76**: 1962–4.

53. Stroncek DF, Clay ME, Herr G et al, Blood counts in healthy donors 1 year after the collection of granulocyte-colony-stimulating factor-mobilized progenitor cells and the results of a second mobilization and collection. *Transfusion* 1997; **37**: 304–8.

54. Tichelli A, Passweg J, Hoffmann T et al, Repeated peripheral stem cell mobilization in healthy donors: time-dependent changes in mobilization efficiency. *Br J Haematol* 1999; **106**: 152–8.

55. Novotny J, Kadar JG, Hertenstein B et al, Sustained decrease of peripheral lymphocytes after allogeneic blood stem cell aphereses. *Br J Haematol* 1998; **100**: 695–7.

56. Dreger P, Glass B, Uharek L et al, Allogeneic transplantation of mobilized

peripheral blood progenitor cells: Towards tailored cell therapy. *Int J Hematol* 1997; **66**: 1–11.

57. Bacigalupo A, Van Lint MT, Valbonesi M et al, Thiotepa/cyclophosphamide followed by granulocyte colony-stimulating factor mobilized allogeneic peripheral blood cells in adults with advanced leukemia. *Blood* 1996; **88**: 353–7.

58. Bensinger WI, Buckner CD, Rowley S et al, Transplantation of allogeneic CD34+ peripheral blood stem cells in patients with advanced hematologic malignancy. *Blood* 1996; **88**: 4132–8.

59. Stroncek DF, Holland PV, Bartch G et al, Experiences of the first 493 unrelated marrow donors in the national marrow donor program. *Blood* 1993; **81**: 1940–6.

60. Buckner CD, Petersen FB, Bolonesi BA, Bone marrow donors. In: *Bone Marrow Transplantation* (Forman SJ, Blume KG, Thomas ED, eds). Blackwell Scientific: Boston, 1994: 259–69.

61. Varas F, Bernard A, Bueren JA, Granulocyte colony-stimulating factor mobilizes into peripheral blood the complete clonal repertoire of hematopoietic precursors residing in the bone marrow of mice. *Blood* 1996; **88**: 2595–601.

62. Glass B, Uharek L, Zeis M et al, Allogeneic peripheral blood progenitor cell transplantation in a murine model: evidence for an improved graft-versus-leukemia effect. *Blood* 1997; **90**: 1694–700.

63. Theilgaard-Mönch K, Raaschou-Jensen K, Andersen H et al, Single leukapheresis products collected from healthy donors after the administration of granulocyte colony-stimulating factor contain tenfold higher numbers of long-term reconstituting hematopoietic progenitor cells than conventional bone marrow allografts. *Bone Marrow Transplant* 1999; **23**: 243–9.

64. Dreger P, Klöss M, Petersen B et al, Autologous progenitor cell transplantation: prior exposure to stem cell-toxic drugs determines yield and engraftment of peripheral blood progenitor cell but not of bone marrow grafts. *Blood* 1995; **86**: 3970–8.

65. Schmitz N, Bacigalupo A, Hasenclever D et al, Allogeneic bone marrow transplantation vs filgrastim-mobilised peripheral blood progenitor cell transplantation in patients with early leukaemia: first results of a randomised multicentre trial of the European Group for Blood and Marrow Transplantation. *Bone Marrow Transplant* 1998; **21**: 995–1003.

66. Ringden O, Hagglund H, Runde V et al, Faster engraftment of peripheral blood progenitor cells compared to bone marrow from unrelated donors. *Bone Marrow Transplant* 1998; **21**(Suppl 3):S81–4.

67. Ringden O, Remberger M, Runde V et al, Peripheral blood stem cell transplantation from unrelated donors: a comparison with marrow transplantation. *Blood* 1999; **94**: 455–64.

68. Weaver CH, Bensinger W, Longin K et al, Syngeneic transplantation with peripheral blood mononuclear cells collected after the administration of recombinant human granulocyte colony-stimulating factor. *Blood* 1993; **82**: 1981–4.

69. Fefer A, Cheever MA, Thomas ED, Bone marrow transplantation for refractory acute leukemia in 34 patients with identical twins. *Blood* 1981; **57**: 421–30.

70. Schmitz N, Dreger P, Suttorp M et al, Primary transplantation of allogeneic peripheral blood progenitor cells mobilized by filgrastim (G-CSF). *Blood* 1995; **85**: 1666–72.

71. Körbling M, Przepiorka D, Engel H et al, Allogeneic blood stem cell transplantation for refractory leukemia and lymphoma: potential advantage of blood over marrow allografts. *Blood* 1995; **85**: 1659–65.

72. Bensinger WI, Weaver CH, Appelbaum FR et al, Transplantation of allogeneic peripheral blood stem cells mobilized by recombinant human granulocyte colony-stimulating factor (rh G-CSF). *Blood* 1995; **85**: 1655–8.

73. Schmitz N, Klein JP, Gratwohl A et al, Prognostic factors for survival after allogeneic peripheral blood progenitor cell transplantation. *Blood* 1998; **92**: Abst.

74. Bensinger WI, Buckner CD, Storb R et al, Transplantation of allogeneic peripheral blood stem cells. *Bone Marrow Transplant* 1996; **17**(Suppl 2): S56–7.

75. Bensinger WI, Appelbaum FR, Demirer T et al, Transplantation of allogeneic peripheral blood stem cells. *Stem Cells* 1995; **13**(Suppl 3): 63–70.

76. Beelen DW, Ottinger HD, Elmaagacli A et al, Transplantation of filgrastim-mobilized peripheral blood stem cells from HLA-identical sibling or alternative family donors in patients with hematologic malignancies: a prospective comparison on clinical outcome, immune reconstitution, and hematopoietic chimerism. *Blood* 1997; **90**: 4725–35.

77. Dreger P, Suttorp M, Haferlach T et al, Allogeneic G-CSF-mobilised peripheral blood progenitor cells for treatment of engraftment failure after bone marrow transplantation. *Blood* 1993; **81**: 1404–7.

78. Arseniev L, Tischler H-J, Battmer K et al, Treatment of poor marrow graft function with allogeneic CD34+ cells immunoselected from G-CSF-mobilized peripheral blood progenitor cells of the marrow donor. *Bone Marrow Transplant* 1994; **14**: 791–7.

79. Molina L, Chabannon C, Viret F et al, Granulocyte colony-stimulating factor-mobilized allogeneic peripheral blood stem cells for rescue graft failure after allogeneic bone marrow transplantation in two patients with acute myeloblastic leukemia in first complete remission. *Blood* 1995; **85**: 1678–9.

80. Redei I, Waller EK, Holland HK et al, Successful engraftment after primary graft failure in aplastic anemia using G-CSF mobilized peripheral stem cell transfusions. *Bone Marrow Transplant* 1997; **19**: 175–7.

81. Körbling M, Huh YO, Durett A et al, Allogeneic blood stem cell transplantation: peripheralization and yield of

donor-derived primitive hematopoietic progenitor cells (CD34+Thy-1) and lymphoid subsets, and possible predictors of engraftment and graft-versus-host disease. *Blood* 1995; **86**: 2842–8.

82. Mackall CL, Granger L, Sheard MA et al, T-cell regeneration after bone marrow transplantation: differential CD45 isoform expression on thymic-derived versus thymic-independent progeny. *Blood* 1993; **82**: 2585–94.

83. Roux E, Helg C, Dumont GF et al, Analysis of T-cell repopulation after allogeneic bone marrow transplantation: significant differences between recipients of T-cell depleted and unmanipulated grafts. *Blood* 1996; **87**: 3984–92.

84. Ottinger HD, Beelen DW, Scheulen B et al, Improved immune reconstitution after allotransplantation of peripheral blood stem cells instead of bone marrow. *Blood* 1996; **88**: 2775–9.

85. Storek J, Witherspoon RP, Maloney DG et al, Improved reconstitution of CD4 T cells and B cells but worsened reconstitution of serum IgG levels after allogeneic transplantation of blood stem cells instead of marrow. *Blood* 1997; **89**: 3891–3.

86. Pavletic ZS, Joshi SS, Pirruccello SJ et al, Lymphocyte reconstitution after allogeneic blood stem cell transplantation for hematologic malignancies. *Bone Marrow Transplant* 1998; **21**: 33–41.

87. Miller JS, Prosper F, McCullar V, Natural killer (NK) cells are functionally abnormal and NK cell progenitors are diminished in granulocyte colony-stimulating factor-mobilized peripheral blood progenitor cell collections. *Blood* 1997; **90**: 3098–105.

88. Bensinger WI, Clift R, Martin P et al, Allogeneic peripheral blood stem cell transplantation in patients with advanced hematologic malignancies: a retrospective comparison with marrow transplantation. *Blood* 1996; **88**: 2794–800.

89. Vigorito AC, Azevedo WM, Marques JFC et al, A randomized, prospective comparison of allogeneic bone marrow and peripheral blood progenitor cell

transplantation in the treatment of haematological malignancies. *Bone Marrow Transplant* 1998; **22**: 1145–51.

90. Jansen J, Goselink HM, Veenhof WFJ et al, The impact of the composition of the bone marrow graft on engraftment and graft-versus-host disease. *Exp Hematol* 1983; **11**: 967–73.

91. Pan L, Delmonte J, Jalonen CK et al, Pretreatment of donor mice with granulocyte colony-stimulating factor polarizes donor T-lymphocytes toward type-2 cytokine production and reduces severity of experimental graft-versus-host disease. *Blood* 1995; **86**: 4422–9.

92. Krenger W, Snyder KM, Byon JHC et al, Polarized type 2 alloreactive CD4+ and CD8+ donor T cells fail to induce experimental acute graft-versus-host disease. *J Immunol* 1995; **155**: 585–93.

93. Rondelli D, Raspadori D, Anasetti C et al, Alloantigen presenting capacity, T cell alloreactivity and NK function of G-CSF-mobilized peripheral blood cells. *Bone Marrow Transplant* 1998; **22**: 631–7.

94. Sugimori N, Nakao S, Yachie A et al, Administration of G-CSF to normal individuals diminishes L-selectin+ T cells in the periphal blood that respond better to alloantigen stimulation than L-selectin− T-cells. *Bone Marrow Transplant* 1999; **23**: 119–24.

95. Mielcarek M, Martin PJ, Torok-Storb B, Suppression of alloantigen-induced T-cell proliferation by CD14+ cells derived from granulocyte colony-stimulating factor-mobilized peripheral blood mononuclear cells. *Blood* 1997; **89**: 1629–34.

96. Majolino I, Saglio G, Scimè R et al, High incidence of chronic GVHD after primary allogeneic peripheral blood stem transplantation in patients with hematologic malignancies. *Bone Marrow Transplant* 1996; **17**: 555–60.

97. Ordemann R, Holig K, Wagner K et al, Acceptance and feasibility of peripheral stem cell mobilisation compared to bone marrow collection from healthy unrelated donors. *Bone Marrow Transplant* 1998; **21**(Suppl 3):S25–8.

98. Sosman JA, Oettel KR, Hank JA et al, Specific recognition of human leukemic cells by allogeneic T cell lines. *Transplantation* 1989; **48**: 486–90.

99. Glass B, Uharek L, Zeis M et al, Graft-versus-leukemia activity can be predicted by natural cytotoxicity against leukemia cells. *Br J Haematol* 1996; **93**: 412–20.

100. Elmaagacli AH, Beelen DW, Opalka B et al, The risk of residual molecular and cytogenetic disease in patients with philadelphia-chromosome positive first chronic phase chronic myelogenous leukemia is reduced after transplantation of allogeneic peripheral blood stem cells compared with bone marrow. *Blood* 1999; **94**: 384–9.

101. Giralt S, Escudier S, Kantarjian H et al, Preliminary results of treatment with filgrastim for relapse of leukemia and myelodysplasia after allogeneic bone marrow transplantation. *N Engl J Med* 1993; **329**: 757–61.

102. Alessandrino EP, Bernasconi P, Bonfichi M et al, Standard chemotherapy and donor peripheral blood stem cell infusion in early relapse after allo-bmt: preliminary results. *Bone Marrow Transplant* 1996; **17**(Suppl 1): S15.

103. Glass B, Majolino I, Dreger P et al, Allogeneic peripheral blood progenitor cells for treatment of relapse after bone marrow transplantation. *Bone Marrow Transplant* 1997; **20**: 533–41.

104. Giralt S, Estey E, Albitar M et al, Engraftment of allogeneic hematopoietic progenitor cells with purine analog-containing chemotherapy: harnessing graft-versus-leukemia without myeloablative therapy. *Blood* 1997; **89**: 4531–6.

105. Slavin S, Nagler A, Naparstek E et al, Nonmyeloablative stem cell transplantation and cell therapy as an alternative to conventional bone marrow transplantation with lethal cytoreduction for the treatment of malignant and nonmalignant hematologic diseases. *Blood* 1998; **91**: 756–63.

106. Hartung G, Uharek L, Zeis M et al, Superior antileukemic activity of murine

peripheral blood progenitor cell (PBPC) grafts mobilized by G-CSF and stem cell factor (SCF) as compared to G-CSF alone. *Bone Marrow Transplant* 1998; 21(Suppl 3):S16–20.

107. Zeis M, Uharek L, Glass B et al, Allogeneic MHC-mismatched activated natural killer cells administered after bone marrow transplantation provide a strong graft-versus-leukaemia effect in mice. *Br J Haematol* 1997; 96: 757–61.

108. Aversa F, Tabilio A, Velardi A et al, Treatment of high-risk acute leukemia with T-cell-depleted stem cells from related donors with one fully mismatched HLA haplotype. *N Engl J Med* 1998; 339: 1186–93.

109. Müller-Ruchholtz W, Wottge HU, Müller-Hermelink HK, Bone marrow transplantation across strong histocompatibility barriers by selective elimination of lymphoid cells in bone marrow. *Transplant Proc* 1976; 8: 537–41.

110. Marmont AM, Horowitz MM, Gale RP et al, T-cell depletion of HLA-identical transplants in leukemia. *Blood* 1991; 78: 2120–30.

111. Cornelissen JJ, Fibbe WE, Schattenberg AV et al, A retrospective Dutch study comparing T cell-depleted allogeneic blood stem cell transplantation vs T cell-depleted allogeneic bone marrow transplantation. *Bone Marrow Transplant* 1998; 21(Suppl 3): S66–70.

112. Dreger P, Viehmann K, Steinmann J et al, G-CSF-mobilised peripheral blood progenitor cells for allogeneic transplantation: comparison of T cell depletion strategies using different CD34+ selection systems or CAMPATH-1. *Exp Hematol* 1995; 23: 147–54.

113. Link H, Arseniev L, Bähre O et al, Transplantation of allogeneic CD34+ blood cells. *Blood* 1996; 87: 4903–9.

114. Bensinger WI, Rowley S, Lilleby K et al, Reduction in graft-versus-host-disease (GVHD) after transplantation of CD34 selected, allogeneic peripheral blood stem cells (PBSC) in older patients with advanced hematologic malignancies. *Blood* 1996; 88(Suppl 1):421a.

115. Urbano-Ispizua A, Rozman C, Martinez C et al, Rapid engraftment without significant graft-versus-host disease after allogeneic transplantation of CD34+ selected cells from peripheral blood. *Blood* 1997; 89: 3967–73.

116. Urbano-Ispizua A, Solano C, Brunet S et al, Allogeneic transplantation of purified CD34+ cells from peripheral blood: Spanish experience of 62 cases. Spanish Group of allo-PBT. *Bone Marrow Transplant* 1998; 21(Suppl 3): S71–4.

117. Bensinger WI, Rowley SD, Mills B, CD34 enriched allogeneic peripheral blood stem cell used for transplantation. *Bone Marrow Transplant* 1998; 21: S102.

118. Schumm M, Lang P, Taylor G et al, Isolation of high purified autologous and allogeneic peripheral CD34+ cells using the CliniMACS device. *J Hematotherapy* 8: 209–18.

119. Handgretinger R, Schumm M, Lang P et al, Transplantation with megadose of haploidentical mobilized stem cells highly purified by magnetic-activated cell sorting. *Blood* 1998; 92(Suppl 1): 688a.

120. Matsuda Y, Hara J, Osugi Y et al, Allogeneic peripheral stem cell transplantation using positively selected CD34+ cells from HLA-mismatched donors. *Bone Marrow Transplant* 1998; 21: 355–60.

121. Uharek L, Zeis M, Steinmann J et al, High lytic activity against human leukemia cells after activation of allogeneic NK cells by IL-12 and IL-2. *Leukemia* 1996; 10: 1758–64.

122. Barrett AJ, Mavroudis D, Tisdale J et al, T cell-depleted bone marrow transplantation and delayed T cell add-back to control acute GVHD and conserve a graft-versus-leukemia effect. *Bone Marrow Transplant* 1998; 21: 543–51.

123. Rooney CM, Smith CA, Ng CY et al, Use of gene-modified virus-specific T lymphocytes to control Epstein–Barr-virus-related lymphoproliferation. *Lancet* 1995; 345: 9–13.

124. Sing AP, Ambinder RF, Hong DJ et al, Isolation of Epstein–Barr virus (EBV)-

specific cytotoxic T lymphocytes that lyse Reed–Sternberg cells: implications for immune-mediated therapy of EBV+ Hodgkin's disease. *Blood* 1997; **89**: 1978–86.

125. Locatelli F, Maccario R, Gerna G, Anticytomegalovirus T-cell clones. *N Engl J Med* 1995; **331**: 601.

126. Craddock CF, Nakamoto B, Andrews RG et al, Antibodies to VLA4 integrin mobilize long-term repopulating cells and augment cytokine-induced mobilization in primates and mice. *Blood* 1997; **90**: 4779–88.

127. Papayannopoulou T, Nakamoto B, Andrews RG et al, In vivo effects of Flt3/Flk2 ligand on mobilization of hematopoietic progenitors in primates and potent synergistic enhancement with granulocyte colony-stimulating factor. *Blood* 1997; **90**: 620–9.

128. Hägglund H, Ringden O, Remberger M et al, Faster neutrophil and platelet engraftment, but no differences in acute GVHD or survival, using peripheral blood stem cells from related and unrelated donors, compared to bone marrow. *Bone Marrow Transplant* 1998; **22**: 131–6.

129. Powles R, Kulkarni S, Mehta J et al, A double-blind randomized study comparing the efficacy of allogeneic marrow versus blood stem cell transplantation. *Blood* 1997; **90**: 254a (Abst).

# Index